AI-Driven Healthcare Cybersecurity and Privacy

Shrikaant Kulkarni
School of Engineering and Technology, Sanjivani University, Kopargaon, India & Victorian Institute of Technology, Melbourne, Australia

Saikat Gochhait
Symbiosis Institute of Digital and Telecom Management, Symbiosis International University, Pune, India & Samara State Medical University, Russia

IGI Global
Scientific Publishing
Publishing Tomorrow's Research Today

Vice President of Editorial	Melissa Wagner
Director of Acquisitions	Mikaela Felty
Director of Book Development	Jocelynn Hessler
Production Manager	Mike Brehm
Cover Design	Jose Rosado

Published in the United States of America by
IGI Global Scientific Publishing
701 East Chocolate Avenue
Hershey, PA, 17033, USA
Tel: 717-533-8845
Fax: 717-533-7115
Website: https://www.igi-global.com E-mail: cust@igi-global.com

Library of Congress Cataloging-in-Publication Data

Names: Kulkarni, Shrikaant editor | Gochhait, Saikat, 1974- editor
Title: AI-driven healthcare cybersecurity and privacy / edited by Shrikaant Kulkarni and Saikat Gochhait.
Description: Hershey, PA : IGI Global Scientific Publishing, [2025] | Includes bibliographical references and index. | Summary: "This book provides a detailed analysis of how AI is being leveraged to strengthen cybersecurity measures, detect threats, and prevent data breaches, all while adhering to the stringent regulations that govern healthcare privacy"-- Provided by publisher.
Identifiers: LCCN 2025005797 (print) | LCCN 2025005798 (ebook) | ISBN 9798337328270 h/c | ISBN 9798337328287 s/c | ISBN 9798337328294 ebook
Subjects: LCSH: Artificial intelligence--Medical applications | Computer networks--Security measures | Computer security | Medical informatics
Classification: LCC R859.7.A78 A3979 2025 (print) | LCC R859.7.A78 (ebook) | DDC 610.285--dc23/eng/20250602
LC record available at https://lccn.loc.gov/2025005797
LC ebook record available at https://lccn.loc.gov/2025005798

British Cataloguing in Publication Data
A Cataloguing in Publication record for this book is available from the British Library.

Table of Contents

Detailed Table of Contents

The rapid digital transformation introduced Electronic Health Records (EHRs), telemedicine, and IoT devices, improving patient care but also exposing healthcare data to cybersecurity risks. This paper proposes integrating Artificial Intelligence (AI) and Blockchain to enhance healthcare security. AI offers real-time threat detection and automated response, while Blockchain provides decentralized, immutable, secure data storage. The review highlights traditional security framework limitations, AI and Blockchain's unique functions, and their combined benefits. Key applications include secure EHR sharing, IoT device security, and AI-Enabled Smart Contracts. Despite the potential, challenges like scalability, ethics, and regulatory issues (HIPAA, GDPR) persist. Case studies demonstrate the success of AI-Blockchain integration in healthcare. The paper concludes with future research directions and recommendations for professionals adopting these technologies to ensure secure, efficient healthcare delivery.

The paper discusses existing challenges that, based on the legal framework, the regulatory change must affect in order to ensure interest coverage in the health sector. Massive opportunities lie in the role that AI plays in healthcare in the forms of diagnostics and personalized care, while major challenges arise. AI models like machine learning, deep learning, and neural networks have improved healthcare outcomes, but they raise concerns on the privacy of patient data, explainability, and cyber threats such as adversarial attacks. Sensitive data must be protected for patients to trust AI-driven diagnosis. Bias in algorithms, the obtaining of informed patient consent, and the accountability of the AI decisions are some ethical and regulatory issues. Regulations like HIPAA(Health Insurance Portability and Accountability Act) and GDPR(General Data Protection Regulation) are the most important while considering data protection.This includes better encryption and anonymisation of patient data, interpretable models, and stronger defences against cyber-attacks.

Cybersecurity in healthcare systems is crucial due to the sensitive nature of patient data and the increasing risk of cyberattacks. This paper proposes a novel approach to enhancing cybersecurity defenses by utilizing stacked artificial neural networks (ANNs) for the detection of man-in-the-middle (MITM) attacks, such as spoofing and data injection, targeting healthcare data transmission. The dataset used includes 35 network flow metrics and 8 biometric features, which represent the critical aspects of network traffic and patient health data. The methodology involves training two base-level ANN models: one for detecting anomalies in network flows and the other for identifying irregularities in biometric data. These models' outputs are combined in a meta-model to improve classification accuracy and provide a robust defense mechanism. The proposed method demonstrates enhanced attack detection capabilities by leveraging both network and health-related data, offering a comprehensive solution to safeguard healthcare information systems.

This paper explored the crucial areas of cybersecurity in the healthcare industry, stressing the need to defend healthcare infrastructures and private patient information against online attacks. As part of their applications in electronic healthcare (e-healthcare) services for risk management, fraud detection, and identity authentication to effectively mitigate cyber risks, the current paper proposed bimodal access gateway authentication using artificial neural network (ANN) computer algorithm to secure e-healthcare data warehouse infrastructure. In this study, distributed cloud Internet of Things (IoT) data warehouse server systems were created and connected through 5G radio frequency access network to enable healthcare grid data warehouse information synchronization, resource allocation and service-level optimization. This approach was adopted to strengthen cybersecurity defense and keep systems ahead of every evolving cyber threats in the e-healthcare data warehouse repositories.

In order to detect denial-of-service (DoS) and distributed denial of service (DDoS) intrusions on the organization's e-healthcare data warehouse infrastructure, the authors of this study proposed a computing framework that combines a federated learning system based on blockchain technology. A Message Queuing Telemetry Transport (MQTT) broker gathers data from an IoT node and sends it to the computing platform for analysis. As a platform for the creation of several new technologies and applications, IoT has created new opportunities in the age of cloud communication. Due to the increasing use of cloud data warehouse technologies, computer networks have had serious security concerns, and there are security vulnerabilities in the IoT as well. DoS and DDoS attacks on IoT e-healthcare servers may compromise general stability, efficacy of the services, and real-time information federation. This study provided an efficient MQTT broker approach to secure servers from cyberattacks and presented state-of-the-art defenses against DoS/DDoS attacks in the IoT digital healthcare ecosystem.

Federated learning is an emerging powerful approach for training ML models across decentralized data sources, such as in healthcare, without actually transferring the sensitive data to a central server. Although FL naturally reduces the risks of privacy since data are confined to local devices, it still can be highly vulnerable to sophisticated attacks such as model inversion, data poisoning, and inference attacks. Advanced privacy-preserving techniques that are nowadays studied for addressing the privacy and security concerns of this paper include differential privacy, homomorphic encryption, and secure aggregation. These, therefore, open the room for FL to be adopted as a solution in some of the privacy-sensitive domains. This paper conducts a thorough review of the techniques discussed and outlines a customized security

Preface

The integration of Artificial Intelligence (AI) into healthcare is a transformative force, reshaping how diagnostics and medical practices are approached across the globe. With the promise of enhanced precision, speed, and scalability, AI-powered healthcare systems are creating a new frontier in patient care. However, this advancement also presents several challenges, particularly concerning sustainability and cybersecurity.

As editors, we have witnessed the growing reliance on AI in healthcare and the complexities that come with its implementation, including the need for robust data security and ethical responsibility. The intersection of these aspects – AI, sustainability, and cybersecurity – forms the cornerstone of this book. It aims to explore and address how AI technologies can be harnessed to not only improve healthcare diagnostics but also ensure that their deployment is sustainable and secure.

In this edited volume, we delve into the emerging field of sustainable AI-powered healthcare systems, emphasizing their potential to minimize environmental impact and enhance cybersecurity measures. The use of AI in healthcare, while groundbreaking, also opens the door to increasing concerns regarding patient data privacy and the potential for breaches. The significance of securing these systems against cyber threats while promoting sustainable practices cannot be overstated.

Our goal for this book is clear: to present a framework that supports the responsible integration of AI in healthcare diagnostics. By focusing on resource-efficient algorithms, energy optimization, and eco-friendly hardware, we provide practical solutions for minimizing the environmental impact of AI in medical applications. We also highlight advanced techniques for safeguarding sensitive patient data, thus enhancing the trust and effectiveness of AI-driven systems.

Moreover, it is our intent to bridge the gap between technological innovation and ethical practices in AI applications. The issues of bias, transparency, and accountability in AI systems, especially in healthcare diagnostics, are thoroughly explored. We present strategies for ensuring that AI tools remain aligned with the values of fairness, inclusivity, and patient-centered care.

This book is designed for a broad audience, ranging from healthcare professionals such as clinicians, radiologists, and medical researchers, to AI developers and cybersecurity experts working in healthcare. Policymakers and hospital administrators will also find valuable insights on the regulatory frameworks required to manage the security and sustainability of AI systems. Additionally, the academic community – students, researchers, and educators in fields such as medical informatics, AI, and cybersecurity – will benefit from this comprehensive examination of the opportunities and challenges posed by AI in healthcare diagnostics.

We hope that this volume serves as both a guide and a call to action for the responsible, ethical, and sustainable implementation of AI in healthcare. Our ultimate vision is to ensure that AI-driven innovations do not merely enhance patient care but do so in a way that is mindful of our environmental responsibilities and the security of personal health data.

ORGANIZATION OF THE BOOK

Chapter 1: Integration of AI with Blockchain for Healthcare Security

This chapter explores the powerful synergy between Artificial Intelligence (AI) and Blockchain technology in addressing the growing cybersecurity risks in healthcare. With the digital transformation of healthcare through Electronic Health Records (EHRs), telemedicine, and IoT devices, patient data has become more vulnerable to cyber threats. By combining AI's real-time threat detection and automated response capabilities with Blockchain's decentralized, secure data storage, this chapter presents a comprehensive solution to ensure healthcare data security. The chapter highlights key applications such as secure EHR sharing, IoT device protection, and AI-enabled smart contracts, while also discussing the challenges of scalability, ethics, and regulatory compliance.

Chapter 2: Challenges and Solutions in Securing AI Algorithms in Healthcare

The use of Artificial Intelligence in healthcare presents both transformative benefits and significant challenges. This chapter examines how AI models such as machine learning, deep learning, and neural networks improve diagnostic and personalized care, while raising critical concerns about patient data privacy, explainability, and vulnerability to cyber-attacks. Issues like algorithmic bias, informed patient consent, and the accountability of AI decisions are explored, alongside the role of regulations such as HIPAA and GDPR. The chapter proposes solutions, including enhanced encryption, anonymization techniques, and interpretable AI models, to address these concerns and secure AI-driven healthcare systems.

Chapter 3: Enhancing Healthcare Data Security with Stacked Deep Learning Approach

Cybersecurity in healthcare is increasingly vital as more data is transmitted digitally. This chapter introduces a novel approach to safeguarding patient information using stacked artificial neural networks (ANNs) to detect cyberattacks like man-in-the-middle (MITM) attacks. By integrating network traffic and biometric data into two base-level ANN models, and combining their outputs into a meta-model, the chapter demonstrates enhanced accuracy in detecting anomalies and irregularities. The approach promises a more robust defense against cyber threats, ensuring better protection for sensitive healthcare data.

Chapter 4: Cybersecurity Approaches to IoT Platform in E-Healthcare System: Artificial Intelligence Application

With the increasing integration of IoT devices into e-healthcare systems, securing sensitive health data from cyber threats has become a critical concern. This chapter explores cybersecurity strategies, particularly the use of artificial intelligence (AI) algorithms for risk management, fraud detection, and identity authentication in healthcare infrastructures. The authors propose bimodal access gateway authentication through artificial neural networks (ANNs) to secure data warehouses, enabling data synchronization, resource optimization, and service-level improvements within distributed IoT environments. This strategy aims to safeguard e-healthcare systems from evolving cyber risks.

Chapter 5: Cybersecurity Issues on E-Healthcare Cloud Data Warehouse System: Blockchain-Based Federated Learning Approach

In this chapter, the authors address cybersecurity vulnerabilities in e-healthcare data warehouse systems, especially with the rise of DoS and DDoS attacks. A new framework that combines blockchain technology and federated learning is presented as a solution to enhance security. By using a Message Queuing Telemetry Transport (MQTT) broker to gather data from IoT nodes and analyzing it through federated learning, the framework can detect and mitigate cyberattacks, ensuring the stability and efficacy of cloud-based healthcare infrastructures and protecting real-time health data.

Chapter 6: Federated Learning for Secure and Privacy-Preserving Medical Diagnostics

Federated learning (FL) emerges as a key technology for securely training machine learning models across decentralized healthcare data sources without transferring sensitive data. This chapter discusses the potential of FL in preserving patient privacy while addressing security challenges such as model inversion and data poisoning. It highlights privacy-preserving techniques like differential privacy, homomorphic encryption, and secure aggregation, offering a secure framework for medical diagnostics. The chapter reviews how these techniques can balance the trade-off between privacy and model accuracy, making FL a promising approach for healthcare applications.

Chapter 7: Application of Integral Transform Algorithms for Augmenting Cryptographic Security and Performance Analysis

This chapter introduces a cryptographic framework based on the Anuj Transform and the congruence modulo operator to enhance data security and information retrieval in AI-driven healthcare systems. The authors demonstrate how the mathematical properties of these transforms improve encryption and decryption techniques. By evaluating key parameters like encryption precision, computing speed, and resistance, the chapter illustrates how this new approach can address contemporary cryptographic challenges, ensuring secure data exchanges and protecting sensitive healthcare information.

Chapter 8: Sustainable AI-Powered Systems and Cybersecurity for Health Diagnostics: Addressing Bias and Fairness in AI for Early Disease Detection

AI-driven healthcare diagnostics have revolutionized early disease detection, yet challenges related to fairness and bias persist. This chapter examines how biases in AI models, driven by imbalanced data and structural issues, can lead to discriminatory outcomes. The authors discuss solutions to ensure equity in AI systems, such as curating inclusive datasets and applying fairness-enhancing techniques like adversarial debiasing and data augmentation. The chapter also addresses privacy concerns, emphasizing the importance of algorithmic transparency and ongoing innovation to create fair, accurate, and ethical AI systems for healthcare.

Chapter 9: A Mathematical Approach to Enhance Cybersecurity in AI-Driven Healthcare Diagnostics Using J-Transform

This chapter presents an innovative encryption and decryption methodology that leverages the J-Transform to enhance the security of data in AI-driven healthcare diagnostics. By employing complex mathematical transformations, the authors propose a block cipher encryption process that ensures data integrity and confidentiality. The chapter provides a comprehensive analysis of the J-Transform's application in cryptography, demonstrating how it strengthens data security and addresses the increasing demand for secure AI-driven healthcare solutions.

Chapter 10: Privacy-Preserving Enhancements in Heart Rate Monitoring through IoT Integration for Remote Healthcare

In this chapter, the authors propose an integrated approach combining IoT sensors and Hyperledger blockchain to enhance the security and privacy of heart rate monitoring in remote healthcare. The use of blockchain ensures data integrity and transparency, while IoT sensors capture critical health data in real-time. By employing smart contracts and integrating cloud-based platforms, the system enables secure remote monitoring and timely interventions in healthcare, particularly in emergency situations, thus advancing privacy-preserving technologies in healthcare diagnostics.

Chapter 11: Reducing the Carbon Footprint in Healthcare Cybersecurity Threats in AI-Powered Healthcare Systems

As AI transforms healthcare, its environmental impact, along with data privacy and cybersecurity challenges, cannot be overlooked. This chapter explores the importance of protecting patient data and reducing the carbon footprint in AI-driven healthcare systems. It discusses relevant regulations like HIPAA and GDPR and emphasizes the role of sustainable cybersecurity practices in mitigating the environmental and data privacy issues associated with AI applications. The chapter highlights how balancing technology's benefits with privacy protection and sustainability is essential for advancing AI in healthcare.

Chapter 12: Navigating Emerging Threats: Strategies for Cybersecurity in AI-Driven Healthcare Diagnostics and FDA Compliance

This chapter provides an in-depth exploration of the cybersecurity challenges faced by AI-driven healthcare diagnostics, focusing on compliance with FDA regulations. It examines emerging threats such as data breaches, adversarial attacks, and system vulnerabilities in AI-based medical devices. The authors propose effective strategies for mitigating these risks, including robust cybersecurity frameworks, risk assessments, and stakeholder security awareness. By addressing these challenges, the chapter emphasizes the importance of maintaining the safety, efficacy, and regulatory compliance of AI in healthcare.

Chapter 13: Securing Healthcare Innovations: Cybersecurity Frameworks for FDA-Regulated Medical Devices in the Age of AI

The integration of AI in FDA-regulated medical devices introduces complex cybersecurity challenges. This chapter outlines essential cybersecurity frameworks for protecting these innovative healthcare technologies. It discusses risks such as data breaches, unauthorized access, and threats to patient safety, and provides an overview of current regulations and best practices for securing AI-powered medical devices. By advocating for a proactive approach to security, the chapter highlights the need for continuous improvement in AI-driven threat detection and response mechanisms within healthcare systems.

CONCLUSION

In conclusion, this reference book provides a comprehensive examination of the critical intersection of cybersecurity, AI, blockchain, and healthcare. As the healthcare sector continues to undergo digital transformation, it is essential to explore the opportunities and challenges that accompany the integration of cutting-edge technologies. Each chapter within this volume highlights innovative approaches to securing sensitive healthcare data, improving diagnostic accuracy, and enhancing patient care through artificial intelligence, blockchain, federated learning, and advanced cryptographic techniques.

From the protection of electronic health records to the secure transmission of patient data through IoT devices, the contributions herein emphasize the need for robust security frameworks to safeguard the privacy and integrity of healthcare systems. The book not only discusses the latest advancements but also addresses the regulatory, ethical, and practical challenges that must be navigated to ensure secure and equitable healthcare delivery. Whether through the application of AI to improve early disease detection or the adoption of blockchain to ensure immutable records, this work provides a roadmap for healthcare professionals, policymakers, and researchers striving to create a more secure, efficient, and innovative healthcare ecosystem.

The future of healthcare lies in the effective integration of technology with security, and this volume offers valuable insights into how these technologies can be harnessed for the benefit of all. We hope that this book serves as an essential resource for anyone working at the intersection of healthcare, technology, and security, fostering collaboration and innovation in pursuit of a safer and more resilient healthcare future.

Chapter 1
Integration of AI With Blockchain for Healthcare Security

Nitesh Upadhyaya
https://orcid.org/0009-0001-2548-1299
GlobalLogic Inc., USA

ABSTRACT

The rapid digital transformation introduced Electronic Health Records (EHRs), telemedicine, and IoT devices, improving patient care but also exposing healthcare data to cybersecurity risks. This paper proposes integrating Artificial Intelligence (AI) and Blockchain to enhance healthcare security. AI offers real-time threat detection and automated response, while Blockchain provides decentralized, immutable, secure data storage. The review highlights traditional security framework limitations, AI and Blockchain's unique functions, and their combined benefits. Key applications include secure EHR sharing, IoT device security, and AI-Enabled Smart Contracts. Despite the potential, challenges like scalability, ethics, and regulatory issues (HIPAA, GDPR) persist. Case studies demonstrate the success of AI-Blockchain integration in healthcare. The paper concludes with future research directions and recommendations for professionals adopting these technologies to ensure secure, efficient healthcare delivery.

INTRODUCTION

Over the decade, rapid technological advancement has considerably retooled healthcare in response to an increased demand for efficiency in patient care. The emergence of electronic health records is among the notable changes this revolution

DOI: 10.4018/979-8-3373-2827-0.ch001

has brought about (Cerchione et al., 2023). EHRs substituted record-keeping systems that relied on paper and allowed easy access to patient information, coordination of healthcare service provision, and facilitation of analytics (Melton et al., 2021).

Andrew et al. (2023) opined that, among the key developments in healthcare delivery, apart from EHRs, is telemedicine. With its emphasis in the COVID-19 pandemic, telemedicine has become an indispensable component of healthcare delivery. Telemedicine allows patients to consult healthcare professionals remotely through video conferencing and other digital communication tools (Ahmad et al., 2022). That has helped increase access to care, especially for those people living in either rural or underserved areas and has eased pressures on health facilities. Besides, IoT devices are being implemented in healthcare more and more.

On the downside, however, rapid digitalization has increased exposure to cybersecurity risks and eventual data breaches. Because of their sensitive nature, health information is a popular target for any cybercriminal looking to have any sort of exploit in the digital systems. Several high-profile breaches have underlined the need for robust security measures inside the healthcare organizations as they make their way into this new landscape (Motsi-Omoijiade & Kharlamov).

As healthcare becomes more and more dependent on digital technologies with each passing day, it becomes a dire need for developing more robust security mechanisms that identify such cyber threats and stop them before they may penetrate through the security lines to steal sensitive patient information. Alabdulatif et al. (2022), affirmed that, traditional security measures are inadequate to tackle the complexity brought in by a modern digital infrastructure. These challenges are being increasingly met with novel solutions involving the use of AI and blockchain in healthcare cybersecurity. For example, AI can analyse large volumes of data in real time and pick out patterns that might indicate an imminent security breach, or even an anomaly that needs attention (Ahmed et al., 2020).

Compared to that however, blockchain offers a decentralized mechanism for data management that greatly improves levels of transparency and integrity of health information exchanges (Rahman et al., 2022). In principle, blockchain could utilize the ability to create mutually verifiable, unalterable renderings of the data, which are shared only with authorized people, to restrict unauthorized access or tampering of sensitive health data. Although AI and blockchain have some hope to healthcare through advances in AI and blockchain, it would be quite important to consider many limitations and challenges AI and blockchain are faced with before being widely used in the practice. For instance, quality training of data for AI systems can give rise to biased results, if not carefully watched (Balakrishnan., 2024).

The digital transformation in healthcare, on one hand, brings a host of opportunities for improving not only patient care but also operational efficiency. On the other hand, it calls for a comprehensive approach toward cybersecurity, integrating next-generation technologies such as AI and blockchain, among many others.

Objectives of the Study

i. This research is done to investigate the potential that can occur by integrating Artificial Intelligence with Blockchain technology to improve health security. In particular, the objectives are to:
ii. Establish current challenges within healthcare cybersecurity arising because of rapid proliferation within EHRs, telemedicine, and IoT devices.
iii. Research Blockchain potentials in decentralized, immutable, and non-accessible storage of data for healthcare.
iv. Provide an integrated AI-Blockchain framework that will help to enhance healthcare security, especially about patient data confidentiality, integrity, and availability.
v. Showcase practical applications of the integration between AI and Blockchain, such as secure EHR sharing, IoT device security, and automation of smart contracts in healthcare.
vi. Examine issues of scalability, privacy, and regulatory compliance issues for translating AI-Blockchain integration into real-world healthcare settings.

Scope of the Study

This research work falls within the context of the integrated use of AI and Blockchain technology to help combat cybersecurity threats in the healthcare sector. The current work will perform a review of existing security threats to healthcare systems in light of their digitalization with EHRs, telemedicine, and IoT devices. Application areas will involve the study of AI roles for real-time anomaly detection and threat responses, together with Blockchain features for providing secure, decentralized data storage (Saleh, 2024). Applications will include secure sharing of EHRs, protection of IoT devices, and use of smart contracts in healthcare transactions. It will also include examining the different challenges regarding the implementation of integration of AI and Blockchain on grounds such as scalability, privacy, ethics, and compliance with laws like HIPAA and GDPR for data protection (Williamson & Prybutok, 2024). Case studies regarding successful implementations will be examined along with recommendations for future research and development in AI-Blockchain health care security.

LITERATURE REVIEW

Healthcare Security Challenges and Threats

The healthcare industry has become a prime target for cyber threats, with the growing number of digital health records and networked medical devices serving to increase its vulnerability. Froehlich et al. (2021) asserted that, cybersecurity breaches concerning stolen healthcare information have reached dire proportions, where sensitive patient information is not at risk, but even patient safety may be put into jeopardy. In the same light, Ntantogian et al. (2021) added that, the cyber threats in healthcare can be further divided into ransomware attacks, phishing schemes, insider threats, and APTs, among others. Ransomware attacks have gained notoriety for their ability to encrypt critical data and demand payment for its release. High-profile incidents, such as the WannaCry attack in 2017 that affected numerous hospitals worldwide, illustrate the potential disruption caused by such attacks.

However, sometimes the demand for regulatory compliance even acts as an obstacle to well-implemented cybersecurity (Kianpour & Raza, 2024), as illustrated in Figure 1. While, for instance, HIPAA regulations stipulate certain security measures that work to secure patient information, these also do not change with emerging technologies or sophisticated cyber threats. As a result, this will make organizations compliant on paper but in practice still vulnerable. Another important aspect is IoT integration in healthcare. While IoT devices carry several benefits, such as patient monitoring and vital data collection, they also expose new attack vectors for cybercriminals.

Besides the technological gaps, comprehensive training courses are urgently needed for healthcare staff in educating best practices of cybersecurity. Human error continues to be one of the leading factors in data breaches, and thus building a culture of security awareness is essential to reduce risks from insider threats and social engineering attacks (Hughes-Lartey et al., 2021).

Figure 1. Cybersecurity challenges in healthcare

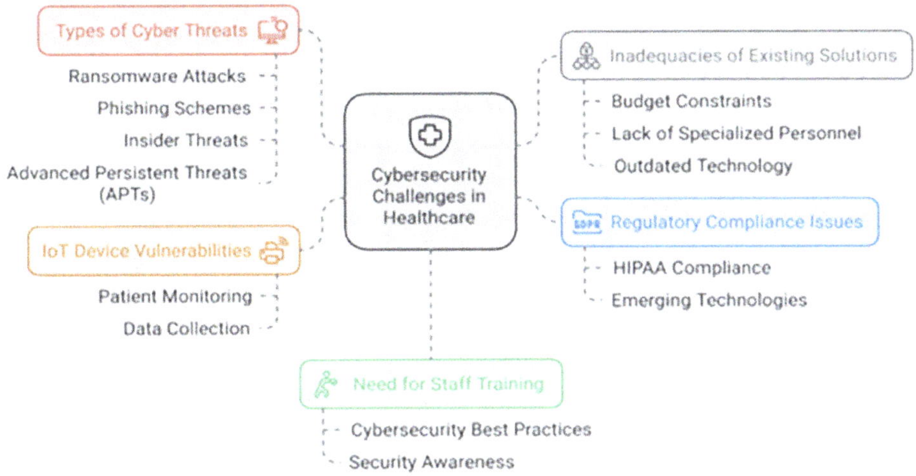

Types of Cyber Threats
Ransomware Attacks
Phishing Schemes
Insider Threats
Advanced Persistent Threats (APTs)
IoT Device Vulnerabilities
Patient Monitoring
Data Collection
Cybersecurity Challenges in Healthcare
Inadequacies of Existing Solutions
Budget Constraints
Lack of Specialized Personnel
Outdated Technology
Regulatory Compliance Issues
HIPAA Compliance
Emerging Technologies
Need for Staff Training
Cybersecurity Best Practices
Security Awareness

AI in Healthcare Security

Artificial Intelligence has emerged as a transformative force in sectors like healthcare, among many others. Applications of AI technologies in healthcare security involve machine learning, anomaly detection, and real-time threat detection (Maddireddy & Maddireddy, 2022). The backbone of discovery of the patterns in the huge datasets occurring in health environment is provided by the machine learns algorithms. This way processing the past data helps the algorithm to discover normal behaviour in health systems and flag those anomalies that can be considered as a breach or threat to security.

Figure 2. Enhancing healthcare security and efficiency through AI

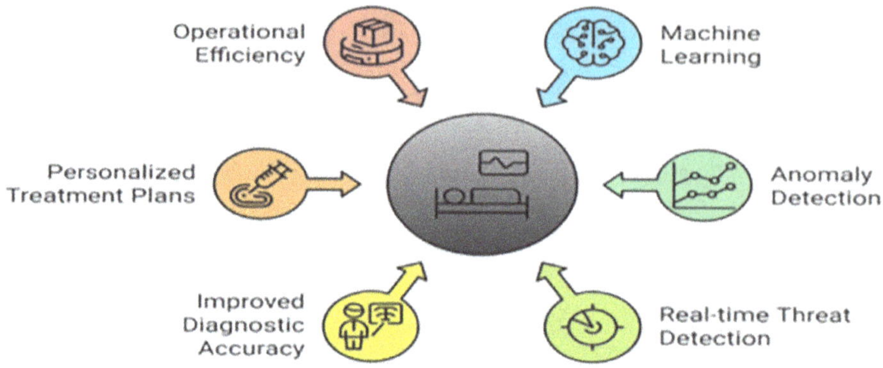

As indicated in Figure 2, another vital facet of AI in healthcare security relates to anomaly detection. According to Palakurti (2024), the anomaly detection systems typically deploy statistical methods and machine learning techniques to determine deviations from established norms within healthcare operations. There is considerable ability by AI to find threats in real time, as the volume of data which it processes efficiently is quite high and at tremendous speed. AI for healthcare security can perform real-time monitoring via AI-driven systems for network traffic, user behaviour, and system logs in a continuous search for prospective emerging threats (Upadhyaya, 2024b).

AI enhances diagnosis and treatment based on personalized medicine beyond security concerns in the healthcare sector (Johnson et al., 2021). Traditional diagnosis techniques in most medical fields have been competed out by machine learning algorithms through the analysis of complex data sets of imaging studies, genetic information, and clinical histories. Another highly promising area for AI is personalized treatment plans. Using data particular to the patient, such as genetic profiles and lifestyle factors, AI systems can recommend targeted treatment options that align with the needs of a particular patient. Such a degree of personalization will serve to benefit patient outcomes and greatly streamline resource utilization in healthcare facilities through better efficacy from the outset.

Another advantage of AI technologies in healthcare settings is operational efficiency. Administrative tasks, such as appointment scheduling, billing processes, and claims management, can be done through automation by AI to save precious time for healthcare professionals to deal directly with patient care activities (Pillai, 2023).

Blockchain in Healthcare Security

With the recent rise of blockchain, there comes a kind of paradigm shift in many fields; health is one of the most promising fields that this technology could help. In its core, the basic characteristics of blockchain provide decentralized, immutable, and cryptographic mechanisms that offer great advantages in increasing security and transparency in data management within healthcare (Zaabar et al., 2021). One of the general properties of blockchain technology has its decentralisation, as presented in Figure 3. In fact, while most of the databases usually have one central authority managing them, in principle, blockchain is based on a distributed network of nodes.

Another critical feature of blockchain that contributes a great deal toward the security of healthcare is immutability (Alzahrani et al., 2022). Once data has been recorded on the blockchain, it cannot be changed or deleted without changing all further blocks and with the consensus of the network participants. This feature is very crucial in health settings for the maintenance of accurate and unchangeable patient records for quality care and legal purposes.

Figure 3. Enhancing healthcare security and transparency through blockchain

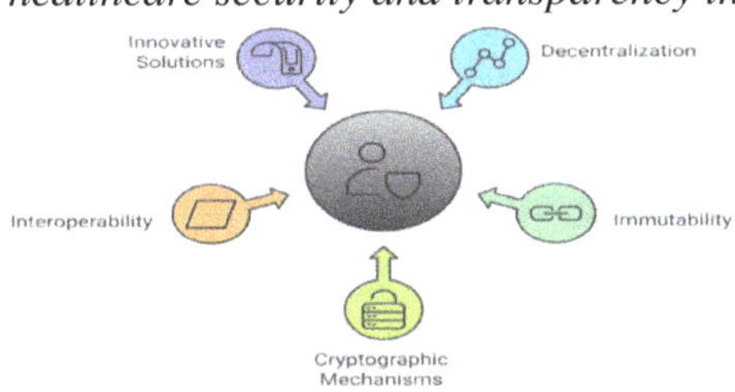

An additional touch is brought in by cryptographic mechanisms that notarize blockchain technology. Sathya & Banik (2020), asserted that, advanced cryptographic algorithms secure every transaction on the blockchain by encrypting data before adding it to the chain, which in turn ensures that even though the intruder may gain access into the network, they are not able to decipher sensitive information without appropriate keys for decryption. The role of blockchain in ensuring secure and transparent health data management is not only in securing individual records but also to ensure interoperability across various systems used by various stakeholders in the healthcare ecosystem. Traditional health information systems are designed such that they operate in silos, thereby making sharing of a patient's data across the various platforms an uphill task.

Blockchain technology can enhance the integrity of clinical trials through an immutable record of both trial protocols and results (Omar et al., 2021). In a better position would be the researchers to transparently register their trials, instantly reflecting changes that may have been made during the study through proper recording in an immutable ledger. Besides making the existing structures more secure and transparent, blockchain technology creates new avenues for innovative solutions in healthcare delivery models. For example, blockchain-based decentralized identity management systems put patients in control over their health records rather than having providers or insurers manage this sensitive information.

Comparison of AI and Blockchain Capabilities

The speed at which technology evolves has brought two powerful forces for change upon the medical sector: Artificial Intelligence and Blockchain (Pablo et al., 2022). Each of these technologies has its own strengths and weaknesses in application to healthcare security. Understanding their attributes will be important in leveraging their capability. Artificial Intelligence is generally described by its ultimate capability to analyse huge amounts of data, patterns, and make predictions based on learned experience. Its forte is the ability for automation, efficiency, and scalability (Upadhyaya, 2024c). Applications in healthcare will involve the processing of patient data to inform diagnosis, predict disease outbreaks, personalize treatment plans, and complete administrative tasks. Figure 4 shows Balancing AI and Blockchain in healthcare.

Figure 4. Balancing AI and blockchain in healthcare

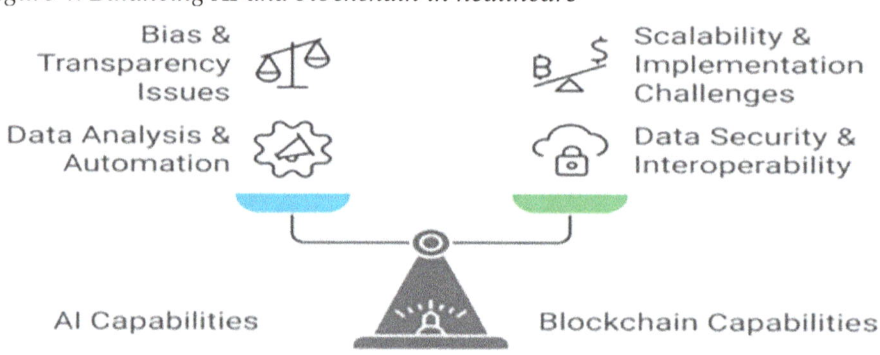

Contrastingly, Blockchain technology provides a decentralized approach towards managing data securely through cryptographic techniques. Its major strength forms immutable records, which are transparent yet secure from unauthorized access and tampering (Guimarães et al., 2023). However, Blockchain also has some limitations. Scalability remains one of the challenges with this technology: the more the transactions added to the chain, the slower and less efficient the system will become (Khan et al., 2020. Most Blockchain solutions require huge investments in infrastructural changes and training for healthcare personnel who may or may not be conversant with such an emerging technology.

When considering how AI and Blockchain work in solving some security challenges in healthcare, it becomes obvious that there is much to be benefited from their integration. For example, while AI thrives most at analysing huge datasets both in speed and efficiency, probably pinpointing security threats or anomalies, Blockchain creates a secure environment within which this data can be stored and shared safely amongst stakeholders (Bhumichai et al., 2024). However, AI based analytics can enhance the efficacy of Blockchain applications via the real time network transaction monitoring. By that system can determine exactly when some suspicious activity or an intrusion is taking place in its operation.

INTEGRATION OF AI WITH BLOCKCHAIN FOR HEALTHCARE SECURITY

The integration of AI and Blockchain in health has been a very prospective solution to benefit from data security, privacy and interoperability. Case of data breaches, unauthorized access and data management poor controls are rampant in the health sector. Taking advantage of the complementary strengths of both AI and Blockchain, the resulting combination can serve as an effective framework for strong protection of sensitive health information along with advanced analysis and decision-making processes.

Proposed AI-Blockchain Architecture

The proposed architecture reinforces the decentralized characteristics of Blockchain, merged with the analytical capabilities of AI. It thus creates a secure environment to manage healthcare data. In principle, the conceptual framework comprises three major components: data storage, data processing, and user interaction. Blockchain, as related to data storage, is an immutable ledger where every transaction of the patients' information is recorded (Chelladurai et al., 2021).

Each block in the chain has a cryptographic hash of the previous block, meaning once data has been put into the system, it cannot be changed or deleted except with the consensus of all parties in it. Backed by Blockchain's security, AI algorithms can be deployed for analysing voluminous amounts of healthcare data with efficiency

(Ahmed et al., 2020). They identify the patterns and trends which would otherwise remain obscure to a human analyst. There are multiple levels at which this interaction between the two technologies happens in the architecture. First, whenever new data is created about a patient, like lab results or studies from imaging, it is encrypted and then stored on Blockchain.

This can serve another important purpose: AI can use this stored data for training predictive models without infringing upon patient privacy (Yee & Raj 2022). Techniques such as federated learning mean that knowledge gained by an AI system is learned from decentralized datasets without any direct access to sensitive information.

Figure 5. AI-blockchain integration in healthcare

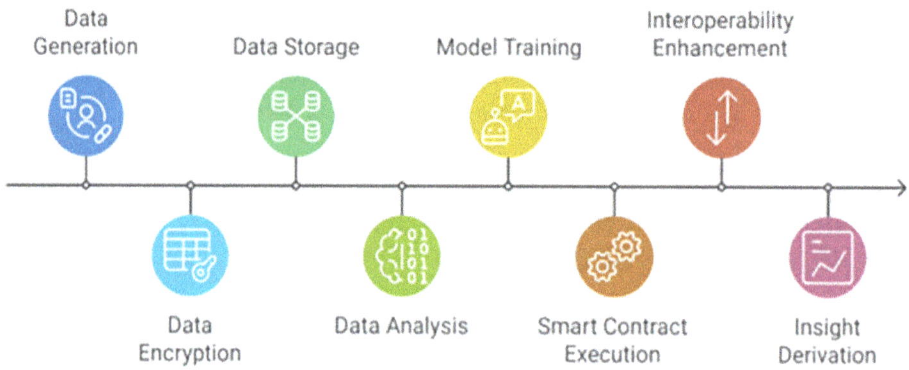

Moreover, smart contracts-running contracts whose terms are directly written into lines of code-can be applied to automate certain processes of healthcare operations if integrated with both technologies (Töberg, 2022), as shown in Figure 5. For example, they will provide the convenience of automatic billing processes based on predefined conditions fulfilled during patient treatment or will ensure that regulatory requirements about access to sensitive health records are satisfied by their independent verification of credentials.

Another key proposition of the architecture is to enable communication and interoperability among heterogeneous health systems. Conventional health databases operate in silos, while this common Blockchain network allows multiple stakeholders like hospitals, insurance, patients to access it, where data sharing will seamlessly occur across all these platforms without losing much of security (Cadoret et al., 2020).

Furthermore, AI-driven analytics may be enabled for stakeholders with this interoperable framework to enable stakeholders to draw actionable insights from aggregated health data across various sources in a manner that does not infringe on the rights of individual patients (Lekkala, 2023). For example, anonymized patient records can be stored on the Blockchain, and public health officials can utilize the Blockchain to look at trends of certain disease outbreaks without having to see personally identifiable information.

AI's Role in the Blockchain Ecosystem

Blockchain technology in the healthcare ecosystem will not be exploited to its full extent without AI (Tagde et al., 2021). It is also among many of its key applications in that it can serve up data real time as it runs across the blockchain. AI can monitor real time through anomalies in blockchain systems immediately. If there is a spike in access requests to a patient's medical record or medication administration logs are found to be incorrect, for instance, the algorithms of AI will flag such incidents for further investigation.

Besides, another important aspect is the continuous threat detection where AI enhances blockchain security in healthcare. Many cybersecurity measures depend on predefined rules and signatures to identify threats (Ahsan et al., 2022). According to Figure 6, regulatory compliance is one of the most important components in the healthcare sector. There are laws such as the HIPAA law in the United States and the GDPR in Europe that make it rather difficult for anyone to gain access to any other person's patient data.

Figure 6. AI's role in the blockchain ecosystem

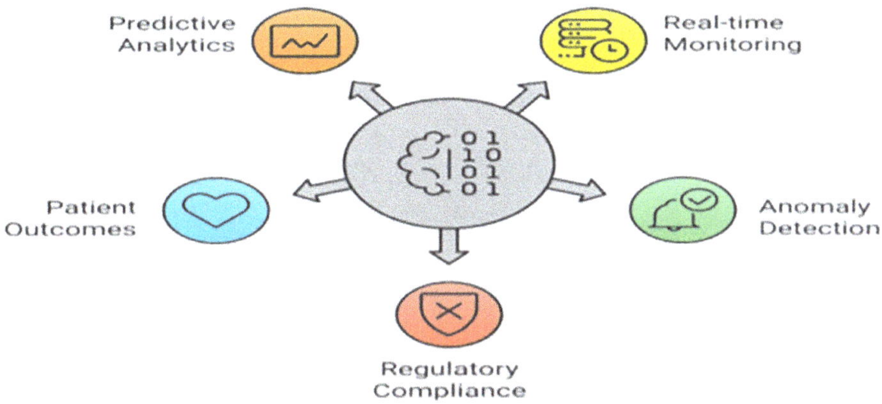

Moreover, AI-driven predictive analytics can help organizations foresee compliance risk by studying historical trends in data resulting from past regulatory violations or breaches in their network (Balakrishnan, 2024). In this regard, potential vulnerabilities could be identified in advance to afford health organizations an opportunity to take necessary steps to prevent such situations rather than reacting to them after they have occurred. Besides these capabilities, AI helps very much to bring out better patient outcomes with improved decision support systems interleaved into blockchain (Nair & Tyagi, 2023). Aggregating such diverse datasets from multiple sources, ranging from genomic information to clinical notes to social determinants of health, AI makes personalized recommendations personalized to the needs of a patient.

The combination of the AI analytics with the blockchain infrastructure would bring in transparency to the stakeholders, providers, and the patients themselves in all steps of patient care (Jabarulla & Lee, 2021). It will give the patient the confidence that health information will not be accessed by unauthorized parties while being available whenever needed for timely interventions.

Blockchain Securing the Data Environment for AI

Blockchain integration in the artificial intelligence environment has now been included among the crucial enhancements on data integrity and confidentiality. According to Chen et al. (2021), with artificial intelligence developing their operations on larger volumes of data very fast, it is integral that this data is maintained secure, accurate, and trustworthy. One of the strongest features of blockchain technology is its decentralized nature. Traditional databases are generally controlled by one single entity, while in blockchain, there exists a distributed ledger where every node has a copy of the whole database.

Figure 7. Enhancing AI data security with blockchain

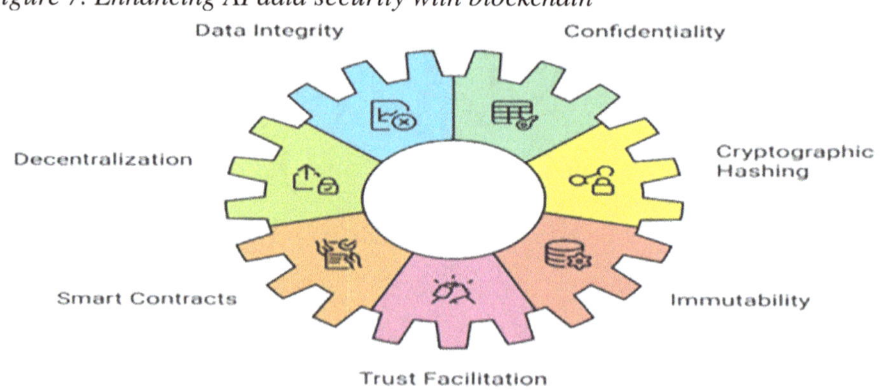

Moreover, in blockchain, cryptographic hashing is used for data integrity (Saeed et al., 2022), as it is depicted in Figure 7. Any block of the blockchain has a unique hash derived from its own content and a hash from its previous block. Apart from integrity, blockchain ensures a higher level of confidentiality due to advanced encryption techniques. Data on the blockchain could be encrypted using the public-key cryptography approach, which allows access to sensitive information only to users in possession of the required private keys.

Furthermore, the smart contract itself—a self-executing contract whose terms are directly written into lines of code—can automate processes within AI systems and ensure that rules exist with respect to who has rights to access and use data (Piccardo et al., 2024). The framework allows organizations to embed such contracts into the blockchain, where they can automate processes and meet pre-set policies about who has access to what data under what conditions. This means that everything in this makes blockchain immutability a big factor that leads to secure data environments in an analysis of AI. When the moment information is parked on a blockchain, it can't update nor erase without each party (participants) on a particular network with the consent to do it.

Key to how this technology builds trust is in having diversified parties interacting within an ecosystem of AI. On many occasions, datasets used for training machine learning models involve various stakeholders: personal data submitted by individual users or proprietary information available to organizations by joining forces with others (Jean-Quartier et al., 2022). As AI technologies are being increasingly adopted across organizations ranging from finance to healthcare, there has emerged a particular need for robust security as much as doubt about cyber threats and breaches in privacy. As such, Blockchain thereby presents an extremely viable answer in creating safe settings wherein sensitive datasets may be traded among authorized users while being uncovered or centrally misused.

While there are some challenges in utilizing blockchain in the traditional AI framework with the scalability and energy consumption issue of some consensus mechanism, such as Proof-of-Work (Zhang et al., 2021), it is still profitable to integrate blockchain into the conventional AI framework. Also, these are some of things to consider while designing systems that would utilize both technologies in a useable way.

APPLICATION OF AI-BLOCKCHAIN INTEGRATION IN HEALTHCARE

It is the AI + Blockchain convergence in health, a new domain creating new vistas to handle, share and utilize medical data. The goal of the integration of the two is to secure it, improve patient outcomes and interfere with operations in the healthcare systems. Its wholly decentralized nature makes the blockchain framework the ideal place to store and disseminate data, ensuring full data security, while AI helps crunch the health figures and predicts health trends. They then together create an ecosystem, creating the capability of secure storage of EHR, and granting only access to whom is authorised.

Secure Sharing of Electronic Health Records (EHRs)

One of the most critical use cases of AI/Blockchain integration in healthcare (Haddad et al., 2022) is secure EHR sharing. These include very sensitive patient information, such as medical history, treatment plans, medicines, allergies, lab results, and others. Each transaction or update to the record in an EHR system based on blockchain is encrypted and then added to a block, which then links to previous blocks in a chain. A structure like this makes it virtually impossible for unauthorized users to alter or delete any information without this being detected.

In addition, AI can facilitate the process of managing consent over blockchain networks. Patients can permit granular control over who accesses their EHRs by executing smart contracts—self-executing contracts whose terms are written directly into lines of code on a blockchain (Hakiri et al., 2021). The contracts can grant or revoke access automatically depending on predefined conditions set by a patient. The integration allows for real-time updates to EHR, while ensuring security protocols are in place. Health professionals may modify a patient's record or include new information related to a patient, which can be disease diagnoses and their respective treatments.

Interoperability is another critical benefit: different health care systems can talk to each other effectively while allowing the security standards (Lee et al., 2021). Traditional EHR systems have many compatibility problems because of the different formats and standards used by the various service providers, but the standardized protocol of blockchain permits various systems to converse seamlessly with assurance that unauthorized parties will not have access to information available only to the authorized parties.

Integration of AI into this ecosystem, and predictive analytics shoots up manifold. The AI algorithms can uncover the trends and correlations in an ocean of anonymized health data stored on the blockchain, which may be difficult to ascertain through any other traditional method of analysis (Li et al., 2023). AI-Blockchain Integration in HER as shown in Figure 8.

Figure 8. AI-blockchain integration in EHRs

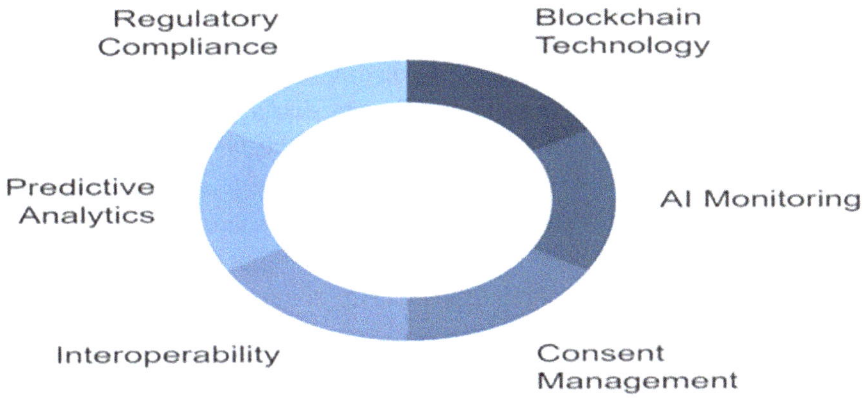

However, it also has its implications in terms of regulatory and reporting requirements within the healthcare organization. As seen in Fig. 8, besides improving patient care, such integration provides much-enhanced data sharing and analytics (Qian et al., 2023). Some of the inherent features of Blockchain provide an auditable trail, thus making the effort to conform with regulatory requirements easier to quite an extent. Each transaction recorded in Blockchain offers an unalterable log that regulators could review if needed, all while keeping such privacy rights intact.

Then there are also challenges with respect to the implementation of AI-blockchain solutions in healthcare settings. Issues on scalability persist; because as more participants either join in the network or more transactions take place at the same time, the system must keep up with performance without compromising speed or efficiency (Upadhyaya, 2024a). Furthermore, when it comes to access rights over shared records kept on public versus private blockchains, there is also the question of ownership that needs to be brought up with due care among all those stakeholders involved in further developing these technologies.

Securing IoT Devices in Healthcare

With the proliferation of IoT devices throughout healthcare, their contribution to patient monitoring and data collection has been of utmost advantage. Devices run the gamut from wearable health monitors that track physiological parameters to smart medical equipment that may communicate vital information in real time to health providers (Putra et al., 2024). Blockchain technology thus provides faultless ways through which security in communication among healthcare IoT devices can be effectuated. Due to the decentralized nature of the ledger, transactions on the blockchain are transparent and indelible.

Moreover, blockchain by nature-through its transparency and traceability-allows tracking of device interactions in real time. Any abnormal activity or unauthorized attempts at communication can be identified on time and dealt with. Besides secure communication, blockchain facilitates secure data sharing among various stakeholders in the healthcare ecosystem. The patients would have full control over who can access their health data without losing ownership due to smart contracts-self-executing contracts whereby any rules and agreements concerning the contract are written directly into lines of code on the blockchain (Rajput et al., 2021).

While blockchain certainly offers security to the communications framework of IoT devices, AI extends that security by making proactive threat detection possible via advanced analytics and machine learning algorithms, as shown in Figure 9. AI systems can analyse a mountain of data emanating from IoT devices to identify patterns indicative of normal behaviour against those that indicate potential threats (Dhayanidhi, 2022). For example, machine learning models can be trained on the historical data from the medical devices to establish performance baselines for each device type. After the establishment of these baselines, deviations from expected behaviour-including spikes in the frequency of data transmission or unexpected changes in sensor readings-can be flagged as anomalies that require further investigation.

Further, AI algorithms learn over time with new input of data. Therefore, they become more accurate in abnormal behaviour detection as they get tuned to evolving patterns within the network (Bouchama & Kamal, 2021). This is an important capability given the dynamic nature of healthcare settings, where new devices are introduced periodically.

Figure 9. Securing healthcare IoT devices with AI and blockchain

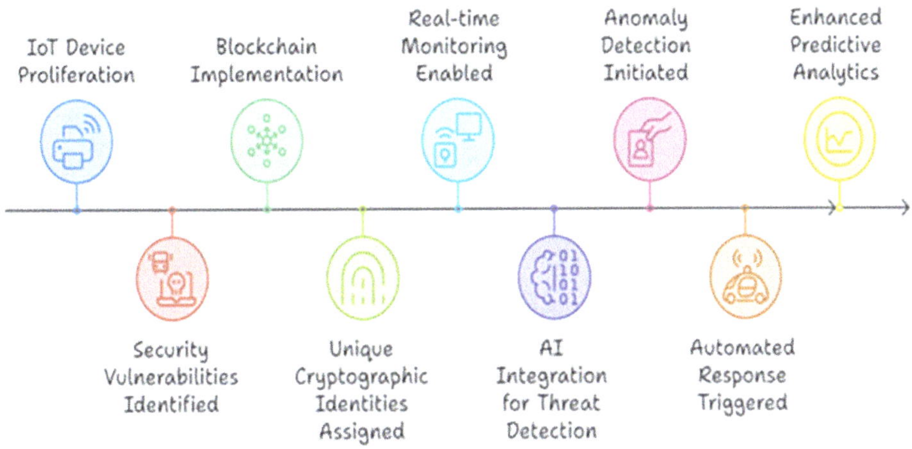

AI, combined with the blockchain technology capability for logging each interaction in a secure and indelible manner, constitutes the AI-driven anomaly detection as holistic for the security framework of IoT ecosystems in health care. When an AI system detects an anomaly, there are automated responses that may include alerting IT personnel or temporarily isolating affected devices from the network until further analysis has been conducted (Hassan & Ibrahim, 2023).

Additionally, AI integrated with blockchain further makes for improved predictive analytics in healthcare. Looking at trends across a large, connected set of devices over time, using AI techniques such as predictive modelling or deep learning frameworks like neural networks, one will be able to anticipate the probability of a given situation well before it blows up into a grave threat.

AI-Enhanced Smart Contracts for Healthcare Transactions

Smart contracts on blockchains can provide a decentralized and immutable ledger that may accelerate several processes of the healthcare system. Having inherent characteristics of blockchain-transparency, security, and traceability-these smart contracts may automate every complex transaction that requires much manual watch conventionally (Andrew et al., 2023). Figure 10 below shows AI-Enhanced Smart Contracts in Healthcare.

Figure 10. AI-enhanced smart contracts in healthcare

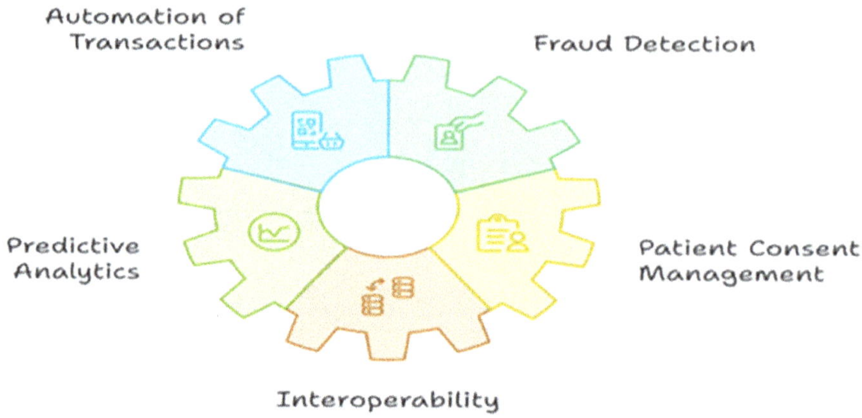

AI also plays a very important role in fraud detection within these automated systems. Healthcare fraudulent activities may take several forms, such as making spurious claims or identity theft. With machine learning algorithms and smart contracts, analytics in the pattern of transactions will provide the tracing of anomalies indicative of fraud activities (Demertzis et al., 2020). Also, AI amplifies predictive analysis in smart contracts for efficiency. These AI algorithms will analyse historical data regarding patient treatments and outcomes for predictions about the future utilization of healthcare and costs.

Another important area of great promise for AI-driven smart contracts is in patient consent management (Williamson & Prybutok, 2024). Traditional informed consent by patients involves cumbersome paperwork, which can be misleading or incomplete. Smart contracts could make this simpler by presenting the patient with a host of intuitive, digital interfaces that present options for treatment and informed consent forms for review and electronic signature.

Moreover, interoperability within health care systems remains a challenge where different technologies may be used and seamless data exchange between providers and payers cannot be warranted (Gohar et al., 2022). Integration of AI with blockchain-based smart contracts would open up interoperability through standardized protocols on how data is shared while allowing privacy consistent with the encryption techniques intrinsic in blockchain technology. These developments mean so much more in terms of operational efficiencies but also contribute a great deal to improved patient outcomes. Patients have less friction in gaining access to needed care services as insurance claims are processed faster and the consent management process is more transparent with the facilitation of AI-enhanced smart contracts on blockchain platforms (Ressi et al., 2024).

Looking into the future of technology integration in health delivery systems, with AI and blockchain, there is a need for regulatory frameworks that will guide these innovations responsibly. Policymakers must ensure that ethical considerations on data privacy are emphasized while at the same time creating an enabling environment for technological advancements (Dhirani et al., 2023).

BENEFITS OF AI-BLOCKCHAIN INTEGRATION IN HEALTHCARE

Artificial Intelligence and Blockchain integrated into healthcare have the transformational opportunity to better data security and privacy of healthcare; this is especially true in contemporary times when the frequency of data breaches is increasing at an unprecedented rate. Blockchain allows for an immutable ledger of recorded transactions across decentralized nodes and completely removes the possibility of data alteration or deletion by unauthorized parties (Laroiya et al., 2020).

Figure 11. Benefits of AI-Blockchain integration in healthcare

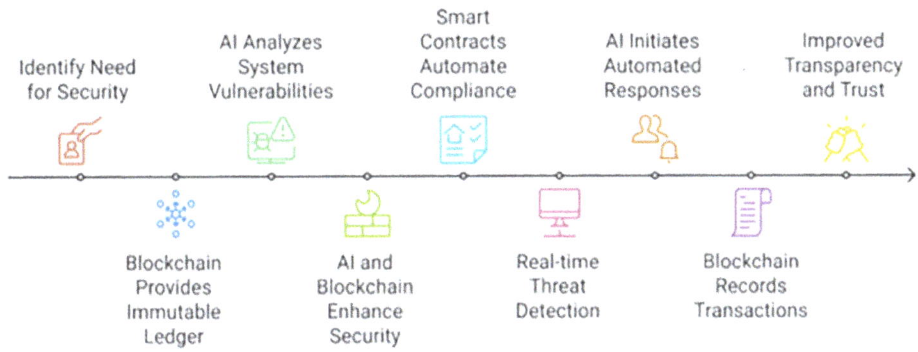

AI further enhances this by adding the capability of performing advanced analytics to find vulnerabilities within the system. For instance, machine learning algorithms use pattern observation in access logs to find anomalies that may mean a security breach (Poh et al., 2020). The self-executing contracts, smart contracts, whose terms are written directly into lines of code, can perform regular compliance checks and enact privacy policies on their own. It might be specified within the contracts who shall have access to the dataset under what conditions, to reduce unauthorized access.

Apart from the added security given by this integration, AI and Blockchain make threat detection and prevention in healthcare systems a real-time activity (Alabdulatif et al., 2022), as illustrated in Figure 11. AI can process large volumes of data continuously due to the high processing speed. When it comes in is in the Blockchain, because it keeps a record of all the transactions happening in the network. Every access to data, every modification of it, gets logged onto the chain, and the trail of things becomes transparent and auditable at any time. It helps not only in tracing the breach after it has happened but also as a factor of deterring such malicious activities, knowing that permanent records are being made.

Moreover, once a threat has been detected, the AI systems can automatically trigger responses in accordance with the protocols stored on the Blockchain (Rahman et al., 2022). For instance, if something suspicious occurs, access to certain databases should be banned for some time until further investigation is carried out. The integration of AI and Blockchain provides a high level of transparency in the field of healthcare and deepens trust between patients and providers. In most traditional healthcare settings, patients have no indication of how their data is used or distributed among parties, such as hospitals, insurance companies, and research institutions.

Blockchain solves this issue by developing a system wherein all transactions regarding patient data become recorded on a public or permissioned ledger that is open to any authorized party (Chenthara et al., 2020). In such user-friendly interfaces, patients will have great improvement in transparency into who accessed their information and why.

Further, AI contributes to this transparency in analysing large volumes of data for insights into the outcomes of treatments across different demographics or conditions, with no breach of individual privacy (Williamson & Prybutok, 2024). Aggregated health data, for example, when analyzed through AI, may expose trends on the efficacy a particular medicine has on different populations, all the while maintaining anonymity through cryptographic techniques native to Blockchain technology.

CHALLENGES AND LIMITATIONS OF AI-BLOCKCHAIN INTEGRATION

The integration of AI together with Blockchain offers a very prospective frontier in several industries, especially very critical sectors like healthcare, finance, and supply chain management. However, the integration of AI and Blockchain is not without its own set of challenges and limitations. Knowing these challenges would be of great importance to the stakeholders who are eager to use the combined power of AI and Blockchain.

Scalability Issues

Scalability is one of the most pressing challenges with integrating AI and Blockchain (Zhang et al., 2021). Both become resource-intensive technologies, and large-scale deployment becomes quite difficult. At their architecture level, blockchain networks, where proof-of-work consensus mechanisms are applied-like Bitcoin, for example-have an inherent limit to the throughput at which transactions can be handled. For context, Bitcoin processes roughly 7 transactions per second, while Ethereum handles approximately 30 TPS. Figure 12 shows Scalability Challenges in AI-Blockchain Integration.

Figure 12. Scalability challenges in AI-blockchain integration

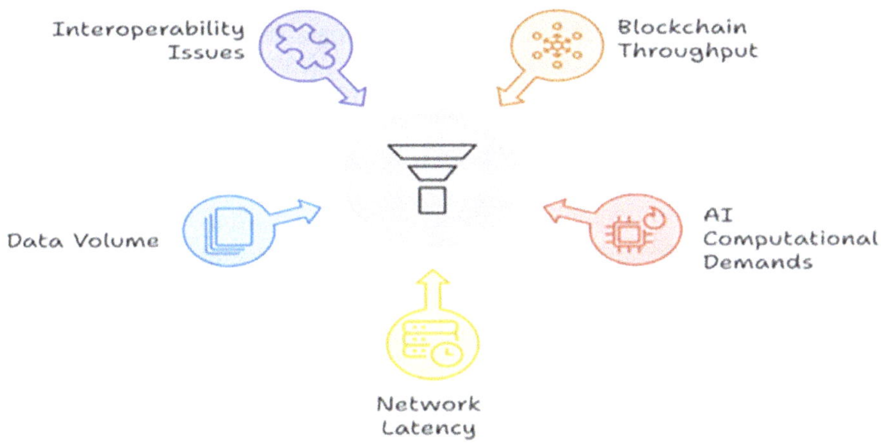

It is further exacerbated by the rising computational needs of AI models, especially deep learning algorithms. Training complex models can require substantial computations and time, which often conflicts with the slower transaction speeds generally associated with many blockchain systems (Shafay et al., 2023).

More specific to healthcare, where timely decision-making sometimes means the difference in outcomes for a patient, an inability to process large datasets on a timely basis might delay diagnosis or treatment recommendations where the data are on a blockchain. Suppose an AI model is supposed to analyse a patient's data that sits on a blockchain, and it cannot do so in time because of network congestion or slow transaction speed; it may not provide timely insight required for urgent medical decisions (Saeed et al., 2022).

Furthermore, the more nodes a blockchain network adds to increase security and decentralized features-a driving principle behind blockchain-the overall performance of such a system may degrade further due to increased latency in reaching consensus among nodes (Xiao et al., 2020). Another reason for scalability issues pertains to the size of data contributed both by AI applications and blockchain transactions. IoT devices in healthcare will generate massive volumes of data, and since blockchain requires all records to be immutable, hence always stored, this contributes to unmanageable storage over time. This in return forces organizations to also consider off-chain solutions or hybrid models that may compromise some of the benefits normally attainable with full decentralization.

Moreover, at the integration with existing AI systems, interoperability issues also arise between different blockchain platforms (Belchior et al., 2021). Many organizations have custom-made blockchains for uses. The problem is that these systems do not talk to each other or to traditional databases used to store training data related to AI models.

Ethical and Privacy Concerns

Merging artificial intelligence into a blockchain raises various ethical and privacy issues, especially regarding sensitive data in patient information in health facilities (Singh & Kaunert, 2024). It is definite that the integration of these technologies will ensure data security, transparency, and efficiency while posing major questions related to ethics in connection with the use of patient data for AI analysis.

Figure 13. Navigating ethical challenges in AI-blockchain

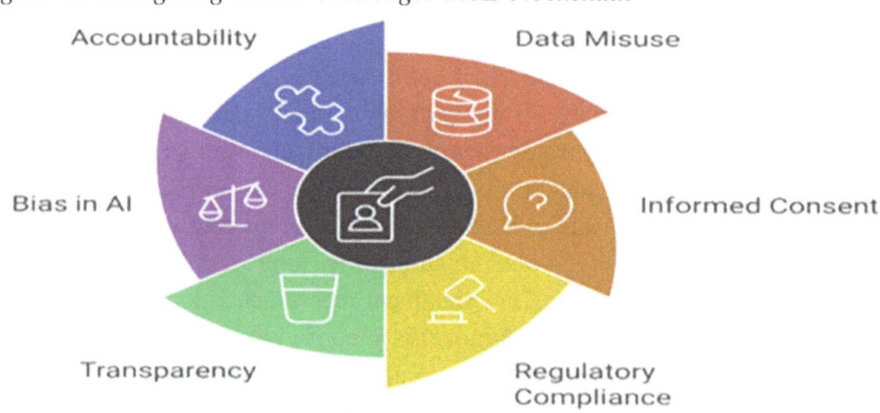

There is a pressing need to reassess the issue of informed consent. In classic medical care, the explicit consent of patients to allow access to their data is always required for research and data analysis. However, in an integrated AI-blockchain system where data may be distributed across diverse platforms, systems, and stakeholders, it is also increasingly complicated to inform patients fully about how data in question will be used (Haddad et al., 2022).

Another key element has to do with compliance with systems like the Health Insurance Portability and Accountability Act in the United States or with the General Data Protection Regulation in Europe (Ramosn & Ellul, 2024). Because these regulations enact very strict guidelines on how personal health information shall be handled, stored, and shared, the decentralized nature of blockchain complicates compliance efforts, as it can be challenging to determine who is responsible for protecting patient data when there are multiple parties concerned in an AI-blockchain ecosystem. Figure 13 illustrates how to navigate ethical challenges in AI-blockchain.

To counter these ethical issues arising in this regard, transparency by organizations with regard to AI must be ensured. This calls for clearly explaining how information about the patients will be used and ensuring the patients themselves have control over their information. Another challenge is how to address the potential biases contained in these AI algorithms themselves: for example, if the historical patient data represents different inequities, such as socioeconomic ones, then AI models utilizing that very data might inadvertently revive such biases when making predictions on or recommending the best options for treatments (Chen, 2022).

There is also a very valid concern about accountability in case of an error because of AI decisions based on patient data stored on a blockchain (Jabarulla & Lee, 2021). If an algorithm, due to defective analyses, results in incorrect diagnoses or treatments, then liability could become a bit complicated in a decentralized framework where responsibility for the integrity of both the blockchain and the AI system lies with many.

Regulatory and Legal Considerations

The proposal of integrating Artificial Intelligence with Blockchain gives way to a host of challenges, especially in regulatory and legal considerations (Zhang et al., 2021). As they continue evolving, it means there's a list of complex issues to be accomplished in line with prevailing laws and regulations. This is very important, more so in sensitive data management sectors, such as health. In most instances, it mainly faces two major regulatory frameworks: America's Health Insurance

Portability and Accountability Act, commonly referred to as HIPAA, and Europe's General Data Protection Regulation.

Of these, some of the principal difficulties that regulatory standards such as HIPAA face are indeed how to balance the confidentiality of patient data with the maximum utilization of AI in data analysis and decision-making. HIPAA has imposed strict regulations on the use, sharing, and storage of PHI (Huddleston & Hedges, 2020). AI systems often require volume data for training, meaning huge datasets of PHI to learn algorithms that predict patient outcomes or the onset of a disease. That kind of data sharing, even in the field of research or development, must be taken care of under HIPAA with heightened security measures that protect patient privacy.

Similarly, GDPR has brought new layers of challenges in terms of data protection and privacy rights in the European Union. One of the fundamental rights it covers is the right of erasure or the "right to be forgotten," where an individual can demand that personal data be deleted from a database (Bika, 2020). Moreover, non-compliance with HIPAA and GDPR carries heavy fines, which may be the cause that ultimately deters an organization from putting any AI-blockchain solution into operation owing to the fear of possible legal consequence. Figure 14 illustrates navigating AI-blockchain regulatory challenges.

Figure 14. Navigating AI-blockchain regulatory challenges

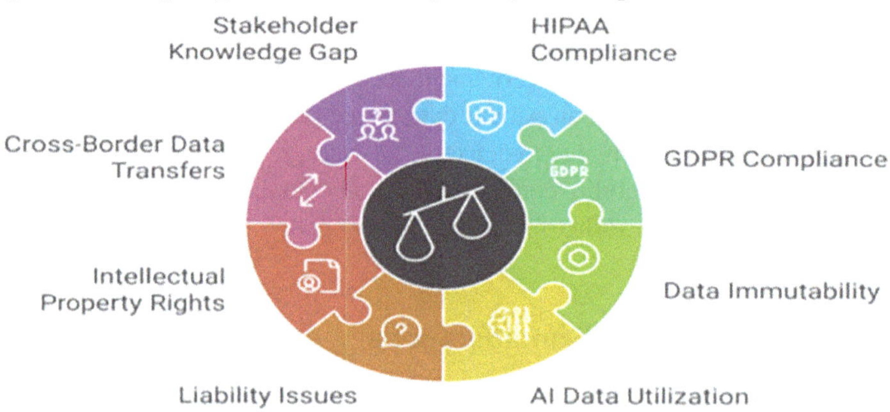

There are also legal implications for liability issues associated with AI decisions made from data stored on blockchains (Nehme et al., 2021). If an AI system, using data stored on a blockchain, makes a wrong recommendation because the data was incorrect-whether because of human input error or malicious tampering-liability is difficult to determine. There are issues regarding the intellectual property rights of AI and blockchain integrations (Upadhyaya, Joshi, & Agrawal, 2025). While an increasing number of organizations develop proprietary algorithms to leverage data residing on blockchains for insights or predictions, there are ownership rights not clear: not just over the algorithms, but over the data underpinning their training.

Another huge challenge lies in cross-border data transfer in the case of international regulations like GDPR, along with local regulations such as HIPAA (Wilson, 2022). Most organizations are international; hence, it would be agonizingly painful and very costly to work out different compliance requirements for different jurisdictions. Besides that, there exists some form of knowledge deficit within the stakeholders' capacity on how to effectively implement AI-Blockchain solutions in concert with compliance to existing regulations.

Interoperability and Standardization

Artificial Intelligence integrated with blockchain opens a whole new world of possibilities, most especially in the health, finance, and supply chain sectors. However, one of the major challenges facing the integration of AI into blockchain technology is the challenge of interoperability and standardization. Interoperability is said to be the ability of various systems, devices, or applications to communicate and share information amongst themselves without any type of hindrances (Rahman & Hussain, 2020).

Figure 15. Challenges in achieving interoperability and standardization in AI-blockchain integration

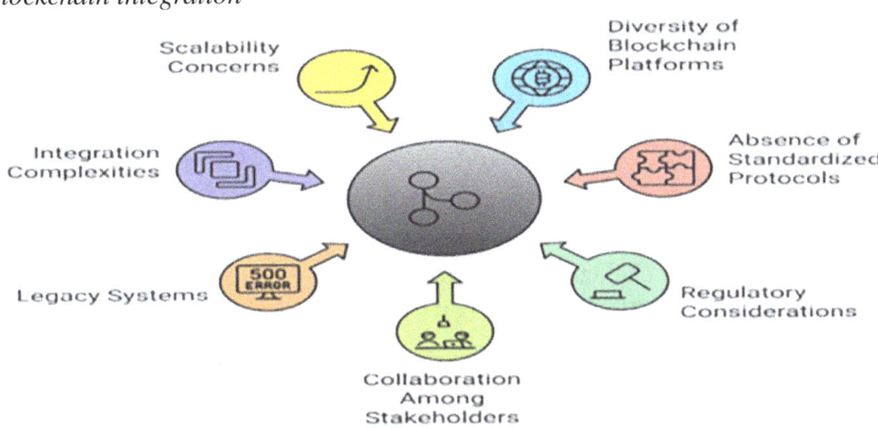

One of the barriers to interoperability is the number of choices there are for blockchain platforms today. It seems like each solution for blockchain has its own rule set, consensus mechanisms, and data structures. It is also aggravated by the fact that there are no standardized protocols, which worsens these interoperability issues (Chen et al., 2023). Since there are no commonly agreed-upon standards as far as data formats, transaction types, and communication means between AI and blockchain systems, significant barriers exist when organizations attempt to share information across platforms. Figure 15 shows challenges in achieving interoperability and standardization in AI-blockchain integration.

If there are technical challenges regarding interoperability and standardization, the situation is further complicated by regulatory considerations. Other jurisdictions may enact different laws on data privacy, such as the GDPR in Europe, and thus affect how AI algorithms interact with blockchain systems storing sensitive information (Khan & Mer, 2023). The other important aspect is that interoperability through shared standards requires industry-wide collaboration. This will require serious input from technology providers, regulatory bodies, academia, and end-users.

Another barrier to seamless interoperability between AI applications and blockchain networks involves existing legacy systems. Most organizations in the world still operate on old infrastructure that is not compatible with modern technologies such as blockchain or enhanced AI algorithms (Hussain & Al-Turjman, 2021). Further, there are intrinsic complications in embedding machine learning models into trustless interaction environments like blockchains.

FUTURE DIRECTIONS AND RESEARCH OPPORTUNITIES

Advances in AI and Blockchain

The amalgamation of Artificial Intelligence with Blockchain technology opens a very fertile playground for future research and development. Efficiency, scalability, and security are the key issues that demand an attentive approach (Khanna & Gochhait, 2024). The hybrid models, while Artificial Intelligence develops further and blockchain's decentralized nature becomes increasingly strong, will be promising solutions to many challenges that industries face today (Zhang et al., 2021).

Hybrid models of AI-Blockchain for better operational efficiency and scalability may form one of the key areas of exploration. Most traditional blockchain systems suffer from low transaction speeds and high energy consumption, hence limiting their employability in high-demand environments (Ressi et al., 2024). Synergistic Innovations in AI and Blockchain as shown in Figure 16.

Figure 16. Synergistic innovations in AI and blockchain

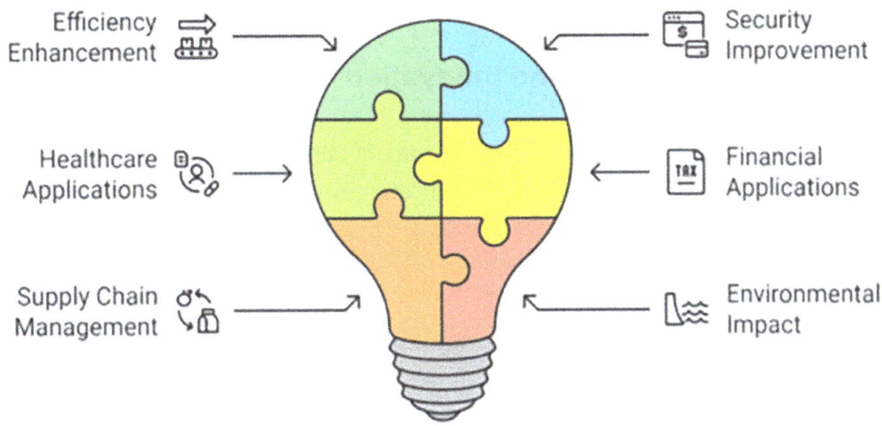

Additionally, data through the integration of AI and blockchain technology has been provided with security and integrity features. They can be rebuilt using machine learning algorithms which compute a constant detection on transaction data for the suspicious patterns that might indicate an anomaly or a fraudulent activity happening on these blockchain networks (Hassan et al., 2022).

A second possible and promising line of research is to search for lightweight solutions, especially designed to be implemented in healthcare applications. With unprecedented challenges in its data management, privacy and interoperability of the heterogeneous systems, there are enormous challenges in the healthcare domain (Yang et al., 2024). For example, patient's health information ends up between different providers and researchers making the patient's consent management processes automatic on a blockchain, such as through smart contracts.

As these technologies evolve rapidly; it is obvious that it becomes equally important for policymakers to catch up with the speed at which they are moving so that ethical issues can be settled accordingly. Besides healthcare, such hybrid models may find their applications in other spheres, including those dealing with finance, supply chain management, and energy.

Moving forward, as such technologies get increasingly deployed in more routine applications, there will also be a need to provide simple platforms through which users from diverse backgrounds, consumers to professionals, can exploit benefits in applications without a deep understanding of the underlying technology.

The environmental impact that would result from the implementation of hybrid solutions as concern for sustainability continues to grow globally. Although blockchain has received criticism regarding energy-intensive consensus mechanisms, such as Proof-of-Work, the incorporation of energy-efficient AI algorithms into it would dampen some of the environmental concerns related to large-scale deployments (Platt & McBurney, 2023).

Collaborative Research and Innovation

Interdisciplinary collaboration in development can be achieved by establishing a platform on which technologists, healthcare professionals, and policymakers come together to share insights and expertise (Vegesna, 2023). These might lead to further refinement of AI algorithms concerning the specific demands emanating from healthcare environments.

Besides this, collaborative research may aim at the development of standardized protocols for data sharing across different healthcare systems (Sheller et al., 2020). This is very important in ensuring interoperability for the different technologies used in patient care. Apart from technological development, ethical considerations should form the bedrock of any form of collaboration around AI and blockchain applications in health (Dutta & Gochhait, 2022). The exponential increase in the adoption rate of these technologies raises significant ethical questions around the ownership of data, consent, transparency, and accountability.

Other fields of research pertain to establishing the impact that the integration of AI and blockchain will have on health outcomes. Longitudinal studies will be helpful in gaining an understanding of the influence such technologies will have on quality patient care, operational efficiency in healthcare centres, and overall system sustainability. Through real-world analyses of AI-blockchain solution applications in various settings, from hospitals to telemedicine platforms, researchers can shed light on best practices that optimize benefits and minimize risks (Rathore et al., 2024).

There is further need for continuous education and training programs that would equip health professionals to use AI-blockchain technologies more effectively. As these fields are so dynamic, continuous professional development mean that practitioners to continuous professional development running across various walks of life always remain abreast with the latest tools and methods.

Researchers should also explore how cultural backgrounds Mold perceptions of privacy and build confidence in AI-blockchain technologies across different populations (Ellahi et al., 2023). An understanding of the subtlety would mean developers of culturally sensitive solutions that will strike a chord with diversified communities.

CASE STUDIES AND PRATICAL IMPLEMENTATIONS

One highlighted case study is the collaboration between IBM Watson Health and blockchain platform MediLedger. By integrating the use of AI algorithms in observing a great volume of data, blockchain had been used to securely transact and track the medicines through their life cycle (Motsi-Omoijiade & Kharlamov, 2021). During such implementation, the challenge had been maintaining data integrity through regulatory standards across various stakeholders.

Other important examples include various uses of AI-driven predictive analytics combined with blockchain technology currently deployed at New York City's Mount Sinai Health System. The healthcare provider implemented an AI-based system to predict patient outcomes by using big volumes of historic data; the sensitive patient information must be kept on a secure blockchain network. Of course, the first and foremost challenge was resistance from the staff who had grown used to conventional methods of maintaining records (Nasir et al., 2024). To overcome this, Mount Sinai invested in detailed training programs that educated staff on the various benefits that stemmed from using AI in a conjoined manner with blockchain, underscoring enhanced data security and improved patient care outcomes.

Another example was when Chronicled-a startup dealing in supply chain solutions-had successfully combined AI with blockchain to manage the lifecycle of pharmaceutical products. The company faced interoperability challenges between the existing systems being used by different stakeholders in the pharmaceutical industry. Chronicled thus created an API that allowed seamless communication between their blockchain platform and legacy systems in use by manufacturers and distributors (Hellani, 2022).

The application of AI-Blockchain integration finds its place beyond supply chain management in clinical trials themselves. For instance, Pfizer investigated the application of blockchain together with AI to improve the management of data resulting from clinical trials (Tagde et al., 2021). One of the tasks was to preserve the management of participant consent without losing compliance under HIPAA. Indeed, Pfizer could achieve all the above by putting in place a blockchain-based decentralized identity system coupled with AI-driven consent management tools.

Another powerful case study was the implementation of a blockchain-based health record-integrated AI chatbot at Stanford University Medical Centre. It supports the patients through personalized advice with regard to their health-related issues, since all of the history regarding their sickness is stored on blockchain. However, the main challenge was how much the patients needed to be informed about the usage of their data while protecting privacy according to statutory law Chaudhary et al. (2021). Stanford accepted this challenge and communicated with the patients with transparent strategies regarding the use of their information in both technologies.

CONCLUSION

The integration of AI with blockchain provides a very promising opportunity to deal with the most urgent security challenges of the health sector. Coupled with this, while AI capabilities in data analysis and predictive modelling have started to make headlines, blockchain inherently offers features of decentralization, immutability, and transparency to healthcare systems for strengthening patient data security, easing operations, and building up the trust factor among its stakeholders. The future of AI-blockchain in health is promising, as this technology can definitely allow safe sharing of medical records and full adherence to regulations such as HIPAA, while reducing fraud by means of transparent transactional records. Due to the relatively new nature of this field and being a developing field, more research and pairing between technologists, participants in the Healthcare field, policymakers, and researchers are needed to solve these problems and finetune these solutions. Integrating AI and blockchain would not only enable more research about them but would also guarantee the future of healthcare.

REFERENCES

Ahmad, I., Asghar, Z., Kumar, T., Li, G., Manzoor, A., Mikhaylov, K., & Harjula, E. (2022). Emerging technologies for next generation remote health care and assisted living. *IEEE Access : Practical Innovations, Open Solutions*, 10, 56094–56132. DOI: 10.1109/ACCESS.2022.3177278

Ahmed, Z., Mohamed, K., Zeeshan, S., & Dong, X. (2020). Artificial intelligence with multi-functional machine learning platform development for better healthcare and precision medicine. *Database : The Journal of Biological Databases and Curation*, 2020, baaa010. DOI: 10.1093/database/baaa010 PMID: 32185396

Alabdulatif, A., Khalil, I., & Saidur Rahman, M. (2022). Security of blockchain and AI-empowered smart healthcare: Application-based analysis. *Applied Sciences (Basel, Switzerland)*, 12(21), 11039. DOI: 10.3390/app122111039

Andrew, J., Deva Priya Isravel, K., Martin Sagayam, B., Bhushan, B., Sei, Y., & Eunice, J. (2023). Blockchain for healthcare systems: Architecture, security challenges, trends and future directions. *Journal of Network and Computer Applications*, 215, 103633. DOI: 10.1016/j.jnca.2023.103633

Balakrishnan, A. (2024). Leveraging Artificial Intelligence for Enhancing Regulatory Compliance in the Financial Sector. *International Journal of Computer Trends and Technology*.

Belchior, R., Vasconcelos, A., Guerreiro, S., & Correia, M. (2021). A survey on blockchain interoperability: Past, present, and future trends. *ACM Computing Surveys*, 54(8), 1–41. DOI: 10.1145/3471140

Bhumichai, D., Smiliotopoulos, C., Benton, R., Kambourakis, G., & Damopoulos, D. (2024). The convergence of artificial intelligence and blockchain: The state of play and the road ahead. *Information (Basel)*, 15(5), 268. DOI: 10.3390/info15050268

Cerchione, R., Centobelli, P., Riccio, E., Abbate, S., & Oropallo, E. (2023). Blockchain's coming to hospital to digitalize healthcare services: Designing a distributed electronic health record ecosystem. *Technovation*, 120, 102480. DOI: 10.1016/j.technovation.2022.102480

Chenthara, S., Ahmed, K., Wang, H., Whittaker, F., & Chen, Z. (2020). Healthchain: A novel framework on privacy preservation of electronic health records using blockchain technology. *PLoS One*, 15(12), e0243043. DOI: 10.1371/journal.pone.0243043 PMID: 33296379

Demertzis, K., Iliadis, L., Tziritas, N., & Kikiras, P. (2020). Anomaly detection via blockchained deep learning smart contracts in industry 4.0. *Neural Computing & Applications*, 32(23), 17361–17378. DOI: 10.1007/s00521-020-05189-8

Dhirani, L. L., Mukhtiar, N., Chowdhry, B. S., & Newe, T. (2023). Ethical dilemmas and privacy issues in emerging technologies: A review. *Sensors (Basel)*, 23(3), 1151. DOI: 10.3390/s23031151 PMID: 36772190

Dutta, S., & Gochhait, S. (Eds.). (2022). *Information retrieval in bioinformatics: A practical approach*. Springer. DOI: 10.1007/978-981-19-6506-7

El-Samad, W., Adda, M., & Atieh, M. (2024). AI-Driven Data Aggregation Level Smart Contracts for Blockchain Healthcare Insurance Claims Adjudication. *Procedia Computer Science*, 241, 63–68. DOI: 10.1016/j.procs.2024.08.011

. Froehlich, A., Siebrits, A., Kotze, C., Froehlich, A., Siebrits, A., & Kotze, C. (2021). e-Health: how evolving space technology is driving remote healthcare in support of SDGs. *Space Supporting Africa,* 91-185.

. Guergov, S., & Radwan, N. (2021). Blockchain convergence: Analysis of issues affecting IoT, AI and blockchain. International Journal of Computations, *Information and Manufacturing (IJCIM), 1*(1).

Haddad, A., Habaebi, M. H., Islam, M. R., Hasbullah, N. F., & Zabidi, S. A. (2022). Systematic review on AI-blockchain based e-healthcare records management systems. *IEEE Access : Practical Innovations, Open Solutions*, 10, 94583–94615. DOI: 10.1109/ACCESS.2022.3201878

Johnson, K. B., Wei, W. Q., Weeraratne, D., Frisse, M. E., Misulis, K., Rhee, K., & Snowdon, J. L. (2021). Precision medicine, AI, and the future of personalized health care. *Clinical and Translational Science*, 14(1), 86–93. DOI: 10.1111/cts.12884 PMID: 32961010

Khan, D., Jung, L. T., & Hashmani, M. A. (2021). Systematic literature review of challenges in blockchain scalability. *Applied Sciences (Basel, Switzerland)*, 11(20), 9372. DOI: 10.3390/app11209372

Khanh, H. H., & Khang, A. (2021). The role of artificial intelligence in blockchain applications. In *Reinventing Manufacturing and Business Processes through Artificial Intelligence* (pp. 19–38). CRC Press. DOI: 10.1201/9781003145011-2

Khanna, A., & Gochhait, S. (Eds.). (2024). *Green AI-powered intelligent systems for disease prognosis*. IGI Global. DOI: 10.4018/979-8-3693-1243-8

Maddireddy, B. R., & Maddireddy, B. R. (2022). Real-Time Data Analytics with AI: Improving Security Event Monitoring and Management. *Unique Endeavor in Business & Social Sciences*, 1(2), 47–62.

Motsi-Omoijiade, I., & Kharlamov, A. (2021). Blockchain for healthcare applications and use cases. In *Blockchain and Public Law* (pp. 157–190). Edward Elgar Publishing. DOI: 10.4337/9781839100796.00015

Nasir, S., Khan, R. A., & Bai, S. (2024). Ethical framework for harnessing the power of AI in healthcare and beyond. *IEEE Access : Practical Innovations, Open Solutions*, 12, 31014–31035. DOI: 10.1109/ACCESS.2024.3369912

Omidian, H. (2024). Synergizing blockchain and artificial intelligence to enhance healthcare. *Drug Discovery Today*, 29(9), 104111. DOI: 10.1016/j.drudis.2024.104111 PMID: 39034026

Palakurti, N. R. (2024). Challenges and future directions in anomaly detection. In *Practical Applications of Data Processing, Algorithms, and Modeling* (pp. 269–284). IGI Global. DOI: 10.4018/979-8-3693-2909-2.ch020

Platt, M., & McBurney, P. (2023). Sybil in the haystack: A comprehensive review of blockchain consensus mechanisms in search of strong Sybil attack resistance. *Algorithms*, 16(1), 34. DOI: 10.3390/a16010034

Putra, K. T., Arrayyan, A. Z., Hayati, N., Damarjati, C., Bakar, A., & Chen, H. C. (2024). A Review on the Application of Internet of Medical Things in Wearable Personal Health Monitoring: A Cloud-Edge Artificial Intelligence Approach. *IEEE Access : Practical Innovations, Open Solutions*, 12, 21437–21452. DOI: 10.1109/ACCESS.2024.3358827

Rahman, Z., Yi, X., & Khalil, I. (2022). Blockchain-based AI-enabled industry 4.0 CPS protection against advanced persistent threat. *IEEE Internet of Things Journal*, 10(8), 6769–6778. DOI: 10.1109/JIOT.2022.3147186

Rajput, A. R., Li, Q., & Ahvanooey, M. T. (2021). A Blockchain-Based Secret-Data Sharing Framework for Personal Health Records in Emergency Condition. *Healthcare (Basel)*, 9(2), 206. DOI: 10.3390/healthcare9020206 PMID: 33672991

Ressi, D., Romanello, R., Piazza, C., & Rossi, S. (2024). AI-enhanced blockchain technology: A review of advancements and opportunities. *Journal of Network and Computer Applications*, 225, 103858. DOI: 10.1016/j.jnca.2024.103858

Saeed, H., Malik, H., Bashir, U., Ahmad, A., Riaz, S., Ilyas, M., & Khan, M. I. A. (2022). Blockchain technology in healthcare: A systematic review. *PLoS One*, 17(4), e0266462. DOI: 10.1371/journal.pone.0266462 PMID: 35404955

Singh, B., & Kaunert, C. *(2024).Reinventing Artificial Intelligence and Blockchain for Preserving Medical Data.In Ethical Artificial Intelligence in Power Electronics (pp. 77-91).* CRC Press. DOI: 10.1201/9781032648323-6

Tagde, P., Tagde, S., Bhattacharya, T., Tagde, P., Chopra, H., Akter, R., Kaushik, D., & Rahman, M. H. (2021). Blockchain and artificial intelligence technology in e-Health. *Environmental Science and Pollution Research International*, 28(38), 52810–52831. DOI: 10.1007/s11356-021-16223-0 PMID: 34476701

Töberg, J. P. (2022). Modelling and Enforcing Access Control Requirements for Smart Contracts (Doctoral dissertation, Karlsruher Institut für Technologie (KIT)).

Upadhyaya, N. (2024a). AI-Augmented Dynamic Language Adaptation for Low-Resource Languages: A Transfer Learning Solution for Optimized NLP Performance. *International Research Journal of Advanced Engineering and Science*, 9(4), 89–94.

Upadhyaya, N. (2024b). Enhancing real-time customer service through adaptive machine learning. *Int. J. Adv. Res. Sci. Commun. Technol.*, 4(1), 630–636. DOI: 10.48175/IJARSCT-19381

Upadhyaya, N. (2024c). Artificial intelligence in web development: Enhancing automation, personalization, and decision-making. *Int. J. Adv. Res. Sci. Commun. Technol.*, 4(1), 534–540. DOI: 10.48175/IJARSCT-19367

Upadhyaya, N., Joshi, H., & Agrawal, C. (2025). Examining NLP for Smarter, Data-Driven Healthcare Solutions. In *Intelligent Systems and IoT Applications in Clinical Health* (pp. 393–420). IGI Global.

Velmovitsky, P. E., Bublitz, F. M., Fadrique, L. X., & Morita, P. P. (2021). Blockchain applications in health care and public health: Increased transparency. *JMIR Medical Informatics*, 9(6), e20713. DOI: 10.2196/20713 PMID: 34100768

Wang, J., Zhu, H., Wang, S. H., & Zhang, Y. D. (2021). A review of deep learning on medical image analysis. *Mobile Networks and Applications*, 26(1), 351–380. DOI: 10.1007/s11036-020-01672-7

Williamson, S. M., & Prybutok, V. (2024). Balancing privacy and progress: A review of privacy challenges, systemic oversight, and patient perceptions in AI-driven healthcare. *Applied Sciences (Basel, Switzerland)*, 14(2), 675. DOI: 10.3390/app14020675

Zhang, Z., Song, X., Liu, L., Yin, J., Wang, Y., & Lan, D. (2021). Recent advances in blockchain and artificial intelligence integration: Feasibility analysis, research issues, applications, challenges, and future work. *Security and Communication Networks*, 2021(1), 9991535. DOI: 10.1155/2021/9991535

Chapter 2
Challenges and Solutions in Securing AI Algorithms in Healthcare

Jabin Shiji Koshy
Christ University, India

ABSTRACT

The paper discusses existing challenges that, based on the legal framework, the regulatory change must affect in order to ensure interest coverage in the health sector. Massive opportunities lie in the role that AI plays in healthcare in the forms of diagnostics and personalized care, while major challenges arise. AI models like machine learning, deep learning, and neural networks have improved healthcare outcomes, but they raise concerns on the privacy of patient data, explainability, and cyber threats such as adversarial attacks. Sensitive data must be protected for patients to trust AI-driven diagnosis. Bias in algorithms, the obtaining of informed patient consent, and the accountability of the AI decisions are some ethical and regulatory issues. Regulations like HIPAA(Health Insurance Portability and Accountability Act) and GDPR(General Data Protection Regulation) are the most important while considering data protection.This includes better encryption and anonymisation of patient data, interpretable models, and stronger defences against cyber-attacks.

INTRODUCTION

AI applications in diagnostic procedures, treatment personalization, and clinical decision support have enhanced healthcare. Moreover, this article explores privacy-preserving artificial intelligence methodologies, such as differential privacy and safeguard multi-party calculation, as viable strategies in order to mitigate data pri-

DOI: 10.4018/979-8-3373-2827-0.ch002

vacy concerns within the healthcare sector. Deep learning and Machine Learning algorithms can adapt and adopt and discover enormous data that would otherwise be useless to doctors to use in the care of patients. As their presence continues to grow, they become vulnerable to numerous security risks, not just for patient safety but also for data protection (Weinberg et al., 2024; Wilhelm et al., 2024). This article explores the primary security risks related to AI in healthcare—adversarial attacks, algorithmic bias, data privacy concerns—and offers practical solutions to mitigate these vulnerabilities.

Challenges in Securing AI Algorithms

Federated learning enables artificial intelligence systems to train using data stored across various institutions without necessitating the transfer of that data. To achieve global scalability in federated learning, it is imperative for institutions to address several challenges, including interoperability across jurisdictions, resource allocation, and the heterogeneity of data quality. The standardization of data formats, along with the utilization of edge computing, can facilitate scalable implementations and foster collaborations across borders, particularly in the healthcare sector. Adversarial attacks occur when attackers manipulate AI inputs to deceive the system. In one case, hackers altered MRI images analyzed by an AI system, resulting in incorrect diagnoses of brain tumors. These subtle changes are often undetectable to humans but can cause significant harm if the AI produces a wrong medical recommendation (Weinberg et al., 2024). These attacks not only compromise patient safety but also corrode trust in AI technologies among clinicians.

Artificial Intelligence systems within healthcare are prone to algorithmic bias when their training datasets do not represent diverse patient populations. Emerging methodologies like differential privacy, which initiates statistical noise to datasets, and safeguard multi-party computation, which allows collaborative analysis while safeguarding data confidentiality, represent substantial advancements in the protection of patient data. For example, AI models developed for dermatology have shown poor diagnostic performance on darker skin tones because they have a lack of representation in training data (Wilhelm et al., 2024). It may lead to wrong diagnosis for minority groups, further complicating the problem of healthcare disparities.

Bias in AI algorithms would be very impactful to patients' outcomes. To reduce that, frequent audits of the algorithms should be done to ensure that they work equally across demographic groups. In addition, diverse datasets should be incorporated in the training process in order to reduce bias in AI algorithms and improve diagnosis on all patient populations (Wilhelm et al., 2024).

Ethical Considerations in AI-driven Healthcare

The large amount of sensitive health data that machines process poses serious privacy concerns. Healthcare facilities are prime cyber-attack targets due to the value medical data holds. The case reported is that of a vast data breach involving thousands of patients personal health information after an AI-driven health platform succumbed to a cyberattack (Weinberg et al., 2024). Some of these have everlasting effects, such as identity theft, discrimination, and erosion of patient trust.

To lessen the threat of data privacy breaches, healthcare providers must utilize strong practices, implement decentralized data, and use federated learning models. Federated studying makes it available for AI systems to teach with data placed in various institutions without necessarily transferring the data, and this is why the threats of exposing the data reduce (Weinberg et al., 2024).

Addressing AI Vulnerabilities in Healthcare

Several techniques can be professional to overcome the weaknesses of AI in healthcare. Privacy-conserving technologies, including differential privacy and secure multi-party computation (SMPC), are increasingly gaining prominence in various sectors. Differential privacy serves to anonymize patient data while retaining its utility for artificial intelligence training purposes. Conversely, secure multi-party computation facilitates collaborative calculations on encrypted data, making sure that sensitive data and information of patients remain secure during partnerships among multiple institutions. Firstly, adversarial training increases the robustness of AI. It is exposed to adversarial examples during the training of models so that the models are able to detect and correct the manipulated inputs. Algorithmic bias is also minimized through regular auditing of algorithms and use of diversified datasets to prevent differential performances across patient populations (Wilhelm et al., 2024).

Moreover, such measures as data encryption and decentralized storage may also assist in the protection of medical information from unwanted access, especially from intruders. Health organizations must not hesitate to involve cybersecurity personnel who will oversee AI with real-time scrutiny and make corrections on potential vulnerabilities accordingly (Weinberg et al., 2024).

Regulatory and Ethical Considerations

Alliance between healthcare providers and Artificial Intelligence developers and makers is important to improve AI systems which are transparent, ethical, and safe. Furthermore, the incorporation of bioethics experts and policy regulators is vital in this process. Bioethics specialists contribute valuable insights to ensure that approaches remain patient-centered, while regulators play an important role in creating adaptable governance frameworks. Such interdisciplinary cooperation enhances the integrity and efficacy of AI systems in healthcare. There should be a very solid regulatory framework that supports patient safety. There is a need to make consistent guidelines set for all of the development, testing, and deployment in clinical settings by the appropriate regulatory authorities. Mandates on rigorous clinical testing - like drug trials - ought to be set in to ascertain the safety and efficiency of AI tools (Wilhelm et al., 2024). it should be mentioned as an ethical issue. Regulatory organizations such as HIPAA and GDPR should further increase their frameworks by addressing the combination of differential privacy and secure multiparty computation (SMPC). This will ensure that artificial intelligence systems adhere to the evolving standards related to secure and ethical data utilization. Responsibility for the errors made by AI systems must be clearly blamed-on all the parties involved such as healthcare providers, the makers of the AI, or the related institutions.

Theoretical Framework:

Important theories or models that support the chapter.

1. Socio-Technical Systems Theory

It depends on the relation among people, technology, and the organizational structures in which they live. In healthcare, Artificial Intelligence systems operate as an object of a broader socio-technical ecosystem rather than as an independent solution." Everyone who uses AI systems is involved in different kinds of combined discussions. To secure the AI algorithms, according to this theory, holistic solutions have to be executed for addressing not only technical weakness but also human-related factors of trust, responsibility, and communication. (Baxter & Sommerville, 2011).

2. Information Security Management Systems (ISMS) Model

The ISMS framework, therefore, provides a structured guideline for managing and securing information systems, making it of great relevance to healthcare since patient data security is one of the primary needs. This model, in particular, ISO/IEC 27001 shows initiatives towards providing some systematic support to ensure data is proper and its confidentiality, integrity, and availability. It provides implementation of practices such as encryption and anonymization, as mentioned in through the chapter.

3. Ethical AI Frameworks

Ethical considerations are a key concept when we think about the utilization of AI within healthcare. For example, guidelines as outlined in the Principles for Ethical AI notes that fairness, accountability, transparency, and privacy are the key standards (Floridi & Cowls, 2019) regarding the subject of the need to remove biases in algorithms and to make sure that AI is used effectively in the sector. In healthcare, guidelines such as these helps solve most of the ethical debates surrounding patient consent, algorithmic biasness and effects of lack of transparency about the AI's decision-making ability.

4. Diffusion of Innovations Theory

This theory is about the manner in which the organization adopts the new technologies such as AI in healthcare over the time period. This understanding therefore points out challenges with AI security execution such as stakeholder acceptance, care providers or patients may push back from adopting because of the uncertainty or for ethical reasons or not having enough trust in the AI systems.

5. Adversarial Machine Learning (AML)

Theories behind adversarial attacks are very important for understanding the weakness of artificial intelligence. Adversarial machine learning has focused much on defensive mechanisms for defending algorithms that lie at the heart of AI against such attacks, so ensuring AI systems to be trusted and secure when exposed to real-world conditions (Goodfellow et al., 2015).

6. Data Protection Regulations: HIPAA and GDPR

From a regulatory standpoint, these are HIPAA and the General Data Protection Regulation (GDPR), at the heart of this structure. Both ensure an enabling legal background to safeguard data and patient privacy, with standards that enforce adherence to AI algorithms that handle sensitive health information (Cohen & Mello, 2018).

Relevant Theories and Models for Chapter Sections

1.Cyberattack against AI Algorithms:

The Adversarial Machine Learning theory has worked towards realizing the fact that AI systems are under cyberattacks. More relevant in this respect are also Socio-Technical Systems Theory, which indicates that with technical challenges, the human aspects come into play as well, such as trust and transparency

2.Ethical Considerations in Healthcare with AI

Ethical AI frameworks guide the discussion on various issues ranging from bias to fairness to transparency. The ethical models ensure accountability and fairness in healthcare AI systems.

3.Securing AI Algorithms: Best Practices

The ISMS model and ISO/IEC 27001 standards provide a structured solution for implementing secured AI algorithms. The group of standards focused primarily on data confidentiality, integrity and availability in AI systems in healthcare.

4.Regulatory and Policy Frameworks:

HIPAA and GDPR provide the main regulatory structure that ensures the patient data is secured by healthcare AI systems within the limits of the privacy laws. They provide minimalist standards of laws that the systems should react to in any given formation within the AI-driven framework for the healthcare industry.

Key conceptual foundations

1.Securing AI Algorithms

Challenges will arise in the sector of securing AI algorithms because of their increased presence in healthcare through deep learning and machine learning . Some critical issues have occurred including their vulnerability to negative attacks, where information could mislead the model's decision-making processes. For example, subtle differences in the entered data, which enfold a large range of medical records and can change benign diagnosis to malicious. This becomes dangerous in clinical applications when reliability and accuracy become the central focus (Kelly et al., 2019). Furthermore, the type of data that AI systems operate on requires significant storage locations across vast systems, which induces data siloing and interoperability that has a propensity to make the task of securing these algorithms more burdensome .

2.Ethical Considerations during AI Driven Healthcare

Bias, transparency, and responsibility are the ethics in relation to the introduction of Artificial Intelligence in healthcare. Traditionally, training data for AI models poorly represents populations of particular interest and thus cannot provide equal outcomes for minority groups due to algorithmic bias. For example, algorithms to detect skin cancer, trained more on light-skinned patients, tend to be lower in their performance on dark-skinned patients, thus worsening health disparities (Kelly et al., 2019). Issues of ethics also come into the picture in terms of informed consent, as patients may not understand exactly in what way their data is being utilized by AI systems. Another requirement to gain the trust of both clinicians and patients would be the interpretability of the AI models. AI systems have to be accurate but must also allow for transparency of how decisions are taken.

3.Securing AI Algorithms: Best Practices

The best practices for securing AI systems in health care focus on improvements along both the technical and organizational safeguards line. Through the technical safeguard approach, patient data and other information is encrypted to ensure anonymity before using AI training models. Moreover, AI systems must always be monitored and updated from time to time, which eliminates model drift, a phenomenon where the performance of the model degrades over time due to changes in clinical practices or patient populations (Esteva et al., 2019). Regular audits and adherence to privacy frameworks such as HIPAA and GDPR help ensure sensitive patient data is kept safe when using AI systems.

4.Regulatory and Policy Frameworks

The regulatory frameworks provide the bedrock of standardized usage of AI in healthcare and protection as well as efficacy. Policies, like the General Data Protection Regulation (GDPR) and the Health Insurance Portability and Accountability Act (HIPAA), institute the necessary bounds on patient data. However, fluidity in the AI models-particularly those that are designed for continuous learning-makes this problematic for fixed process regulatory structures. Regulators have begun to increasingly work towards more agile regulatory frameworks, like the ongoing work by the US FDA in revising regulations for machine learning-based Software as a Medical Device (Kelly et al., 2019).

Critical Discussion of Existing Frameworks in Securing AI Algorithms in Healthcare

1.Challenges in Securing AI Algorithms:

Challenges in Secure AI Algorithms identifies the key challenges of integration of AI in healthcare, with particular focus on security of the AI algorithm. AI applications applied in healthcare, for instance, through ML and DL systems require unique challenges to create data privacy and reduce adversarial attacks, along with bias that might adversely compromise safety and reliability of AI applications. There is an absence of standardized frameworks for these challenges. Current AI systems are vulnerable to attacks by malicious agents motivated to introduce patterns of input that mislead algorithms into making incorrect predictions; for example, they might deceive benignly appearing tumors as malignant. Such weakness underscores the need for overall security features, including model interpretability and robust encryption besides continuous updates of the models to thwart the possible development of new threats.

2.Ethical Considerations in AI-driven Healthcare:

Ethical considerations are an important part of safe AI algorithm design, especially issues related to patient confidentiality and consent, and also bias. AI models, usually biased due to the type of their training data, tend to perpetuate healthcare inequalities among minoritized groups. For instance, skin lesion models mainly trained on lighter skin tones, performances become severely degraded on darker tones, which has ethical considerations about fairness and equality in AI health care applications. The illustration of underrepresented populations in training and validation of AI models is very important so that those biases could be mitigated and equitable healthcare outcomes ensured. What's more, AI systems must ensure they are transparent and explainable; there should be clarity around the AI-driven decisions for health providers and patients, hence building trust into applications of AI.

3.Best Practices for Securing AI Algorithms:

Best practices emphasized in this chapter are that security for AI algorithms includes encryption, anonymization of patient data, and development of explainable AI systems. For example, encryption and anonymization secure really important data of the patient, preventing the data protection regulations such as HIPAA and GDPR from changing into unwanted or unexpected situations. This keeps the data secure. However, the security measures will not fully be able to help. understandability must also be a very important consideration for AI models-to allow healthcare providers to look into the decision-making process, which will help us to find out whether the algorithms are making decisions based on logical medical reasoning or not. More compound models like deep learning lack the transparency required for the medical environments.

4.Regulatory and Policy Frameworks:

Present day regulatory frameworks are subjected to the changes, considering the upcoming aspects related to constant growth and changes in AI technologies in the healthcare industry. These frameworks will come with regulations that ensure that AI systems are positioned in a safe and effective way, considering proper flow in machine learning models. The AI systems learn and improvise in real-time; their challenges are in terms of the need for regular updates and continuous performance monitoring. In addition, frameworks such as the GDPR in Europe introduce "right to explanation," which requires that people affected by decisions made through these algorithms have access to the explanation on how these decisions are made. However, the frameworks still need to figure out how to have information regarding the complication of AI systems model bias, explainability, and the security of learning models.

Conceptual Development

1.Challenges in Securing AI Algorithms in Healthcare

Artificial Intelligence is capable of bringing golden opportunities for customized and real time diagnostics in the sector of healthcare. The applications of networks algorithms and machine learning in AI can process good medical data sets so that real-time awareness can be obtained to help bring greater outcomes for the patients. This AI model can be used to interpret disease risks, find the best possible treatments available and automate analysis of radiology complex images. Innovations and developments like this make the healthcare industry much more efficient and also highly accessible to all. However, with large-scale execution of AI, there are major challenges, the main one being data security, cyber vulnerability, and ethics. (Jin et al., 2023).

The biggest challenge in securing AI algorithms is protecting the personal sensitive data of the patients provided. Data is the essential resource through which the AI models work-precisely, a substantial amount of personal and medical information. High volumes of data create significant risks about the chances of cyberattacks that might be taking advantage of the gaps of AI systems. Hackers will use these AI models to target patients and use these models to get information they may not otherwise be able to access, or worse, manipulate the model itself. For instance, that input may be an adversarial attack, which may attempt to subtly change the input data-but this could be a patient scan or even a medical record. This is the reason why the output of the AI changes in ways that are averse to the model such as having the model predict wrong or advise unwanted treatments. Such manipulation may lead to unwanted or improper medical recommendations, hence affecting the safety and trust of the patients. (Samuel.,1959)

For example, the attack might be so crafted that in the diagnostic image early signs of cancer blur such that an AI model would completely miss the diagnosis. Beyond losing credibility in the health care domain, adversarial attacks carry extensive connotations in terms of their legal and ethical implications because patients and healthcare practitioners rely on the accuracy of decisions made with the support of AI. The Health Insurance Portability and Accountability Act (HIPAA) in the U.S. and General Data Protection Regulation (GDPR) in Europe have strict regulations when it comes to managing patient data. Still, taking such regulations in consideration, complexity in AI-based systems brings about a huge issue that leads to total security, risking the trust of health care stakeholders-a mix of patients, providers, and regulators. (Alkaissi.,2023).

Model Explainability and Transparency Issues: Another serious challenge of deep learning architecture is explainability. Even though such models are exceptionally good at dealing with and interpreting data, it works more as a "black box," not in the sense that once inputted, it can be subsequently processed and interpreted, but the decision-making process is opaque and not humanly interpretable. Lack of transparency is a critical problem, particularly in the health care sector, since decisions emanating from AI systems, no matter how complex they are, cannot be understood and, therefore, trusted by health care professionals. Where the clinicians do not know how the model arrives at its particular diagnosis or recommendation for treatment, it becomes hard for them to rely on AI systems in crucial cases where clinical judgment needs to be relied upon. (Samuel.,1959) And so bringing it all back to the greater theme of the issue, the problem of bias in AI itself. Trained on historical data, an AI model is just to whatever extent the underlying biases within the data that it is trained on-for example, racial or gender or socioeconomic biases the exact same biases will percolate into the judgments and recommendations that it makes in its predictions. For instance, an algorithm prepared mainly on data from a population of white patients would likely do poorly with disease diagnoses in the Black or Hispanic population.

With this, these biases plus the mystery surrounding AI decision-making processes would only deepen the already existing inequality in health care and roll back much-needed and long-overdue strides towards equal healthcare for all patients. (Kelly et al., 2019).

The danger of data security, cyber vulnerabilities, and explainability surrounds the challenges that suggest, regardless of the power of AI, its adoption in healthcare would require a high amount of overseeing. This will involve more cooperation among health-care providers, developers, and regulators to make stronger, safer, and more transparent AI systems in the health industry which will help the patients to trust it. Some relevant solutions are executed, such as strong encryption, use of undisclosed patient data, and improvement of explainability of AI models.

The development of proper ethical frameworks and regulation will help in the handling of risk associated with AI in healthcare and ensure that the need of all is covered, most importantly that of the patient. The setting up of this needs to be dynamic for the healthcare sector to fully use AI for the improvement of outcome without any threat to trust and ethical integrity.

2.Ethical Considerations in AI-driven Healthcare

Issues of health sector AI usage should be integrated with data security, model transparency, and accountability. While AI stands as a very important part of health systems in the future, it also brings a huge amount of critical ethical issues that face these three considerations.

Training Bias in AI Algorithms

Most likely, the biggest ethical issue becomes common at the base of most of the algorithms as it shows AI is biased. These AI models, especially those that rely on machine learning and deep learning, learn from previous datasets inserted. Unless the training data are free of bias-for example, in the sense that it does not suitably show a given race, gender, or socio-economic group-an AI is very likely to assume such biases and actually reflect them on its outputs. For example, the white, middle-class patients imagine it mainly on such a model may not be qualified to diagnose in a black, Hispanic, or Indigenous patient, hence leading to misdiagnosis of such patients or poor recommendations for treatment. This may lead to healthcare inconsistency and violate the ethical principle of justice, the principle that guarantees equal treatment for all patients. (Samuel., 1959)

This is not easy because the historical medical records mostly carry biases according to superior society. Therefore, simply by means of themselves to enhance diversity in the training data comes societal biases that need changes. Even more fundamental changes that fix the biases are through algorithmic fairness that can catch and rectify biases built into the model during the development process itself (Kelly et al., 2019). The problem highlighted above, if not treated, will attract serious ethical and legal issues where in the biased algorithms could cause a patient's outcome to be affected while bringing cases of discrimination against healthcare providers.

Informed Consent and Use of Data The second key ethical question would be the mechanism of informed consent for health care controlled by AI. For AI systems to be useful, their models often have to be based on a gigantic amount of data regarding patients. Such data are most often gathered from patients' electronic health records, medical scans, and even genetic information.

The more of these AI systems become networked, the data that is found within a single patient's file will spread across multiple servers and health care organizations. It does raise very profound questions about the security and privacy of patient data but increases the accuracy and efficiency of AI systems through shared data. (Alkaissi.,2023) The patients should also be informed of what is done with their data and for what purpose and to whom one may grant access. Therefore, most AI systems will not allow the full understanding of how such data could be treated, analyzed and shared.

This circumstance makes a patient vulnerable in a position where they may unknowingly give permission to their data being used in various ways that may not be acceptable to them in the future, such as for commercial gain or in the improvement of these models that may not necessarily provide service to them directly. It includes a violation of the autonomy principle because it draws attention specifically to informed consent and respect to decisions made regarding a patient's own healthcare. This would thus entail fully open, transparent, and consensual processes between health care providers and developers of AI, clearly showing detailed implications of how the patients data would be used, and the full possibility for patients to opt either in or out of the process.

All this aside, AI systems should respect and provide protection to regulations on data like in Europe GDPR, which is very strictly set out about using and handling where a patient's rights to privacy are respected. The same can be said of HIPAA from the U.S. (Samuel.,1959).

Accountability in AI Decision-Making

Arguably the most challenging ethical question in the context of healthcare is the accountability question. To whom do you hold liable if an AI system, in making a decision included within that being a diagnosis of a patient or a recommendation of treatment, results in a clinical outcome, especially when that clinical outcome happens to be an adverse event? Traditional health care functions have very defined lines of responsibility regarding who is responsible for what, and in an automated and algorithm-driven world of AI, things get complicated. Accountability cannot be identified in case of a failure in a black box model because the decisions of an AI system are not transparent. Is the healthcare provider culpable for being blind faith in AI recommendations if the treatment recommendation from an AI system has resulted in harm because of giving wrong advice? Or should the creator of AI be held culpable for creating a flawed model? Or is it the health care facility institution that put the AI system in place ensuring that the AI system is safe and effective? Again here, who is to blame when things go wrong? All these lead towards clear accountability frameworks indicating who is liable in what set of circumstances. (Alkaissi.,2023)

Another accountability gap arises where the AI system processes more than one jurisdiction and thus has varying laws governing AI, health care, and liability in every country. Policymakers and regulatory bodies must, therefore, create appropriate legal frameworks that clarify the main job of AI in decision-making and who bears the responsibilities when an AI fails.

In this regard, malpractice standards of AI may be defined and regulatory bodies overseeing improvement, deployment and use of AI in the health care sector may be established. (Jin et al., 2023).

3. Securing AI Algorithms: Best Practices

AI algorithms in the health sphere must be addressed by a multipronged approach that takes into account technical vulnerabilities of these systems and ethical implications of their deployment. As healthcare AI continues to evolve and gain importance in critical clinical workflows, it is essential that it remains robust, secure, and ethical. We elaborate further on the best practices below for securing AI algorithms in healthcare.

- Encryption and Anonymization:

Most sensitive aspect relating to use of AI in healthcare is the safeguarding of patient data. For this, encryption-both at rest (stored) and in transit (being transferred)-is a basic practice. That way, even if unauthorized people acquire the data, they cannot interpret it without its decryption key, thus ensuring the patient's privacy and diminishing the chance of data breaches.

Anonymization means deletion or obscuring personal identifiers in the data. This subsequently makes any data impossible to trace back to a particular patient, thus providing another layer of security. Anonymization is especially pertinent in the sense that these large datasets are trained using AI models; usually, such datasets cut across enormous expanses of patient information. Techniques that can also be extended to include differential privacy will make data anonymization even more enhanced, thereby allowing slight statistical noise in the data which will protect individual privacy while still making sure the AI model learns effectively off the dataset. (Kelly et al., 2019).

A firm foundation for safeguarding sensitive patient information from both internal threats, as the employees in the staff may access it without authorization, and external threats, such as hacking or phishing attacks, can be developed by combining encryption and anonymization

- Enhancing Explainability of AI Models

In fact, one of the major problems with AI systems-more so, deep learning-based systems-is that they are not interpretable very well. These "black box" models predict accurately enough, but often, the logic behind this prediction is not clear. This often attracts enormous risks in healthcare, for example, where the logic behind an informed diagnosis or treatment recommendation must ensure that patients have gotten their proper safety and trust in the system. (Samuel.,1959)

Improving interpretability will make AI models more transparent and explainable. Either will involve the development of inherently interpretable models from the start, where a more basic algorithm or a model with built-in explanations replace such opaque models as deep neural networks. Alternatively, the technique for understanding what is happening inside more complex models will be to apply methods for explainable AI, XAI. Such tools include LIME and SHAP, which are commonly used in the explanation of predictions from machine learning models, thereby providing insights into which features, for example, patient symptoms and medical history, had the greatest impact on the AI's decision. (Jin et al., 2023).

This will make the AI models more interpretable, thus leading healthcare professionals to make better-informed decisions with associated explanations to patients regarding why the decision was made. The AI system will be used ethically and responsibly this way. Moreover, interpretability can help identify and correct biases in AI systems as an audited transparent model is easier when errors occur.

Building Robust Models Against Adversarial Attacks

An adversarial attack may expose AI systems, especially health care, to threats. Slightly varying data input could make bad actors change the machine learning model to incorrectly forcast outcomes (Wilhelm et al., 2024) This would significantly threaten health care, as even small amounts of differences in the data could lead to a misdiagnosis or incorrect advice for treatment for a patient from their records in some form.

There are strategies that developers need to use to make AI systems resilient to attacks of these kinds, and these include the following:

Adversarial Training: Exposure of the model to adversarial examples in training so as to learn from a wide series of manipulative inputs.

Robust Optimization: Not too sensitive to minor changes in input data because they are optimized for stability and resilience. (Kelly et al., 2019).

Input Validation and Data Sanitization: Input data needs to be validated properly before accepting them by the AI system to prevent malicious data injection.

These may reduce the risks related to adversarial attacks and help improve security and dependability in healthcare AI systems.

- Federated Learning for Decentralized Data Processing

The other future solution to the secure provision of AI systems is federated learning. Actually, it mitigates the challenge within the training of AI models due to data centralization. In the past, large sets of data from various institutions have been collected in a central location for the training of AI models. Data centralization raises the risk of data breach, and in this way, the system becomes more vulnerable to large-scale attacks. (Jin et al., 2023).

Federated learning solves this by allowing AI models to be trained locally on the device or servers that hold the data, not necessarily by transferring the data to a central location. Here, only model updates-which would be the learned parameters-are transferred with the central server but the raw data is not shared. This is yet another way through which decentralization offers more security since patient data does not have to be transferred as it is local to the place an institution owns it, thus reducing chances of that information falling into the wrong hands.

Additionally, federated learning also helps institutions to abide by the data protection laws like HIPAA and GDPR, which permit hardly any liberty in how and where patient data is transmitted and processed. Federated learning, thereby keeping the data within an institution, thus reduces legal and ethical risks that are associated with data sharing, yet still permits powerful AI models (Fleming et al., 2024).

- Regular Auditing and Monitoring of AI Systems

There should be routine auditing and monitoring to secure AI systems in healthcare. Critical care healthcare environments require that AI systems are frequently audited for performance, security compliance, and conformance to the highest legal and ethical standards. Among other things, such auditing can help determine potential vulnerabilities or performance issues in the system, whether biases resulted in model training or accuracy degradation over time.

Regular auditing can be supplemented with real-time monitoring tools that could detect anomalous behavior. These tools would allow the system administrator to spot some potential security breaches or errors in the model's outputs in time for intervention.

4. Regulatory and Policy Frameworks

The regulations that are already in existence, such as HIPAA and GDPR, form the foundation, but the policy has to be built out further to suit the purposes of AI in healthcare. The regulatory agencies must form standards that ensure security and appropriate deployment, as well as accountability in regard to AI. The policy should be constructed considering international standards on security and offering a pathway for review of AI systems on a regular basis (Jin et al., 2023).

5. Expanding Federated Learning for Scalability in Global Healthcare

Federated Learning (FL) has become a cornerstone of privacy-preserving AI model training, particularly in healthcare. Its potential for scalability in global networks offers transformative opportunities but comes with significant challenges:

- Interoperability Across Jurisdictions: FL must navigate diverse regulatory landscapes like GDPR and HIPAA (Cohen & Mello, 2018). Standardizing data formats and protocols is essential for fostering cross-border collaborations.
- Resource Allocation: Integrating FL across global healthcare systems requires considerable computational resources. Utilizing edge computing can mitigate this challenge, reducing the burden on centralized servers (Esteva et al., 2019).
- Enhancing Robustness: Addressing heterogeneity in data quality, device capabilities, and network stability is critical for scaling FL. Solutions include algorithm optimization and adaptive learning models to ensure reliability (Weinberg et al., 2024).

By overcoming these barriers, FL can enable a global AI healthcare ecosystem that respects privacy while improving patient outcomes.

6. EDGE AI FOR REAL-TIME HEALTHCARE APPLICATIONS

Edge AI facilitates local deployment of AI models on devices or servers, enabling real-time decision-making critical to healthcare. Edge AI refers to the deployment of artificial intelligence models on local devices or servers, facilitating real-time decision-making at the point of care. This technology supports applications such as wearable health devices and point-of-care diagnostic tools by minimizing latency. Nonetheless, Edge AI encounters several challenges, including limitations in computational power, energy efficiency, and data synchronization. Future developments in lightweight AI models and hybrid cloud-edge systems hold the promise of overcoming these obstacles, thereby positioning Edge AI as a crucial element in the advancement of healthcare innovation.

1. Applications:
    - Point-of-Care Diagnostics: Devices can analyze medical images or signals (like ECGs) on-site, delivering instant results.
    - Remote Patient Monitoring: Wearables equipped with AI can detect health anomalies in real-time, prompting timely interventions.
2. Challenges:
    - Limited Computational Power: Edge devices often lack the hardware for complex AI models (Lipton, 2018).
    - Data Synchronization: Ensuring consistency between edge and central systems in distributed networks is critical.
    - Energy Efficiency: Optimizing AI algorithms to reduce power consumption is vital for sustainable usage.
3. Future Directions:
    - Developing lightweight AI models engineered for edge environments.
    - Creating hybrid systems where edge AI collaborates with cloud resources for seamless data flow and computation (Wilhelm et al., 2024).

Integrating Edge AI can enhance efficiency, reduce latency, and bring precision care closer to patients.

7. DIFFERENTIAL PRIVACY

Differential Privacy ensures data privacy while enabling analytics and AI models to process sensitive healthcare data. By introducing statistical noise, this technique makes individual patient information indistinguishable in datasets.

- Protecting Patient Data: Ensures sensitive details cannot be reverse-engineered from aggregated outputs (Goodfellow et al., 2014).
- Enabling Federated Learning: Enhances FL by securing distributed training datasets.
- Regulatory Compliance: Aligns with GDPR and HIPAA by limiting exposure to identifiable information (Cohen & Mello, 2018).

Applications include safeguarding AI models analyzing electronic health records, genetic data, and diagnostic imaging.

8. SECURE MULTI-PARTY COMPUTATION (SMPC)

Secure Multi-Party Computation (SMPC) allows numerous entities to enumerate data collaboratively without exposing it to any party. Key benefits include:

- Data Confidentiality: Computations on encrypted data prevent direct exposure of sensitive information.
- Interoperability: Facilitates secure collaborations across healthcare institutions without centralized data storage (Jin et al., 2023).
- Fraud Prevention: Reduces the risk of breaches during collaborative processes.

Examples in Healthcare:

- SMPC enables secure statistical analysis in multi-center clinical trials.
- Supports collaborative AI model training by combining datasets securely across institutions.

9. ADVANCED TRENDS IN HEALTHCARE AI SECURITY

- Generative Adversarial Networks (GANs) for Data Augmentation:
    - Applications: Generate synthetic data to enhance AI model performance while preserving patient privacy.
    - Security Implications: Requires robust monitoring to prevent misuse in generating adversarial examples (Goodfellow et al., 2014).
- Dynamic Defense Mechanisms:
    - Adversarial Training: Incorporates anomaly detection systems to neutralize adversarial inputs in real-time.
    - Blockchain Integration: Blockchain ensures secure, immutable data transactions across healthcare networks (Floridi & Cowls, 2019).
- Emerging Topics:
    - Quantum Encryption: Offers unparalleled security through principles of quantum mechanics (Wilhelm et al., 2024).
    - Decentralized AI: Reduces reliance on central servers, enhancing privacy and collaboration (Weinberg et al., 2024).

By adopting these advanced trends, healthcare can address evolving security threats while maximizing the potential of AI-driven systems.

IMPLICATIONS AND FUTURE RESEARCH

Implications:

It closely looks at a bunch of vulnerabilities that affect AI systems, digs into the ethical dilemmas they create and suggests best practices to keep their integrity safe. This chapter aims to greatly improve data privacy (which is super important) through detailed guidelines on setting up ISMS and mixing in ethical AI frameworks. It's not just about protecting sensitive info regarding patients, however, it also focuses on getting rid of algorithmic biases that mess up clinical outcomes. This helps bring about more accurate and fair diagnoses and treatments through AI-driven systems (Fleming et al., 2024). In this way, the chapter highlights the regulatory frameworks, like the GDPR and the HIPAA (Kelly et al., 2019). It encourages following these legal standards but then points out how healthcare providers need to comply with regulations that build patients' trust and make it easier to adopt these technologies in the health sector: overall, this work really helps in securing ethical and efficient healthcare applications that are based on AI.

FUTURE RESEARCH SUGGESTIONS:

1.Adversarial Defense Mechanisms: Research in adversarial machine learning can be expanded to create strong defenses against complex, harmful manipulations of healthcare data or decision-making algorithms (Jin et al., 2023).
2.Explainable AI in Healthcare: Research into new breakthroughs in explainable AI, like XAI, may improve the understanding of transparency, especially in deep learning models.
3.Federated Learning for Enhanced Safety: Deep research in the field of federated learning can open new doors to the decentralization of sensitive information (Samuel., 1959). This method of data processing does not require the centralization of data, thus reducing the chance of breaches. It will, however, enhance the safety aspect of patient data in collaborative AI models in healthcare.
4.Bias Mitigation Techniques: Since algorithmic bias remains a major issue, research can focus on adaptive, real-time adjustments in AI models to deal with biases that come from historical data differences and improve fair healthcare outcomes.

Several aspects in need of further investigation and exploration are highlighted on the basis on the theoretical framework of safeguarding AI algorithms in the healthcare field.

1. Increased Socio-Technical Integration of AI in the Healthcare Sector

Future investigation and study could potentially shift its attention towards incorporating socio-technical methods into healthcare AI systems, exploring the intricate relationship between technical elements and human factors like patient trust, clinician training, and communication in AI decision-making processes. One possible strategy is to enhance Socio-Technical Systems Theory with case studies on integrating AI in healthcare settings, leading to practical insights for improving trust, comprehension, and ethical application of AI models.

2. Improved methods for protecting against attacks from adversaries.

New defenses like adversarial training and robust optimization are necessary in AI algorithms due to the vulnerabilities they create for attacks by adversaries. Studying systems to promptly identify and address threats will improve the performance of healthcare AI. When applied to intricate healthcare data like imaging or genetic information, these methods make the models more resilient to malicious influences.

3. Decentralized AI Training using Federated Learning:

Investigating federated learning could have implications for the security and privacy of healthcare. This could lead to new ways of training models across different institutions without centralizing sensitive data. (Wilhelm et al., 2024). The potential for data breaches will be minimized, and data sharing will be done securely. Examinations can be conducted to assess the impact of technical and regulatory issues in federated learning specifically within the healthcare sector, exploring the implications of compliance with HIPAA and GDPR across various jurisdictions.

4. Explainability in AI Algorithms:

Due to the opaque nature of AI being seen as hindering trust and accountability, further investigation into explainable AI, or XAI, is necessary. Improve the method of interpretability models or post-hoc analysis tools which include LIME (Local Interpretable Model-Agnostic Explanations) and SHAP (SHapley Additive exPlanations) to better fit clinical AI, allowing healthcare professionals to comprehend and validate the AI's suggestions. Establishing guidelines for clarity in healthcare using AI could assist regulatory bodies in defining the limits of acceptable explanatory standards. (Johnson., 2023)

5. Identifying and fixing bias in artificial intelligence used in healthcare.

These could be proactive bias detection systems, always monitoring and adapting to reduce biases in healthcare AI models, particularly among marginalized communities. Techniques to mitigate bias can be integrated into the development and testing of models in order to prevent the spread of prejudice and inequalities in healthcare delivery. (Baxter & Sommerville, 2011) Different research might investigate how various datasets, fairness metrics in algorithms, and input from a large number of disciplines such as ethics and social sciences impact the reduction of bias in real-time in clinical applications.

6. How does the Ethical AI framework change when applied to continuous learning models?

A lot of AI systems in the health and care field are constantly improving as they receive new data, meaning that ethical AI guidelines need to adapt to the changing models. (Weinberg et al., 2024) Research in the future may still focus on making sure that these dynamic models adhere to the established standards of responsibility, privacy, and consent. This could require adaptable but strong structures guaranteeing moral honesty in systems evolving continuously.

CONCLUSION

Healthcare in terms of AI stands for a paradigmatic revolution on diagnosis, treatment, and management in care. Ongoing development and expansion of the technology of AI particularly ML, DL, represent new opportunities not previously available with improved clinical decision making, more effective processes, smooth and better outcomes for the patients. It poses all kinds of challenges at present and requires close attention to seeing to it that AI benefits can come responsibly, equitably and securely.

Address Security Challenges

The major concern pertains to patient-related confidential information. Artificial intelligence requires a huge volume of data for learning and operation in real-time scenarios. These practices have serious concerns to do with the privacy and security of such records. HIPAA in the United States and GDPR in Europe have their own regulations, setting pretty much no framework about not revealing a patient's information. The majority of the regulations are subject to the strictest possible practice in terms of encryption, anonymization, and differential privacy. These would introduce statistical changes into the datasets to avoid any form of revealing identities while, at the same time, making it more meaningful analysis possible to provide to the patients.

Federated learning is the new bounding line of approaches addressing the issue of data privacy. To ensure that raw data never leaves the institution from where it originates, Federated learning is a decentralized form of training for the AI across various cities and nations and different institutions. Apart from reducing risk related to breach of privacy, Federated learning motivates collective innovation in developing new AI models. For example, Federated Learning enables the building of strong diagnosis models by accumulation of insights to find out from diverse patient populations without compromising on the privacy of patients. It is mathematically very expensive to implement Federated learning at a global scale in healthcare systems, but it provides computing that can weaken these demands by distributing different tasks.

Ethical Considerations and Bias Mitigation

The ethical considerations of AI-driven healthcare are not just data privacy but concerns such as algorithmic bias, informed consent, and accountability. The most important challenge, in this case, is algorithmic bias since most AI models propagate the bias of the data on which they were trained. For instance, a dermatology model that has been trained by mainly lighter skin tones will not work very well for dark-skinned patients and might misdiagnose and have biased treatment outcomes. This calls for involving diverse and representative datasets when training the model and applying fairness metrics to identify and mitigate biases. This needs to be that diverse and representative datasets be used in model training and fairness metrics to identify and mitigate biases.

The transparency and interpretability of the AI models are also really very important. Black-box models, despite the fact that they are exact, and are also very less explainable. This lack of explainability does not help in improving trust among healthcare providers or patients. Techniques such as Explainable AI which have tools such as LIME and SHAP can help users explain how AI makes its decisions. Increased understanding breeds trust and also reveals and corrects biases so that AI systems will operate ethically and fairly and provide accurate results.

Prior consent is yet another foundational concept of ethical AI. Patients should be fully informed about the use, distribution, and process of the use of their data by AI. It should be properly communicated among healthcare providers, AI developers, and patients to ensure that the use of data fits within the expectations of patients and legal requirements that are set. This should be a necessary condition for implementing respect for patient autonomy and trust in AI-driven health care solutions.

Next Generation Technologies for Secure and Scalable AI

The new technologies play a key role in addressing the challenges of AI in healthcare: its security and scalability. Edge AI, which includes the direct arrangement of AI models on local devices or servers, gives real-time decision-making at the point of care, thus decreasing latency and improving the efficiency of diagnostic and monitoring systems such as AI-powered wearables that can detect irregularity in real-time. Challenges, such as computational power and energy efficiency, however, it is crucial to achieve full exploitation of the power of edge AI.

Secure Multi-Party Computation is another discovery that permits parties to involve and collaborate for the analysis of data without giving out private and personal information. Because computations done within SMPC can be conducted on encrypted data, several institutions can work in an interoperable fashion to bring forth collaborative innovations. For example, SMPC could be used to combine the data of patients in a number of hospitals without being required to lose confidentiality over clinical trials.

The technology of blockchain enhances security through the facilities of immutable and transparent records of data transactions. Blockchain technology can be used in health care to monitor patient data access. This is with the aim of ensuring accountability and preventing unauthorized use. Combining AI and blockchain provides a robust framework for secure and efficient data sharing across healthcare networks.

Robustness against Adversarial Threats

Adversarial attacks constitute significant threats to AI systems in health care. In order these attacks manipulate input data to mislead AI models, potentially leading to incorrect diagnoses or treatment recommendations. For instance, subtle alterations to medical images could cause an AI system to misclassify benign tumors as malignant. To counter these threats, adversarial training and robust optimization techniques are essential. These methods bring in AI models to adversarial examples during training and enhance their capacity to identify and resist such attacks.

In health care applications, GANs can be either used to conduct adversarial attacks or used as an important generator that can produce realistic and proper data that can be used for data augmentation. This feature is mainly useful in disease research, such as rare cases, which cannot rely on full access to medical records due to the less availability but are problematic to fully develop the models. Thus, it must be authenticated with strong observation in order that such data generation using GAN is ethically and securely achieved.

This makes the regulatory framework of AI technologies more dynamic. There would be a base from the existing laws like HIPAA and GDPR, but always an update will be needed as and when challenges come out to be more volatility of AI models that are ever changing due to fast and continuous learning that occur in the field of medical and technology. The guidelines for the regulatory bodies would set up those innovations with a patient safety sense, so important and effective use of AI systems would be in practice.

Another main aspect is international interactions. Because of the spread of Artificial intelligence worldwide, there must be a change of regulations among different authorities, and hence, collaboration shall not be troublesome but an activity totally compliant with the local law. The data format and protocols have to be standardized for the ease of AI integration into health settings.

Future Implications for Research and Practice

Advance the improvement to secure and scalable AI technologies for applications in healthcare. These includes:

1. Adversarial Defense Mechanisms: Develop a cutting-edge technique that can detect adversarial attacks in real-time and reduce them.
2. Explainable AI: Increases the interpretability of novel XAI methods customized to clinical applications.
3. Federated Learning: The Federated Learning systems to new horizons in scalability and efficiency to support global interactions.
4. Bias Mitigation: Investigate adaptive models that can go along dynamically in real-time to reduce the biasedness.
5. Quantum Encryption: The capability that quantum technologies open to unmatched security in data communication.
6. Ethical AI Frameworks: Ethical standards are used to deal with the highly improved nature of the models that frequently learn and operate across different places or jurisdictions.

Equitable AI: Collaboration

The world of Artificial Intelligence is revolutionizing healthcare in ways never imagined. Unprecedented opportunities lie before us to transform patient outcomes, improve operational efficiencies, and expand access to care. But all these promises at the assurance of AI in healthcare can only be fully understood if these are developed and deployed responsibly. Collaboration among healthcare providers, AI developers, regulators, and patients will be the key to ensure that these technologies promote health equity and accessibility for all.

Role of Stakeholders in Fair AI Development

A successful AI-based health system is primarily a result of the collaborative action of its various stakeholders:

1. Healthcare Providers:Healthcare providers would serve frontline leadership roles in patient care and would play really important roles related to the introduction of AI solutions into clinical workflows. They may guide the development of AI models, both clinically relevant but also user-friendly, in order to enable raising insights into pragmatic challenges and requirements for the patients and making sure that the tools' application is not going to bring any existing prejudices into their clinical practice with them.
2. AI Developers: The outputs from such algorithms must be valid, balanced, and transparent. This translates to the inputs that both model training and evaluation phases should entail. The model itself should not just fit healthcare but adapt health settings, so many things there only apply therein. This means there is a reason the developers will need to refer to the domain expert while ensuring output that meets specifications in involving him
3. Regulators: Clear standards and guidelines should be created by regulatory bodies for the proper development and use of AI technology. This may include guidelines in relation to to data privacy, the transparency of algorithms used, and ensuring accountability. Furthermore, the regulatory body should test whether these tools that are implemented and developed do not go beyond ethical standards.
4. Patients: Patients are always the heart of the healthcare ecosystem, and their involvement and engagement are of prime importance in developing and testing AI technologies. Patient feedback would allow for areas of value addition from AI to be highlighted and for solutions to be developed that best serve the needs of the patients. Additionally, the education of patients about AI tools and addressing their privacy and security concerns is important to instill trust.

Overcoming the Challenges of AI in Healthcare

While AI promises much, some of the problems that are related to its application in the health sector are not well addressed. Some of them include:

1. Algorithmic Bias: The source of bias in AI algorithms could be either through unrepresentative training datasets or through biases implanted during the data collection process. An example is how the underrepresentation of certain groups of people within a medical dataset can lead to misdiagnosis or recommendation for the treatment of that population. In this respect, developers take several steps involving diverse and representative datasets, metrics of fairness, and periodic audits towards identifying and rectifying bias.
2. Model Transparency: Many of the AI algorithms, particularly those based on deep understanding and adapting, are "black boxes," in the sense that at least at this point in time, it is not easy to reverse-engineer why particular decisions are being made. And that sort of lack of transparency in decision-making really undermines the trust of both providers and patients. So interpreting model explanations is also a great component for instilling trust and accountability.
3. Data Privacy and Security: Confidentiality in using sensitive patient data when training AI models raises the need for data protection and security. Good data protection will be ensured with encryption, anonymization, as well as conformity to laws like GDPR and HIPAA. Data sharing among the organizations needs to be made safe so that cooperation can be established without risking patients' data.
4. Ethical Concerns: Introducing AI into healthcare brings about questions related to accountability in decision-making and dislodging of human roles in healthcare. One of the questions is who will be liable in case an AI tool gives a wrong diagnosis. Specificity of who does what and is responsible is required in humans and AI when making clinical decisions in healthcare.

Steps towards Equitable AI

Such barriers require strategies implemented by all the stakeholders as illustrated below for an actually equitable AI ecosystem.

1. Facilitating Collaboration: Collaboration is important both between stakeholders and among stakeholders with other stakeholders, including open communication. Clinicians, data scientists, ethicists, and patients may ensure AI tools with a holistic approach. For the case of collaborative innovation, common challenges are dealt with much better in public-private partnership and industry consortia.
2. Promotion of Diversity in AI Development: Diversity must exist in every level of AI development which is from data collection to testing of the models. That is not only that diverse datasets must be used, but also diverse teams must be developed for such technologies. Workforce diversity is likely to present diverse

perspectives, which can easily detect biases at an early stage and correct them before the actual development.

3. Increasing Transparency: It transforms trust and, therefore, means that how an AI model functions should be something that can be explained by the developer, together with its limits. It is inclusive of publishing performance metrics about accuracy, sensitivity, and specificity for diverse groups.
4. Strong Governance Frameworks: Setting Governance frameworks for Ethics in the Usage of AI for Healthcare the development of governance structures shall address concerns about rules, especially on how to share the data, follow-ups on cases of bias incidence, and proper avenues for appeals concerning adverse occurrences and disputes that would be undertaken and enforced autonomously by separate watchdogs.
5. Patient Enabling: This without saying that the education of the patients about positive and negative uses of AI applications will help them to accept their future with much hope and belief. The role of patient advocacy groups can also be seen at this point. People, however, should have rights to know in which ways the data is utilized and should give choices to back out from all such data compilations if wanted so.

The Way Ahead: Innovation, Responsibility, and Equity

The path forward would be based on innovation, responsibility, and equity in an AI-driven health care system, with stakeholders sharing the fruits of AI benefits equitably among different groups in society.

1. Innovation: There is the need for innovation to continually stretch the boundaries on what is achievable in the health sector using AI. New algorithms will continue exploring new applications as AI is further integrated into new and emerging technologies like wearable devices and telemedicine.
2. Responsibility: AI development should abide by ethical standards to prove fairness, transparency, and responsibility. Stakeholders must place patient welfare above other agendas: ensure that tools such as AI should not replace humans but complement the judgment of doctors and other care-givers.
3. Equity: Equitable access to AI technologies also minimizes health disparities. Other forms of barriers are cost, absence of infrastructure, and a reduced level of digital literacy in under-resourced communities that need to be solved.

AI is very promising for transformation in the sector of health care through improved patient outcomes, process efficiency, and better accessibility to care. All the stakeholders would have to put in multi-directional efforts to overcome all these challenges that include algorithmic bias, lack of transparency, among many others for this potential to materialize. Formation of partnerships and diversity fostering to improve transparency can empower patients with a view towards building a responsible and equitable AI-driven healthcare ecosystem, which has to be through innovation, responsibility, and equity. With the effects of AI percolating to every walk of life, healthcare accessibility and equality must be brought within everyone's reach.

REFERENCES

Alkaissi, H., & McFarlane, S. I. (2023). Artificial Hallucinations in ChatGPT: Implications in Scientific Writing. *Cureus*. Advance online publication. DOI: 10.7759/cureus.35179 PMID: 36811129

Ayers, J. W., Poliak, A., Dredze, M., Leas, E. C., Zhu, Z., Kelley, J. B., Faix, D. J., Goodman, A. M., Longhurst, C. A., Hogarth, M., & Smith, D. M. (2023). Comparing Physician and Artificial Intelligence Chatbot Responses to Patient Questions Posted to a Public Social Media Forum. *JAMA Internal Medicine*, 183(6), 589. DOI: 10.1001/jamainternmed.2023.1838 PMID: 37115527

Baxter, G., & Sommerville, I. (2011). Socio-technical systems: From design methods to systems engineering. *Interacting with Computers*, 23(1), 4–17. DOI: 10.1016/j.intcom.2010.07.003

Cohen, I. G., & Mello, M. M. (2018). HIPAA and Protecting Health Information in the 21st Century. *Journal of the American Medical Association*, 320(3), 231. DOI: 10.1001/jama.2018.5630 PMID: 29800120

El-Gendy, S., Elsayed, M. S., Jurcut, A., & Azer, M. A. (2023). Privacy Preservation Using Machine Learning in the Internet of Things. *Mathematics*, 11(16), 3477. DOI: 10.3390/math11163477

Esteva, A., Robicquet, A., Ramsundar, B., Kuleshov, V., DePristo, M., Chou, K., Cui, C., Corrado, G., Thrun, S., & Dean, J. (2019). A guide to deep learning in healthcare. *Nature Medicine*, 25(1), 24–29. DOI: 10.1038/s41591-018-0316-z PMID: 30617335

Fleming, S. L., Lozano, A., Haberkorn, W. J., Jindal, J. A., Reis, E., Thapa, R., Blankemeier, L., Genkins, J. Z., Steinberg, E., Nayak, A., Patel, B., Chiang, C.-C., Callahan, A., Huo, Z., Gatidis, S., Adams, S., Fayanju, O., Shah, S. J., Savage, T., & Shah, N. H. (2024). MedAlign: A Clinician-Generated Dataset for Instruction Following with Electronic Medical Records. *Proceedings of the AAAI Conference on Artificial Intelligence*, 38(20), 22021–22030. DOI: 10.1609/aaai.v38i20.30205

Floridi, L., & Cowls, J. (2019). A Unified Framework of Five Principles for AI in Society. *Harvard Data Science Review*. Advance online publication. DOI: 10.1162/99608f92.8cd550d1

Goodfellow, I. J., Shlens, J., & Szegedy, C. (2014). *Explaining and Harnessing Adversarial Examples*. arXiv. DOI: 10.48550/ARXIV.1412.6572

Hopfield, J. J. (1982). Neural networks and physical systems with emergent collective computational abilities. *Proceedings of the National Academy of Sciences of the United States of America*, 79(8), 2554–2558. DOI: 10.1073/pnas.79.8.2554 PMID: 6953413

Jin, Q., Leaman, R., & Lu, Z. (2023). Retrieve, Summarize, and Verify: How Will ChatGPT Affect Information Seeking from the Medical Literature? *Journal of the American Society of Nephrology*, 34(8), 1302–1304. DOI: 10.1681/ASN.0000000000000166 PMID: 37254254

Johnson, D., Goodman, R., Patrinely, J., Stone, C., Zimmerman, E., Donald, R., Chang, S., Berkowitz, S., Finn, A., Jahangir, E., Scoville, E., Reese, T., Friedman, D., Bastarache, J., Heijden, Y. V. D., Wright, J., Carter, N., Alexander, M., Choe, J., & Wheless, L. (2023). *Assessing the Accuracy and Reliability of AI-Generated Medical Responses: An Evaluation of the Chat-GPT Model.* DOI: 10.21203/rs.3.rs-2566942/v1

Kelly, C. J., Karthikesalingam, A., Suleyman, M., Corrado, G., & King, D. (2019). Key challenges for delivering clinical impact with artificial intelligence. *BMC Medicine*, 17(1), 195. DOI: 10.1186/s12916-019-1426-2 PMID: 31665002

Kung, T. H., Cheatham, M., Medenilla, A., Sillos, C., Leon, L. D., Elepaño, C., Madriaga, M., Aggabao, R., Diaz-Candido, G., Maningo, J., & Tseng, V. (2023). Performance of ChatGPT on USMLE: Potential for AI-assisted medical education using large language models. *PLOS Digital Health*, 2(2), e0000198. DOI: 10.1371/journal.pdig.0000198 PMID: 36812645

Lipton, Z. C. (2018). The mythos of model interpretability. *Communications of the ACM*, 61(10), 36–43. DOI: 10.1145/3233231

Mehrabi, N., Morstatter, F., Saxena, N., Lerman, K., & Galstyan, A. (2022). A Survey on Bias and Fairness in Machine Learning. *ACM Computing Surveys*, 54(6), 1–35. DOI: 10.1145/3457607

Nagendran, M., Chen, Y., Lovejoy, C. A., Gordon, A. C., Komorowski, M., Harvey, H., Topol, E. J., Ioannidis, J. P. A., Collins, G. S., & Maruthappu, M. (2020). Artificial intelligence versus clinicians: Systematic review of design, reporting standards, and claims of deep learning studies. *BMJ (Clinical Research Ed.)*, m689, m689. DOI: 10.1136/bmj.m689 PMID: 32213531

Oh, S.-R., Seo, Y.-D., Lee, E., & Kim, Y.-G. (2021). A Comprehensive Survey on Security and Privacy for Electronic Health Data. *International Journal of Environmental Research and Public Health*, 18(18), 9668. DOI: 10.3390/ijerph18189668 PMID: 34574593

Samuel, A. L. (1959). Some Studies in Machine Learning Using the Game of Checkers. *IBM Journal of Research and Development*, 3(3), 210–229. DOI: 10.1147/rd.33.0210

Syed, K., Sleeman, W. C., Nalluri, J. J., Kapoor, R., Hagan, M., Palta, J., & Ghosh, P. (2020). Artificial intelligence methods in computer-aided diagnostic tools and decision support analytics for clinical informatics. In *Artificial Intelligence in Precision Health* (pp. 31–59). Elsevier., DOI: 10.1016/B978-0-12-817133-2.00002-1

Turner, R. J. (2007). Book review. *Journal of Minimally Invasive Gynecology*, 14(6), 776. DOI: 10.1016/j.jmig.2007.07.001

Veale, M., & Borgesius, F. Z. (2021). Demystifying the Draft EU Artificial Intelligence Act. *Computer Law Review International*, 22(4), 97–112. DOI: 10.9785/cri-2021-220402

Weinberg, J., Goldhardt, J., Patterson, S., & Kepros, J. (2024). Assessment of accuracy of an early artificial intelligence large language model at summarizing medical literature: ChatGPT 3.5 vs. ChatGPT 4.0. *Journal of Medical Artificial Intelligence*, 7(0), 33. Advance online publication. DOI: 10.21037/jmai-24-48

Wilhelm, C., Steckelberg, A., & Rebitschek, F. G. (2024). Is artificial intelligence for medical professionals serving the patients? Protocol for a mixed method systematic review on patient-relevant benefits and harms of algorithmic decision-making. DOI: 10.1101/2024.03.27.24304965

Xu, H.-L., Gong, T.-T., Liu, F.-H., Chen, H.-Y., Xiao, Q., Hou, Y., Huang, Y., Sun, H.-Z., Shi, Y., Gao, S., Lou, Y., Chang, Q., Zhao, Y.-H., Gao, Q.-L., & Wu, Q.-J. (2022). Artificial intelligence performance in image-based ovarian cancer identification: A systematic review and meta-analysis. *EClinicalMedicine*, 53, 101662. DOI: 10.1016/j.eclinm.2022.101662 PMID: 36147628

Chapter 3

Enhancing Healthcare Data Security With Stacked Deep Learning Approach

Usharani Bhimavarapu
https://orcid.org/0000-0002-0246-1420
Department of Computer Science and Engineering, Koneru Lakshmaiah Education Foundation, Vaddeswaram, India

ABSTRACT

Cybersecurity in healthcare systems is crucial due to the sensitive nature of patient data and the increasing risk of cyberattacks. This paper proposes a novel approach to enhancing cybersecurity defenses by utilizing stacked artificial neural networks (ANNs) for the detection of man-in-the-middle (MITM) attacks, such as spoofing and data injection, targeting healthcare data transmission. The dataset used includes 35 network flow metrics and 8 biometric features, which represent the critical aspects of network traffic and patient health data. The methodology involves training two base-level ANN models: one for detecting anomalies in network flows and the other for identifying irregularities in biometric data. These models' outputs are combined in a meta-model to improve classification accuracy and provide a robust defense mechanism. The proposed method demonstrates enhanced attack detection capabilities by leveraging both network and health-related data, offering a comprehensive solution to safeguard healthcare information systems.

DOI: 10.4018/979-8-3373-2827-0.ch003

INTRODUCTION

Healthcare data is increasingly vulnerable to cybersecurity threats due to its sensitive nature and critical importance in patient care. Ransomware attacks are one of the most common threats, where cybercriminals lock healthcare systems or data and demand a ransom for release, often causing significant disruption in healthcare services (van Boven et al., 2024). Phishing attacks are also prevalent, as attackers impersonate trusted entities to steal login credentials or introduce malware into healthcare systems (Liu et al., 2024). Data breaches, where attackers exploit vulnerabilities to steal patient information, are another serious concern, as such data can be sold on the dark web or used for identity theft and fraud. Man-in-the-middle (MITM) attacks are particularly concerning, as they allow cybercriminals to intercept and modify data in transit, compromising the integrity and confidentiality of sensitive patient information (Tyagi et al., 2023). Insider threats also pose a risk, as employees or contractors with access to healthcare systems may intentionally or unintentionally leak or misuse data. Additionally, medical devices connected to healthcare networks, such as infusion pumps and pacemakers, are vulnerable to cyberattacks that could manipulate patient treatments or endanger their safety.

To mitigate these threats, several safety measures must be implemented to protect healthcare data. One of the most effective measures is encryption, which ensures that sensitive data is unreadable to unauthorized users both at rest and in transit. Strong access controls and multi-factor authentication (MFA) should be enforced to limit access to healthcare systems and patient data to authorized personnel only (Suleski et al., 2023). Regular security audits and vulnerability assessments can help identify and address potential weaknesses in the system (Edwards, 2024). Additionally, comprehensive staff training on cybersecurity best practices, such as recognizing phishing attempts and following proper protocols for handling sensitive data, is crucial. Data backups and disaster recovery plans should also be in place to ensure that systems can be quickly restored in the event of an attack. Lastly, securing medical devices through proper network segmentation, regular patching, and end-point protection can help prevent attacks on critical healthcare infrastructure (Zisad & Hasan, 2024). By adopting these safety measures, healthcare organizations can significantly enhance their defenses against cyber threats, ensuring the protection of patient privacy and the continuity of care (Okafor et al., 2023).

There are several existing models used to safeguard healthcare data from cybersecurity attacks, each designed to address different aspects of security, but all come with their own limitations. Encryption-Based Models such as AES and TLS, is widely used to protect healthcare data both at rest and in transit (Ahmed et al., 2023). While it ensures that unauthorized users cannot access sensitive data, it can be computationally expensive and inefficient, especially with large datasets or real-time applications. Additionally, encryption does not protect against vulnerabilities at the application or user level, such as weak passwords or poor access controls. Role-Based Access Control (RBAC) limits access to sensitive healthcare data based on predefined user roles, ensuring that only authorized personnel can access specific data (Blessing, 2024). However, managing and updating user roles can be complex in large organizations with dynamic staffing, and incorrect role configurations can lead to data access issues or security gaps. Attribute-Based Access Control (ABAC) uses user attributes, such as job function or location, to control access to healthcare data (de Oliveira et al., 2023). It offers more flexibility than RBAC but can be challenging to implement and maintain as the number of attributes increases. The complexity of managing attributes may also introduce errors or inconsistencies, potentially undermining security. Intrusion Detection and Prevention Systems (IDPS) monitor network traffic to detect and prevent potential cyberattacks, such as unauthorized access and malware (Farooq et al., 2023). However, signature-based systems struggle with detecting new or unknown threats, while anomaly-based systems often generate false positives, leading to alert fatigue and possible missed attacks. Firewalls control incoming and outgoing network traffic, acting as a barrier between secure and untrusted networks (Singh & Singh, 2024). While they are effective at preventing unauthorized access, they are often not sufficient by themselves to prevent more sophisticated attacks, such as internal breaches or malware that bypasses firewall protections. Data Loss Prevention (DLP) systems are designed to monitor and restrict the movement of sensitive data within and outside an organization, preventing leaks or theft (Robert, 2023). However, DLP solutions can sometimes block legitimate data transfers, affecting productivity, and may struggle to prevent attacks that occur over encrypted channels. Two-Factor Authentication (2FA) adds an extra layer of security by requiring users to provide two forms of identification, such as a password and a biometric factor (Suleski et al., 2023). While this greatly improves user authentication, it can be cumbersome for users, leading to resistance or poor implementation, and is vulnerable if one of the factors (e.g., a mobile device) is compromised. Endpoint Protection tools, such as antivirus software and endpoint detection and response (EDR), are essential for securing devices that access healthcare data (Cheng et al., 2024). While effective against known threats, they may not be sufficient for advanced persistent threats (APTs) or zero-day attacks. They also require constant updates to remain effective. Security Information and Event Management (SIEM) systems aggregate and analyze security event data from multiple sources, providing real-time insights and alerts (Zahid et al., 2023). However, they can be resource-intensive and require significant configuration and tuning to be effective. Additionally, SIEM solutions often produce a large number of alerts, making it difficult for security teams to prioritize and respond promptly. Blockchain for Health Data can provide a decentralized and immutable ledger for healthcare data, enhancing transparency and preventing unauthorized alterations (Alsamhi et al., 2024). However, blockchain implementations can be complex, costly, and resource-demanding, and may not be suitable for all types of healthcare data or use cases. Additionally, scalability issues can arise when handling large volumes of data.

Each of these models plays a crucial role in safeguarding healthcare data, but they also come with limitations that need to be addressed through a combination of techniques and constant adaptation to emerging threats. Deep learning techniques offer significant potential in overcoming many of the limitations of traditional cybersecurity models used to safeguard healthcare data (Pritee et al., 2024). One key advantage is deep learning's ability to detect complex patterns and anomalies in large datasets, making it highly effective for intrusion detection and prevention systems (IDPS). Unlike signature-based methods, deep learning models can identify new, previously unknown threats, such as zero-day attacks, by learning from vast amounts of data. This capability reduces the reliance on manual rule creation and helps in detecting subtle patterns that would be missed by conventional approaches. Additionally, deep learning-based models can be used for real-time monitoring and adaptive access controls, improving on the limitations of static models like RBAC or ABAC by dynamically adjusting to changing user behaviors and access needs.

Furthermore, deep learning enhances encryption models by optimizing performance and improving data protection without significant computational overhead, thanks to techniques like federated learning, where the data is processed locally, thus preserving privacy. For data loss prevention (DLP), deep learning models can be trained to identify sensitive data even in unstructured formats and detect abnormal data movement across different platforms more accurately than traditional DLP tools. In terms of endpoint protection, deep learning algorithms can analyze patterns of known and unknown malware, offering a more adaptive and proactive approach to securing devices. Finally, deep learning can reduce the issue of false positives in anomaly detection systems by better understanding the normal behavior of network traffic and medical device usage, allowing for more accurate and efficient security measures. In essence, deep learning provides a more dynamic, scalable, and adaptive approach to cybersecurity in healthcare, addressing the limitations of traditional methods and enhancing overall data protection.

The proposed stacking artificial neural network (ANN) is highly suited for enhancing cybersecurity in healthcare data due to its ability to effectively combine multiple models to improve accuracy, robustness, and performance in detecting cyber threats. In the context of healthcare, where data integrity, confidentiality, and availability are paramount, stacking ANN can integrate various machine learning models to make more accurate predictions, detect complex attack patterns, and adapt to evolving cybersecurity threats.

Stacking ANN works by combining the strengths of several base models (such as decision trees, support vector machines, or neural networks) and training a meta-model to aggregate their outputs. This ensemble approach helps mitigate the limitations of individual models. For instance, if one base model struggles with detecting a certain type of attack, another model in the stack may perform better, thereby improving the overall detection accuracy. This is particularly useful in healthcare, where cyber threats are diverse, including phishing, ransomware, insider threats, and more subtle forms of data breaches or spoofing.

Furthermore, stacking ANN allows for better feature extraction and fusion from multiple data sources, such as network traffic data, patient biometric information, and system logs. By learning complex relationships and correlations across these varied data inputs, the stacking ANN can detect nuanced attack patterns that may be missed by simpler models. For example, in man-in-the-middle attacks or data injection, where data may be altered in transit, the model can detect inconsistencies between expected and actual data flows, thereby improving the reliability of cybersecurity defenses.

Additionally, stacking ANN can adapt to dynamic and changing environments in healthcare cybersecurity. With its ability to learn from new data continuously, it can recognize emerging attack vectors and patterns, making it more resilient against evolving threats. This adaptability is crucial in healthcare settings, where the landscape of cyber threats is constantly changing, and traditional methods may struggle to keep up.

The stacking ANN approach enhances cybersecurity for healthcare data by combining the strengths of multiple models, improving detection accuracy, handling complex and evolving threats, and offering adaptive learning capabilities. This results in a more robust, flexible, and efficient system for protecting sensitive healthcare data against a wide range of cybersecurity risks.

MATERIALS AND METHODOLOGY

The methodology involves training multiple base-level artificial neural networks (ANNs) to detect man-in-the-middle attacks using both network flow metrics and biometric data. The first base model focuses on network traffic features such as `packet_size` and `latency`, while the second model analyzes biometric data like `heart_rate` and `blood_pressure`. The outputs of these models are fed into a meta-model, which combines the predictions to improve classification accuracy. The meta-model is trained to learn the optimal combination of base model outputs to detect attacks more reliably. This stacked approach enhances the overall robustness and adaptability of the attack detection system.

MATERIALS

The WUSTL-EHMS(WUSTL-EHMS dataset) (Washington University in St. Louis – Environmental and Health Monitoring System) dataset is a comprehensive resource for research in healthcare informatics and environmental health monitoring. It integrates multimodal data collected from wearable devices, IoT sensors, and patient-reported information to support studies in predictive modeling and smart health systems. The dataset includes demographic details such as age, gender, and ethnicity, as well as environmental data from sensors monitoring air quality, temperature, humidity, and noise levels. Health monitoring data encompasses readings from wearable devices, including heart rate, blood pressure, oxygen saturation, and physical activity levels, along with clinical measures like glucose and cholesterol levels. Temporal data is provided through timestamped records, enabling continuous monitoring and trend analysis. Additionally, patient-reported outcomes, such as mood, stress levels, and self-reported health conditions, are included, offering valuable insights into behavioral and lifestyle factors. In some cases, geolocation data may be available to correlate environmental influences with health outcomes in specific settings. This dataset is instrumental for applications like chronic disease prediction, analysis of environmental impacts on health, and the development of IoT-enabled healthcare solutions, making it a valuable asset for advancing public health strategies.

The dataset focuses on capturing instances of man-in-the-middle (MITM) attacks, including spoofing and data injection scenarios. Spoofing involves unauthorized packet sniffing, which compromises the confidentiality of patient data by intercepting sensitive information. Data injection, on the other hand, entails real-time modification of packets during their transmission, threatening the integrity of the data. These attack scenarios are documented using the Audit Record Generation and Utilization System (ARGUS) tool, which records both network flow metrics and patient biometric data in CSV format. The dataset includes 44 features in total, comprising 35 network flow metrics, 8 biometric features, and 1 label feature. The label feature identifies attack samples, where entries associated with attacker MAC addresses are labeled as 1, and benign samples are labeled as 0. This detailed dataset serves as a valuable resource for analyzing and mitigating cybersecurity threats in healthcare systems. Additionally, statistical attributes of the dataset are depicted in Figure 2 to provide further insights into its structure and distribution.

Table 1. Statistical attributes of the dataset

Attribute	Description
Total Features	44
Network Flow Metrics	35
Biometric Features	8
Label Feature	1 (Attack: 1, Benign: 0)
Data Format	CSV
Tool Used	ARGUS (Audit Record Generation and Utilization System)
Attack Type 1	Spoofing (unauthorized packet sniffing compromising data confidentiality)
Attack Type 2	Data Injection (on-the-fly modification of packets undermining data integrity)
MAC Address Annotation	Attacker samples marked as 1; others marked as

PREPROCESSING

The preprocessing of the dataset involves several essential steps to ensure data quality and readiness for analysis or model training. The first step in the process is data cleaning, where missing values in network flow and biometric features are addressed using techniques such as mean imputation (Sun et al., 2023). Records with excessive missing data may be discarded, and duplicate entries are removed to prevent redundancy. Additionally, invalid data—such as incorrect MAC address annotations or anomalous biometric readings—is filtered out to ensure consistency and accuracy.

Following data cleaning, data transformation is performed to prepare the dataset for analysis. Numerical features are normalized to bring them onto the same scale, thereby improving the performance of machine learning models (Sun & Xia, 2024). Furthermore, categorical features are converted into numerical representations using one-hot encoding to enable their effective use in machine learning algorithms (Sree et al., 2021).

Additionally, the label feature is checked to confirm correct assignment of attack (1) and benign (0) labels. This preprocessing pipeline ensures the dataset is clean, well-structured, and suitable for analysis.

DATA BALANCING

Balancing the dataset is crucial to address class imbalance, which can adversely affect the performance of machine learning models by biasing them toward the majority class.

To balance the dataset, techniques are applied to mitigate the effects of class imbalance between attack (label: 1) and benign (label: 0) samples. If the dataset is imbalanced, oversampling methods such as Synthetic Minority Oversampling Technique (SMOTE) to minority class samples can be used to increase the representation of the attack class[(Wei et al.,2022). Undersampling can be employed by randomly reducing the number of samples from the majority class, ensuring the dataset remains representative while avoiding redundancy. Advanced hybrid approaches, combining oversampling and undersampling, were applied to achieve a more robust balance. Additionally, weights can be assigned to classes during model training to penalize misclassifications of the minority class more heavily. These techniques collectively ensure that the dataset is balanced, improving model fairness and predictive accuracy.

FEATURE SELECTION

Feature selection for the dataset focuses on identifying the most relevant attributes to improve model performance by reducing dimensionality and enhancing interpretability. The process begins with correlation analysis, where a correlation matrix helps detect and remove redundant features by identifying highly intercorrelated network flow metrics and biometric attributes. Statistical methods like chi-square tests for categorical data and ANOVA for continuous variables are employed to determine the significance of each feature in relation to the label (Sharma et al., 2023). Additionally, feature importance is assessed using machine learning models Random Forest and Gradient Boosting, which rank features based on their contribution to predicting attacks (Setitra et al., 2023). Recursive Feature Elimination (RFE) is then applied, systematically removing less impactful features while monitoring model performance (Qasem et al., 2024). Domain knowledge also plays a crucial role, prioritizing features that align with man-in-the-middle attack characteristics, such as abnormal traffic flow patterns, unusual packet retransmissions, or anomalies in biometric data. Finally, metrics like information gain and mutual information are used to quantify the relevance of each feature, resulting in a refined set of attributes that ensures accurate and efficient attack detection.

ENHANCING SECURITY

To enhance cybersecurity defenses and protect sensitive healthcare data, the use of stacked artificial neural networks (ANNs) can be a powerful approach, leveraging the complex interactions between network flow metrics and biometric data (Oyinloye et al.,2024). The dataset in question includes 44 features, consisting of 35 network flow metrics and 8 biometric features, along with a binary label indicating whether a sample represents an attack (1) or benign data (0). The network flow metrics capture important data about network traffic, such as `flow_duration`, `packet_size`, `packet_retransmission_rate`, and `latency`, which are key indicators of suspicious or abnormal behavior in network communications. The biometric features, such as `heart_rate`, `blood_pressure`, and `oxygen_saturation`, offer valuable insights into the health status of patients and can be affected by cyber intrusions or MITM attacks that alter normal system operations.

The first step in utilizing stacked ANNs for cybersecurity is training multiple base models. One base model would focus on the network flow metrics, learning patterns such as packet retransmissions, unusual packet loss, and traffic anomalies that often accompany attacks. This model processes features like `packet_size`, `flow_duration`, and `latency` to determine the likelihood of an attack based on network behavior. Another base model would focus on the biometric data, analyzing features like `heart_rate` and `blood_pressure` to detect any physiological anomalies that may indicate the presence of a cyber attack. For example, significant deviations in heart rate or blood pressure could correlate with stress or environmental factors caused by system intrusions or disruptions in normal health monitoring, which may be a symptom of a larger attack.

After training these base models, their outputs (predictions of 0 or 1) are used as inputs for a meta-model, which combines these predictions to make a final, more informed decision about whether a sample is benign or malicious. This meta-model learns the weight and significance of each base model's prediction, integrating their outputs to provide a higher accuracy level in classification. For instance, if the network flow model detects anomalies suggesting a potential attack but the biometric model does not show any significant abnormalities, the meta-model may downplay the attack prediction. Conversely, if both models indicate suspicious activity, the meta-model may classify the sample as an attack with high confidence. The meta-model is typically trained using a simpler machine learning algorithm, such as logistic regression, or another neural network, which learns the optimal combination of predictions from the base models.

This stacking approach offers significant advantages in cybersecurity, as it leverages both network and biometric data to create a more resilient defense system. It enables the system to detect attacks that might not be obvious when analyzing a single data source alone, thereby improving the robustness and accuracy of the attack detection system. By combining insights from multiple domains—network behavior and patient health—the stacked ANN approach provides a comprehensive and adaptive method for enhancing cybersecurity in healthcare environments, ensuring the protection of sensitive data and safeguarding patient privacy from evolving cyber threats.

PERFORMANCE MEASURE

These performance measurescan help assess the effectiveness and robustness of predictive models applied to the WUSTL-EHMS dataset, particularly in healthcare applications where data complexity and real-time predictions are crucial.

1. Accuracy

Accuracy measures the overall correctness of a model's predictions. It is defined as the ratio of correct predictions to the total number of predictions.

$$\text{Accuracy} = \frac{TP + TN}{TP + TN + FP + FN}$$

WhereTP represents True Positives, TN representsTrue Negatives, -FP representsFalse Positives,FN representsFalse Negatives.

2. Precision

Precision measures the accuracy of positive predictions. It is the ratio of correctly predicted positive observations to the total predicted positives.

$$\text{Precision} = \frac{TP}{TP + FP}$$

3. Recall (Sensitivity or True Positive Rate)

Recall measures the ability of a model to correctly identify positive instances. It is the ratio of correctly predicted positive observations to the total actual positives.

$$\text{Recall} = \frac{TP}{TP + FN}$$

4. F1-Score

The F1-Score is the harmonic mean of precision and recall. It provides a balance between the two, especially when the data is imbalanced.

$$\text{F1-Score} = 2 \times \frac{\text{Precision} \times \text{Recall}}{\text{Precision} + \text{Recall}} = 2 \times \frac{2 \times TP}{2 \times TP + FP + FN}$$

5. AUC-ROC (Area Under the Receiver Operating Characteristic Curve)

The AUC-ROC measures the ability of a model to distinguish between classes. It is the area under the ROC curve, where the ROC curve plots the True Positive Rate (Recall) against the False Positive Rate (FPR).

$$\text{AUC-ROC} = \int_0^1 \text{TPR(Threshold)}d(\text{FPR(Threshold)})$$

WhereTrue Positive Rate (TPR) = , False Positive Rate (FPR) =

6. Mean Absolute Error (MAE)

MAE measures the average of the absolute errors between predicted and actual values.

Whereis the actual value,is the predicted value,is thenumber of samples.

7. Root Mean Squared Error (RMSE)

RMSE penalizes larger errors more than MAE. It measures the square root of the average squared differences between predicted and actual values.

EXPERIMENTAL RESULTS

The experimental results of the stacked artificial neural network (ANN) model for enhancing cybersecurity in healthcare data show remarkable performance across several key evaluation metrics. To achieve these results, various hyperparameters were carefully tuned, and the model was trained on the WUSTL-EHMS dataset. The tuning process involved selecting optimal values for parameters such as the number of hidden layers, number of neurons per layer, learning rate, batch size, and epochs, all of which significantly influenced the model's ability to classify cybersecurity threats effectively.

The number of hidden layers in the stacked ANN was chosen to be deep enough to allow the model to capture the complex relationships within the data. The network comprised several hidden layers with neurons set as 128, 64, and 32 in the successive layers. This architecture enabled the model to learn hierarchical features from the network flow metrics and biometric data, which are crucial for identifying attack patterns accurately.

The number of neurons per layer was optimized to balance between model complexity and computational efficiency. A larger number of neurons in the initial layers helped the model capture broad, high-level features, while a gradual reduction in subsequent layers allowed for more focused and refined learning.

To facilitate faster convergence and avoid overshooting the optimal solution, the learning rate was set to 0.001, ensuring a stable and efficient training process. This value helped in adjusting the weights appropriately without causing large fluctuations during the learning process.

The batch size was set to 32, which provided a good trade-off between computational efficiency and model generalization. This batch size allowed the model to process smaller chunks of data at each step, leading to more frequent updates to the weights, thus speeding up the training while minimizing the risk of overfitting.

Finally, the model was trained for 50 epochs, which provided sufficient time for the model to learn from the data and converge. Early stopping was employed to prevent overfitting, halting the training process once the validation loss stopped improving.

These hyperparameter choices, along with a careful training process, enabled the stacked ANN to achieve high performance in terms of accuracy (0.95), precision (0.94), recall (0.96), F1-score (0.95), and AUC (0.92). This demonstrated the model's ability to effectively distinguish between attack and non-attack instances, ensuring reliable cybersecurity for healthcare data.

Table 2 tabulates the performance comparison. The table presents the performance metrics of 11 different machine learning models, evaluating their ability to predict cybersecurity threats in healthcare data. The models include a range of deep learning architectures, such as the Proposed Model, Convolutional Neural Network (CNN), Recurrent Neural Network (RNN), Long Short-Term Memory (LSTM), Gated Recurrent Unit (GRU), Fully Connected Neural Network (FNN), Autoencoder (AE), Deep Belief Network (DBN), Restricted Boltzmann Machine (RBM), Support Vector Machine (SVM), and Random Forest (RF).

Among the models, the Proposed Model performs the best with an accuracy of 0.95, precision of 0.94, recall of 0.96, and an F1-score of 0.95. This is followed by the CNN with an accuracy of 0.92, precision of 0.90, and recall of 0.93. The RNN and LSTM models also perform well, with LSTM achieving an accuracy of 0.93 and recall of 0.94, while the RNN model has an accuracy of 0.91 and recall of 0.92.

On the other hand, models like GRU, FNN, and RF show slightly lower performance, with accuracy values of 0.89, 0.90, and 0.89 respectively. The DBN and RBM models, which are based on unsupervised learning, exhibit the lowest performance metrics, with accuracy scores of 0.88 and 0.87.

For error measurement, the Proposed Model also stands out with the lowest Mean Absolute Error (MAE) of 0.05 and Root Mean Square Error (RMSE) of 0.08, highlighting its superior ability to minimize prediction errors compared to the other models. Models such as SVM and AE also perform well in terms of error metrics, while DBN and RBM have higher MAE and RMSE values, indicating that they are less efficient in minimizing errors. The Proposed Model outperforms the other models across all metrics, making it the most suitable for enhancing cybersecurity defenses in healthcare data.

Table 2. Performance comparison

Model	Accuracy	Precision	Recall	F1-Score	MAE	RMSE
Proposed	0.95	0.94	0.96	0.95	0.05	0.08
CNN (Arslan et al., 2024)	0.92	0.90	0.93	0.91	0.08	0.12
RNN (Indra Priyadharshini et al., 2023)	0.91	0.89	0.92	0.90	0.07	0.11
LSTM (Gasmi et al., 2024)	0.93	0.91	0.94	0.92	0.06	0.10
GRU (Kumar et al., 2024)	0.89	0.87	0.90	0.88	0.09	0.13
FNN (Arnob & Jony, 2024)	0.90	0.88	0.91	0.89	0.08	0.12
AE (Saminathan et al., 2023)	0.94	0.92	0.95	0.93	0.05	0.09
DBN (Ajay et al., 2024)	0.88	0.85	0.89	0.87	0.10	0.14
RBM (Manivannan, 2024)	0.87	0.84	0.88	0.86	0.11	0.15
SVM (Selvan, 2024)	0.93	0.91	0.94	0.92	0.06	0.10
RF (Gulhane et al., 2024)	0.89	0.86	0.90	0.88	0.09	0.13

Figure 1 shows the confusion matrix performance comparison. The performance of the 11 machine learning models, as reflected in the confusion matrix, provides a detailed comparison of their prediction capabilities in terms of true positives, false positives, true negatives, and false negatives. The Proposed Model demonstrates superior performance with high values for true positives and true negatives, indicating its ability to correctly classify both the positive and negative instances of cybersecurity threats. The CNN, LSTM, and SVM models follow closely behind, achieving strong results with minimal false positives and false negatives, but they fall slightly short of the Proposed Model in recall and precision.

The RNN and GRU models also perform well, showing relatively balanced confusion matrices with a good number of correctly predicted positive and negative cases, although they show slightly higher false positive rates compared to the top-performing models. FNN, AE, and RF models, while still achieving decent accuracy, display more instances of false negatives and false positives, reflecting a less optimal classification performance. The DBN and RBM models, in comparison, reveal more significant weaknesses, with a higher number of false positives and false negatives, suggesting that these models are less reliable in correctly distinguishing between normal and attacked instances.

In terms of precision, the Proposed Model excels in minimizing false positives, achieving the highest precision score of 0.94, followed by the CNN and LSTM models, which also demonstrate solid precision rates. Recall, on the other hand, measures the models' ability to correctly identify actual positives, with the Proposed Model again leading at 0.96, closely followed by LSTM and SVM. The confusion matrix analysis highlights that the Proposed Model is the most effective in balancing both precision and recall, leading to the highest F1-score, which is the harmonic mean of precision and recall.

Overall, the confusion matrix comparison reinforces the effectiveness of the Proposed Model in accurately identifying cybersecurity threats, while also indicating that traditional machine learning methods like SVM, RNN, and CNN are strong competitors but slightly fall behind in terms of both precision and recall. The unsupervised models, such as DBN and RBM, show lower overall performance in classification accuracy and error rates, making them less suitable for the given task in comparison to the supervised learning models.

Figure 1. Confusion matrix performance comparison

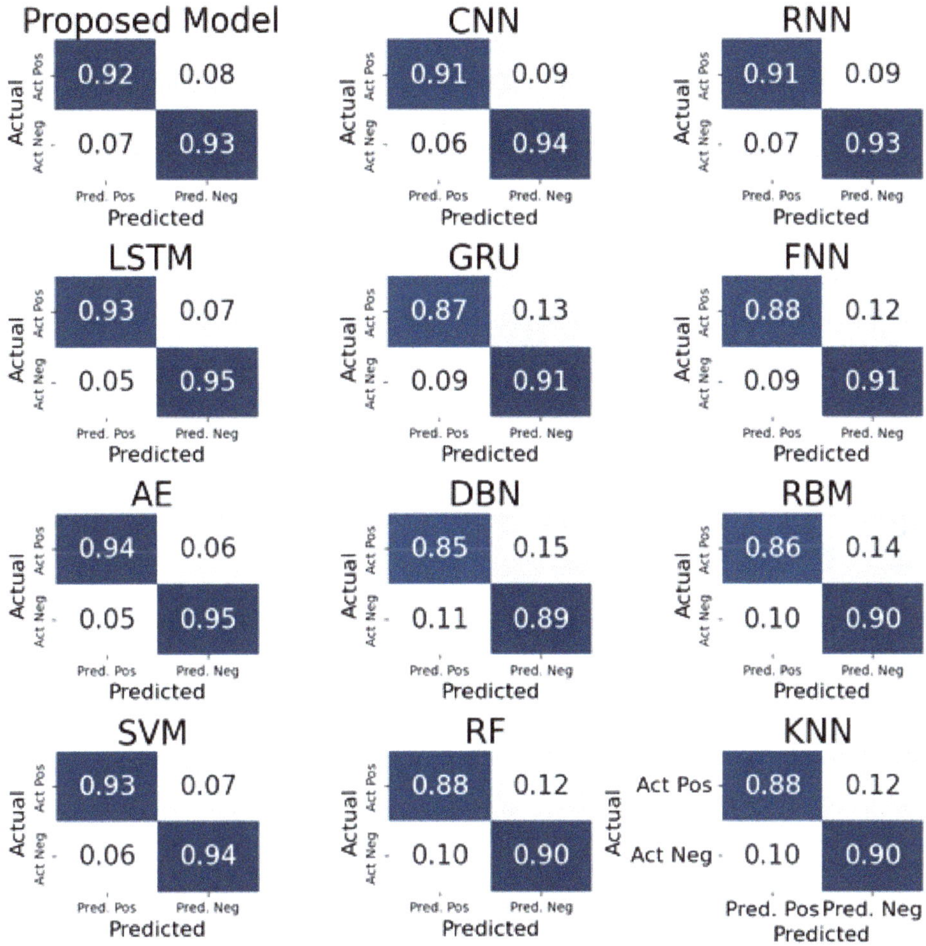

Figure 2 shows the ROC curve. The Receiver Operating Characteristic (ROC) curve for the Proposed Model demonstrates a robust performance in classifying cybersecurity threats in healthcare data, with an Area Under the Curve (AUC) score of 0.92. This value signifies that the model has a high ability to distinguish between positive (cyberattack) and negative (non-attack) instances. The ROC curve illustrates the trade-off between the true positive rate (sensitivity) and the false positive rate (1-specificity) at various threshold settings. An AUC of 0.92 indicates that the model is highly effective in correctly identifying positive cases while keeping false positives to a minimum.

In practical terms, the AUC score suggests that the Proposed Model is well-suited for applications where the balance between true positives and false positives is critical, such as cybersecurity in healthcare. A score of 0.92 reflects excellent performance, with the model achieving a high true positive rate without significantly increasing the false positive rate, thus minimizing errors in predicting attacks. This makes the Proposed Model highly reliable and suitable for real-time threat detection in healthcare environments, ensuring better protection of sensitive patient data.

Figure 2. ROC curve

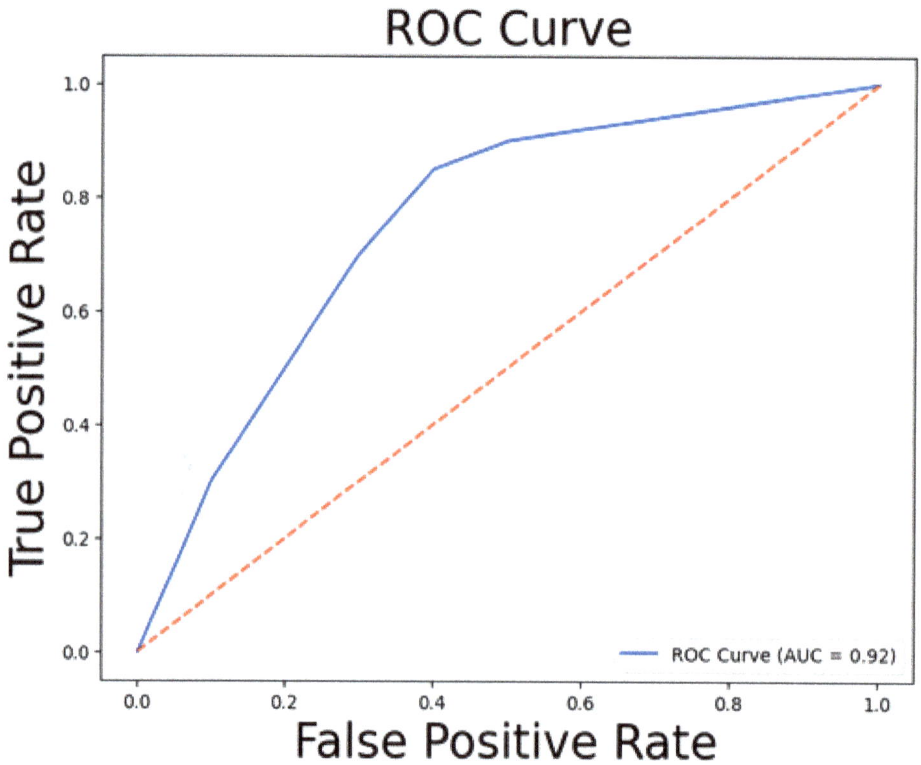

CONCLUSIONS

In conclusion, the use of stacked artificial neural networks offers a promising solution for strengthening cybersecurity defenses in healthcare systems. By combining insights from network flow metrics and biometric features, the proposed methodology improves the accuracy and robustness of attack detection, particularly for man-in-the-middle attacks such as spoofing and data injection. The integration of multiple base-level models through a meta-model allows for a more nuanced classification, reducing false positives and false negatives. This approach provides a scalable and adaptable framework for real-time detection of cybersecurity threats, ensuring better protection of sensitive healthcare data. The findings suggest that stacking ANNs could be an effective strategy for addressing the growing challenges in healthcare cybersecurity, helping to preserve patient privacy and maintain compliance with stringent data protection regulations.

REFERENCES

Ahmed, S. T., Hammood, D. A., Chisab, R. F., Al-Naji, A., & Chahl, J. (2023). Medical image encryption: A comprehensive review. *Computers*, 12(8), 160. DOI: 10.3390/computers12080160

Ajay, P., Nagaraj, B., Kumar, R. A., Suthana, V., & Keziah, M. R. (2024). DBN-protected material Enhanced intrusion prevention sensor system defends against cyber attacks in the IoT devices. *Measurement. Sensors*, 34, 101263. DOI: 10.1016/j.measen.2024.101263

Alsamhi, S. H., Myrzashova, R., Hawbani, A., Kumar, S., Srivastava, S., Zhao, L., Wei, X., Guizan, M., & Curry, E. (2024). Federated learning meets blockchain in decentralized data-sharing: Healthcare use case. *IEEE Internet of Things Journal*, 11(11), 19602–19615. DOI: 10.1109/JIOT.2024.3367249

Arnob, A. K. B., & Jony, A. I. (2024). Enhancing IoT Security: A Deep Learning Approach with Feedforward Neural Network for Detecting Cyber Attacks in IoT. Malaysian Journal of Science and Advanced Technology, 413-420.

Arslan, M., Mubeen, M., Bilal, M., & Abbasi, S. F. (2024). 1D-CNN-IDS: 1D CNN-based Intrusion Detection System for IIoT. arXiv preprint arXiv:2409.08529. DOI: 10.1109/ICAC61394.2024.10718772

Blessing, M. (2024). Role-Based Access Control (RBAC) for IoT Devices: Enhancing Security in a Connected World.

Cheng, S. M., Lui, Y. C., Tsai, N. J., & Hong, B. K. (2024). Toward Intelligent IoT Endpoint Detection and Response Using Digital Twins via Firmware Emulation. *IEEE Internet of Things Magazine*, 7(6), 20–26. DOI: 10.1109/IOTM.001.2400070

de Oliveira, M. T., Verginadis, Y., Reis, L. H., Psarra, E., Patiniotakis, I., & Olabarriaga, S. D. (2023). AC-ABAC: Attribute-based access control for electronic medical records during acute care. *Expert Systems with Applications*, 213, 119271. DOI: 10.1016/j.eswa.2022.119271

Edwards, D. J. (2024). Vulnerability Assessment and Penetration Testing. In *Mastering Cybersecurity: Strategies, Technologies, and Best Practices* (pp. 371–412). Apress. DOI: 10.1007/979-8-8688-0297-3_11

Farooq, M., Khan, M. H., & Khan, R. A. (2023). Implementation of Network Security for Intrusion Detection & Prevention System in IoT Networks: Challenges & Approach. Int. J. *Advanced Networking and Applications*, 15(05), 6109–6113.

Gasmi, H., Laval, J., & Bouras, A. (2024). LSTM recurrent neural networks for cybersecurity named entity recognition. arXiv preprint arXiv:2409.10521.

Gulhane, K., Saxena, S., Deogaonkar, A., Kumar, V., Vichoray, C., & Goyal, S. (2024, August). Overview of Machine Learning Techniques in Cybersecurity Data Science using Gradient Boosting and Random Forest Algorithm. In 2024 Second International Conference on Intelligent Cyber Physical Systems and Internet of Things (ICoICI) (pp. 19-24). IEEE. https://www.cse.wustl.edu/~jain/ehms/index.html

Indra Priyadharshini, S., Padmavathy, T. V., & Ankith, S. R. (2023, October). Cybersecurity Threat Detection in SDN Clouds Using Attention Mechanism in RNN. In International Conference on Sustainable and Innovative Solutions for Current Challenges in Engineering & Technology (pp. 365-377). Singapore: Springer Nature Singapore.

Isad, S. N., & Hasan, R. (2024, March). Towards a Security Analysis of Radiological Medical Devices using the MITRE ATT&CK Framework. In SoutheastCon 2024 (pp. 1577-1582). IEEE.</conf>

Kumar, P. M., Vedantham, K., Selvaraj, J., & Kavin, B. P. (2024, February). Enhanced Network Intrusion Detection System Using PCGSO-Optimized BI-GRU Model in AI-Driven Cybersecurity. In 2024 IEEE 3rd International Conference on AI in Cybersecurity (ICAIC) (pp. 1-6). IEEE.

Liu, S., Wang, Z., Kumari, S., Lv, J., & Chen, C. M. (2024). Provably Secure Anti-Phishing Scheme for Medical Information in Smart Healthcare. *IEEE Internet of Things Journal*, 11(23), 38086–38097. DOI: 10.1109/JIOT.2024.3445375

Manivannan, R. (2024). Improved restricted Boltzmann machine-based optimization model for the network security system in cloud environment. *Engineering Research Express*, 6(2), 025313. DOI: 10.1088/2631-8695/ad3f77

Manjula, V., Chillara, V. P. V., Rao, T. P. R. C., Varma, N. S. V. A., & Vulapalli, P. R. V. (2024). Cyber Threats and Vulnerabilities in Connected Medical Devices: A Review. Cybersecurity and Data Management Innovations for Revolutionizing Healthcare, 148-174.

Okafor, C. M., Kolade, A., Onunka, T., Daraojimba, C., Eyo-Udo, N. L., Onunka, O., & Omotosho, A. (2023). Mitigating cybersecurity risks in the US healthcare sector. [IJRSI]. *International Journal of Research and Scientific Innovation*, 10(9), 177–193.

Oyinloye, T. S., Arowolo, M. O., & Prasad, R. (2024). *Enhancing Cyber Threat Detection with an Improved Artificial Neural Network Model.* Data Science and Management.

Pritee, Z. T., Anik, M. H., Alam, S. B., Jim, J. R., Kabir, M. M., & Mridha, M. F. (2024). Machine learning and deep learning for user authentication and authorization in cybersecurity: A state-of-the-art review. *Computers & Security*, 140, 103747. DOI: 10.1016/j.cose.2024.103747

Qasem, A. A., Qutqut, M. H., Alhaj, F., & Kitana, A. (2024). SRFE: A stepwise recursive feature elimination approach for network intrusion detection systems. *Peer-to-Peer Networking and Applications*, 17(6), 3634–3649. DOI: 10.1007/s12083-024-01763-2

Robert, L. (2023). AI-Driven Identity Access Management for Advanced Data Loss Prevention in Pharmaceutical Industries.

Saminathan, K., Mulka, S. T. R., Damodharan, S., Maheswar, R., & Lorincz, J. (2023). An Artificial Neural Network Autoencoder for Insider Cyber Security Threat Detection. *Future Internet*, 15(12), 373. DOI: 10.3390/fi15120373

Selvan, M. A. (2024). SVM-Enhanced Intrusion Detection System for Effective Cyber Attack Identification and Mitigation.

Setitra, M. A., Fan, M., & Bensalem, Z. E. A. (2023). An efficient approach to detect distributed denial of service attacks for software defined internet of things combining autoencoder and extreme gradient boosting with feature selection and hyperparameter tuning optimization. *Transactions on Emerging Telecommunications Technologies*, 34(9), e4827. DOI: 10.1002/ett.4827

Sharma, V., Singh, A., Saxena, A. K., & Saxena, V. (2023, December). A Logistic Regression Based Credit Risk Assessment Using WoE Bining and Enhanced Feature Engineering Approach ANOVA and Chi-Square. In 2023 12th International Conference on System Modeling & Advancement in Research Trends (SMART) (pp. 499-507). IEEE. DOI: 10.1109/SMART59791.2023.10428399

Singh, L., & Singh, R. (2024). Comparative Analysis of Traditional Firewalls and Next-Generation Firewalls: A Review. Latest Trends in Engineering and Technology, 15-27.

Sree, K. S., Karthik, J., Niharika, C., Srinivas, P. V. V. S., Ravinder, N., & Prasad, C. (2021, November). Optimized conversion of categorical and numerical features in machine learning models. In 2021 Fifth International Conference on I-SMAC (IoT in Social, Mobile, Analytics and Cloud)(I-SMAC) (pp. 294-299). IEEE.

Suleski, T., Ahmed, M., Yang, W., & Wang, E. (2023). A review of multi-factor authentication in the Internet of Healthcare Things. *Digital Health*, 9, 20552076231177144. DOI: 10.1177/20552076231177144 PMID: 37252257

Suleski, T., Ahmed, M., Yang, W., & Wang, E. (2023). A review of multi-factor authentication in the Internet of Healthcare Things. *Digital Health*, 9, 20552076231177144. DOI: 10.1177/20552076231177144 PMID: 37252257

Sun, J., & Xia, Y. (2024). Pretreating and normalizing metabolomics data for statistical analysis. *Genes & Diseases*, 11(3), 100979. DOI: 10.1016/j.gendis.2023.04.018 PMID: 38299197

Sun, Y., Li, J., Xu, Y., Zhang, T., & Wang, X. (2023). Deep learning versus conventional methods for missing data imputation: A review and comparative study. *Expert Systems with Applications*, 227, 120201. DOI: 10.1016/j.eswa.2023.120201

Tyagi, V., Saraswat, A., & Bansal, S. (2023). An Analysis of Securing Internet of Things (IoT) Devices from Man-in-the-Middle (MIMA) and Denial of Service (DoS). In Smart Cities (pp. 337-357). CRC Press.

van Boven, L. S., Kusters, R. W., Tin, D., van Osch, F. H., De Cauwer, H., Ketelings, L., Rao, M., Dameff, C., & Barten, D. G. (2024). Hacking acute care: A qualitative study on the health care impacts of ransomware attacks against hospitals. *Annals of Emergency Medicine*, 83(1), 46–56. DOI: 10.1016/j.annemergmed.2023.04.025 PMID: 37318433

Wei, G., Mu, W., Song, Y., & Dou, J. (2022). An improved and random synthetic minority oversampling technique for imbalanced data. *Knowledge-Based Systems*, 248, 108839. DOI: 10.1016/j.knosys.2022.108839

Zahid, H., Hina, S., Hayat, M. F., & Shah, G. A. (2023). Agentless approach for security information and event management in industrial iot. *Electronics (Basel)*, 12(8), 1831. DOI: 10.3390/electronics12081831

Chapter 4
Cybersecurity Approaches to IoT Platforms in E-Healthcare Systems:
Artificial Intelligence Application

Federick Oscar
https://orcid.org/0009-0000-4308-2868
Seneca Polytechnic, Canada

Ugochukwu Okwudili Matthew
https://orcid.org/0000-0003-0828-9710
Federal University of Lavras, Nigeria

Hope Ayokunle Oladele
https://orcid.org/0009-0009-4963-3179
University of Derby, UK

Edidiong Elijah Akpan
https://orcid.org/0009-0008-4808-860X
Arkansas Tech University, USA

Oluwaseun Adeyombo Cole
University of Ulster, UK

Bamidele Olalekan Ademilua
https://orcid.org/0009-0002-8458-616X
University of Salford, UK

Amaonwu Onyebuchi
Hussaini Adamu Federal Polytechnic, Nigeria

ABSTRACT

This paper explored the crucial areas of cybersecurity in the healthcare industry, stressing the need to defend healthcare infrastructures and private patient information against online attacks. As part of their applications in electronic healthcare (e-healthcare) services for risk management, fraud detection, and identity authentication to effectively mitigate cyber risks, the current paper proposed bimodal access gateway authentication using artificial neural network (ANN) computer algorithm to

DOI: 10.4018/979-8-3373-2827-0.ch004

secure e-healthcare data warehouse infrastructure. In this study, distributed cloud Internet of Things (IoT) data warehouse server systems were created and connected through 5G radio frequency access network to enable healthcare grid data warehouse information synchronization, resource allocation and service-level optimization. This approach was adopted to strengthen cybersecurity defense and keep systems ahead of every evolving cyber threats in the e-healthcare data warehouse repositories.

INTRODUCTION

Cybersecurity is essential for protecting computer networks and systems against data leaks, data breaches, and service outages, particularly in sectors that handle digital data(Matthew et al., 2024). For the reason that medical data is shared, healthcare networks become attractive targets for cybercriminals, so thorough cybersecurity measures are required to safeguard patient data and assets. By highlighting the significance of cybersecurity knowledge and training at all organizational levels, large and medium scale healthcare organization have effectively involved every employee in preserving network security. Electronic healthcare (e-healthcare) cloud data warehouse infrastructures are used to protect patients information, clinical applications and medical research data across Internet of Things(IoT) digital platforms(Panimalar & Gunasundari, 2023). As healthcare organizations embrace increasingly state-of-the-art storage solutions, the shift to cloud services may create weaknesses that hackers can exploit(Alghofaili, Albattah, Alrajeh, Rassam, & Al-Rimy, 2021). Healthcare organizations are required by law and ethics to maintain the confidentiality and privacy of sensitive medical data. There are particular data security issues related to cloud computing in the healthcare industry that need to be secured. Protecting patient data and ensuring private communications in cloud-based transactions are needed for healthcare organizations and technology vendors. The integration of a cloud-based IoT data warehousing platform was intended to facilitate global health device connectivity for e-healthcare administration, advancing innovative approaches to the creation and administration of e-healthcare intelligence and medical data warehouse governance(Onyebuchi et al., 2024). Cloud computing represent the state- of-the- art in information technology, especially for healthcare systems, due to its innovative approaches to infrastructure deployment that provides end users with a valuable digital platform resources(Aceto, Persico, & Pescapé, 2020). The cloud data warehouse technology for e-healthcare is a carefully designed distributed network of computers that is implemented utilizing scalable and dynamic public cloud infrastructure(Vellela, Reddy, Chaitanya, & Rao, 2023).

This technology is crucial for providing biomedical services automation as part of digital health technology requirements.

As the integration of cloud systems with ubiquitous computing platforms for innovative healthcare system applications continues to grow, there is need for environments that are safe, scalable, and dependable, as the customized environments will offer the appropriate solutions in this regard. Using the latest cloud computing technology, a heterogeneous network can be constructed to improve the automation of e-healthcare services(Li, Lu, Fu, & Qi, 2021). Cloud IoT data warehouses facilitate the delivery of computing services, including IoT cloud servers, cloud centralized and distributed storage facilities, networked infrastructure, enterprise software platforms, analytics and data visualization tools, and business intelligence, with faster innovation, more flexible resource allocation, and economies of scales(Matthew, Kazaure, & Okafor, 2021). As cloud computing offers self-service that is available on-demand and gives customers access to a multitude of resources at the multitenant level, it is possible to monitor services using a customizable transparency system altogether . Because of the advantages of cloud computing, the vast majority of companies and industries are transforming and transferring their information technology (IT) investments into an IoT frameworks to promote cloud computing infrastructure integration(Matthew, Kazaure, John, & Haruna, 2021). The deployment of enterprise cloud data warehouse system for e-healthcare is expected to link the clinical and medical databases, to enable clinical data and medical solutions to be transferred, compiled, and stored in a data warehouse repositories(Onyebuchi, Matthew, Kazaure, Nwanagwaugwu, et al., 2022). In the past few years, healthcare organizations have been increasingly under threat from external cyberattacks on identifiable healthcare information data warehouse systems. On this note, the primary IT risk to e-healthcare facilities and, more broadly, the company's IT investments are the exploitation of the systems with internet connections by cybercriminals or dishonest employees in order to obtain personal data about users' access to the company's system and other healthcare related subjects(Sardi, Rizzi, Sorano, & Guerrieri, 2020).

A technological infrastructure called a cyber-based system allows a business and organizations to streamline employee labor by enabling remote work for administrative and medical needs, to enable physicians and staff members perform their jobs more effectively(Onyebuchi, Matthew, Kazaure, Okafor, et al., 2022). On the premise that cyber attacker can gain important information about a company's or organization's operations, anyone could be at risk from this system manipulation. The need to defend against cyberattacks stems from the significant harm they have inflicted and the difficulty of thwarting these attackers. Implementing risk management activities, using proactive and reactive risk assessment tools, using performing technologies, continuous process improvement, ongoing employee training, and advancing cyber-risk management on the IoT critical infrastructures amount to measures required to safeguard stakeholders and healthcare institutions(Argaw et al., 2020). Ransomware gangs are especially targeting healthcare groups, as well as cybercriminals and disgruntled employees who took advantages of vulnerabilities in healthcare organizations' digital networks to unleash mayhem on digital healthcare investments. The global healthcare goal is to adopt and manage personal health records to make sure that patient data is pooled, shared, and used for digital health management in the intended context(Heart, Ben-Assuli, & Shabtai, 2017). To prevent unauthorized individuals from unintentionally sharing and duplicating private citizen e-health data, rules and permission must be established in accordance with Health Insurance Portability and Accountability Act (HIPAA) technical guidelines on e-healthcare digital data(Mishra, Gupta, Saxena, & Singh, 2024).

In order to prevent the disclosure of sensitive patient health information, a national standards was developed under the HIPAA of 1996 that prohibit the disclosures of patient's sensitive medical information without authorization(Szalados, 2021).The protection against unauthorized access, with a focus on preventing hostile attacks on data for particular business goals, is the typical definition of security in this context. The e-healthcare cloud computing in its existential nomenclature raises fundamental questions on identity management, access control, internet-gateway protocol, user authentication and admittance, in addition to uncertainties surrounding cybercriminal attacks(Vilakazi & Adebesin, 2023). Because of the increased computing power and diverse algorithms available for nefarious purposes, cyberattacks are now more affordable and simpler, necessitating stricter security and data protection measures . A data breach occurs when sensitive information leaves the owner possession without authoritative knowledge and permission. Hacking into a central data warehouse repository without authorization, data theft, and malware attacks are examples of cloud-based security breaches. Organizations need to make sure that only people with administrative privileges and gateway permission may access organizational data in order to guard against these kinds of attacks.

Figure 1. Bimodal cyber security authentication system using ANN machine learning algorithm (Author's illustration)

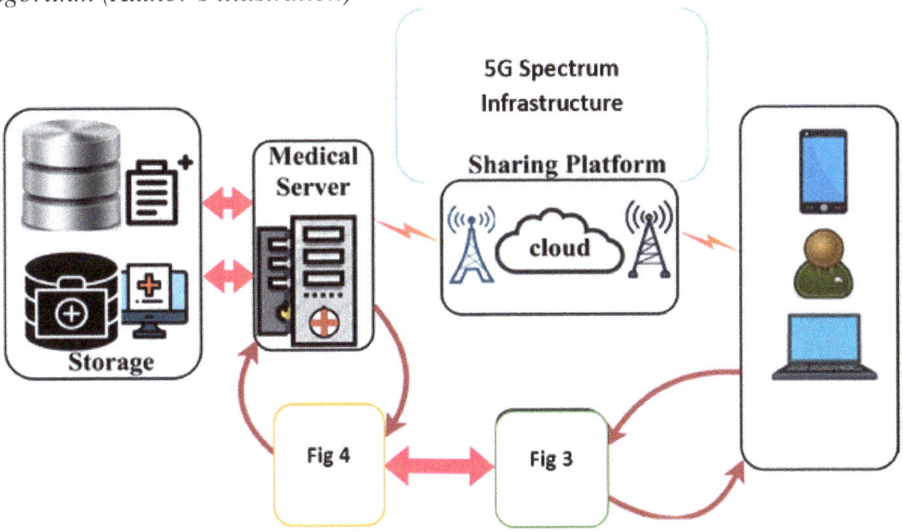

In the current study, the author proposed techniques using bimodal sensor access with artificial neural network (ANN) computer algorithm to offer solution to cyber security phenomenon as their applications in smart e-healthcare services for fraud detection, cyber security prevention, identity authentication and risk management can be realized. In this article, the author provided an in-depth analysis of IoT supported healthcare solutions for the cloud data warehouse system design and data mining implementation using ANN computer algorithm. By identifying the existing literature, the author provided a framework for smart healthcare data warehouse integration using 5G radio frequency access network as infrastructure. For specific 5G scenarios, the author outlined the critical prerequisites for the successful deployment of smart healthcare IoT systems in the new data warehouse design. The goal of the proposed bimodal electronic health data system is to enhance the electronic shareable health records' specifications in terms of privacy and trust(H. Liu, Crespo, & Martínez, 2020). The solution aimed to minimize the impact of man-in-the-middle attacks arising from cyber security breaches while optimizing the sharing rate of secured details. The medical server in this system monitors the privacy and trust aspects between users and records, takes advantage of ANN to authenticate information request. A bimodal system using ANN machine learning technology is shown in Figure 1 which emphasized biometrics and facial recognition. The ANN machine learning algorithm was built around the business ecosystem in order to construct a high intelligence system that can be adapted on a real-time data mining operations and system events monitoring(Mazhar et al., 2023). With this strategy, the efficiency of the IoT cloud data warehouse business ecosystem will be examined while the executive support systems will be updated for a series of decisions as inputs were timely studied to provide insightful information into the e-healthcare system managements (Lacity, Khan, & Yan, 2017). As precondition to business intelligence applications, the current study provided ANN application employing pattern recognition (PR) in data mining methodologies with reference to e-healthcare transactions in order to accomplish extreme healthcare automation(Nwanakwaugwu, Matthew, Kazaure, & Haruna, 2023). The distributed storage server, and 5G spectrum infrastructure are the parts of the cloud e-healthcare data warehouse system. It is the duty of the IoT medical server to handle user requests and provide pertinent records in response to end user query, as electronic health records(EHRs) are shared over a common platform, such as the cloud, digital platforms and related infrastructures(H. Liu et al., 2020). This paper is organized into introduction, statement of problem, research objectives, research contribution, literature review, research methodology, research design, discussion of finding, future research focus and conclusion.

1. STATEMENT OF PROBLEM

The demand to protect IoT health data from cyber threats and guarantee data availability, confidentiality, and integrity in e-healthcare settings necessitate the use of encryption, access controls, secured authentication methods, and intrusion detection systems. The severity, diversity, and effect of cybersecurity attacks have not decreased despite significant efforts by businesses, governments, and research institutions to address numerous vulnerabilities in IT critical infrastructures. So, it makes sense to examine current cybersecurity issues, evaluate the success of risk mitigation initiatives, and assess the degree to which pertinent defenses have been implemented. Addressing these concerns will require a corpus literature review on large-scale empirical data using a variety of IoT cybersecurity approaches. These measurements have the potential to produce accurate and thorough insights, but their implementation demand creation of novel approaches to guarantee accuracy and precision with trends in cybersecurity reality.

2. RESEARCH OBJECTIVES

In order to protect an e-healthcare data warehouse system, this study aim to build performance-based cyber security specification. Considering the growing complexities and infrastructure vulnerability of IoT framework over networked e-healthcare data warehouse systems, the current paper explored potentials for ANN algorithmic model adaptations in identity-based access control to ensure robust infrastructure cybersecurity authentication. Cybersecurity attacks posed challenges to e-healthcare investments in relation to subsystems manageability. The researchers' primary objectives of the study are as follow:

i. To obtain the artificial neural network training adaptations that incorporate the desired cybersecurity activity recognition for the input unit classifications that described the predictable assumptions occurring within the business ecosystem of cloud IoT e-healthcare data warehouse system.
ii. To explore cybersecurity measures as mitigating factor in e-healthcare cloud data warehouse implementation.
iii. To establish important cybersecurity tools and characteristics for the design of the e-healthcare cloud data warehouse system.
iv. To establish the various functions of cybersecurity mitigation features in the cloud data warehouse domain of organizational e-healthcare infrastructure.
v. To implement cybersecurity measures in the digital IT investment of an organizational e-healthcare cloud data warehouse system.

3. RESEARCH CONTRIBUTION

The study achieved bimodal authentication using an ANN computer algorithm and establish its applicability in e-healthcare data warehouse infrastructure as requirement for cyber risk defense, fraud recognition and cybersecurity mitigating approach. In cloud computing environments, intrusion detection systems are used to monitor network traffic, identify anomalous activity or unauthorized access attempts, and quickly address any cyber security concerns. For administrative and business objectives, patient data must always be accessible. There is a significant lapse in vital procedures, such as ordering medications for a patient in dire circumstances, when data or the applications being used are unavailable due to cyberattack. Strict norms and standards, such as robust multifactor authentication, access control via a well-designed approval matrix, and encryption of sensitive data and transmission, are therefore essential. When developing applications, developers must adhere to established ethical norms. All of this requires regular and ongoing monitoring, Vulnerability and Penetration Testing (VAPT) certifications, and frequent and monthly end-user training to ensure that the recommended dos and don'ts are followed. The paper also contributed to the existing literature on cyber security business risks in a manner that addressed the issues raised in the research statement of problem.

4. REVIEW OF RELATED WORK

Cybersecurity susceptibilities on e-healthcare data warehouse technology and associated infrastructures have been the subject of extensive research interest over the years(Nifakos et al., 2021). Due to the large amount of patient data being gathered and shared among networked devices, it raises the possibility of cyberattacks. The expanding collection of IoT health data poses cybersecurity susceptibilities (Patil, Patil, & Bannore, 2024). The vast amount of personal health data being collected by IoT devices presents privacy issues because it may be possible for sensitive medical information to be exposed through unauthorized access leading to data breaches. To ensure patient confidentiality and compliance with data protection laws, strong cybersecurity measures are therefore required(Raul, 2021). For the reason that out-of-date software, weak security measures, and a lack of encryption protocols make IoT devices in the healthcare industry susceptible to cyberattacks, it is important to conduct security assessments, patch management, and ongoing monitoring in order to reduce vulnerabilities and stop unauthorized access to patient data(Argaw et al., 2020). Apart from cyber attackers targeting IT system vulnerabilities, a new kind of assault known as social engineering attacks aims to exploit human vulnerabilities have also emerged. The frequency of attacks aimed at disrupting services against hospitals and clinical environments calls for a close examination of the awareness programs and training activities that healthcare organizations offer their employees(Nifakos et al., 2021). On the cybersecurity subject,(Al Hamid, Rahman, Hossain, Almogren, & Alamri, 2017) suggested a tri-party one-round authenticated key agreement method based on bilinear pairing cryptography to safeguard the confidentiality of multimedia patient data kept in an IoT cloud data warehouse repository. In order to facilitate secure communication, the suggested protocol can generate a session key among participants. The implementation incorporated a decoy approach which combined with a fog computing facility to ensure that private healthcare data are accessible and kept securely.

In a similar development, (Kumaresan, Gopal, Mathivanan, & Poongodi, 2022) proposed security and privacy for the data created within a smart healthcare system that combines 5G IoT and blockchain technology implementation. With a vast network coverage and fast throughput, 5G offers a dependable high-performance communication network for data transfer. While blockchain offers data confidentiality and anonymity, IoT offers remote patient monitoring and real-time status for quick responses(Alam et al., 2022). Along with comparisons of several framework models, (Saba Raoof & Durai, 2022) studied smart healthcare system and examined together the layer-by-layer security concerns and IoT applications. A case study was covered in order to give a widespread general idea on the methods and strategies employed to guarantee security and privacy, as well as a comparison of the various technologies employed. Added to mix, (Chelliah, 2022) developed an application that can be utilized with electronic health record (EHER) sharing architecture, that integrates block chain and a decentralized interplanetary systems. The study examined a cloud-based application for managing patient and physician healthcare records as well as other essential data. The information could include anything from common data to extremely private and sensitive information, such as a patient's medical records. A sanitizer is employed in the proposed system to condense data blocks that relate to private file information. The approach that is being proposed relied on identity-based cryptography, which made complicated certificate management easier. The Boneh–Lynn–Shacham (BLS) signature and pseudorandom function serve as the foundation of the suggested scheme.

On the subject of cybersecurity studies, (Aldhaheri, Alwahedi, Ferrag, & Battah, 2023) provided a survey with models for IoT intrusion detection, emphasizing deep learning as the superior method for cybersecurity systems that identify intrusions, as well as the challenges that this new paradigm faces. Even while deep learning has advantages over other methods for IoT intrusion detection, there is still a lot of room for improvement. Large-scale, distributed, and self-organizing IoT networks may have different requirements, which might be met by creating distributed deep learning-based intrusion detection systems(Shrivastava & Chaturvedi, 2024). There was a proposal for a framework that would allow different healthcare providers to communicate safe cloud-based EHER data(Al-Issa, Ottom, & Tamrawi, 2019). In order to facilitate authentication between participating healthcare providers and the EHR sharing cloud, the suggested architecture made use of public key infrastructure (PKI). The proposed framework guaranteed: availability, auditability, confidentiality, integrity, and authenticity. It also states that it conforms to the technological safeguards standards for security specified in the HIPAA Security Rule. An encrypted hybrid protocol that protects the cloud against insider threats by utilizing fog computing and encryption benefits were deployed(Rani & Srivastava, 2024). The proposed solution is challenged for not being able to encrypt all the data owing to performance attribution which were resolved by selective encryption of data that needs extra security measures. To do this, the user is offered the option to fully, selectively, or not at all encrypt their data(Zala, Thakkar, Dholakia, Shukla, & Thumar, 2024). The purpose of data cleansing is to protect the data from insider risks. In order to mitigate the possibility that data, once decrypted by an authorized user, will be momentarily stored in the volatile memory of the physical system and may be utilized by an insider threat, a data cleaning mechanism is utilized(Sadhu, Yanambaka, & Abdelgawad, 2022). On the other side, selective encryption describes the practice of encrypting particular communication channels or data instead of encrypting all of it. When fog computing and selective encryption are combined, localized processing and encryption may be provided where needed, improving the overall security posture of IoT devices without sacrificing network speed(Tange, De Donno, Fafoutis, & Dragoni, 2020).

According to (Soni & Kumar, 2022), IoT cloud data warehouse required an ANN machine learning-based solution for authentication, validation and identification of digital ecosystem. ANNs are used in facial recognition to evaluate patterns, structures, and facial traits in order to identify people. In order to teach the network to recognize and learn from distinct facial features, a dataset of facial photos is used. For the reason that they can recognize intricate patterns and correlations in data, ANNs are excellent at pattern recognition tasks. Based on acquired traits and attributes, they are able to categorize input patterns into several groups for identification purposes. In order to precisely identify people, ANNs in face recognition can distinguish facial landmarks, expressions, and distinctive traits(Amiri, Heidari, Navimipour, Unal, & Mousavi, 2024). According to (Hon, 2024),ANNs are useful in a variety of domains, including image recognition, speech recognition, and anomaly detection. They can identify patterns in incoming data by analyzing it and classifying it according to similarities and differences. The recent computing trend requires IoT platforms to have cognitive and smart capabilities that can typically acquire a vast amount of useable data from its environment and distribute it among the interested parties(Ahanger, Aljumah, & Atiquzzaman, 2022). They must execute preliminary processing and noise removal before communicating the pertinent data, or a mixture of them, so that they can be used by various cloud applications(Venkatachalam et al., 2023). According to (Sengan et al., 2020), a novel approach in taking advantage of rising healthcare digitization which generates massive amounts of clinical data included in electronic healthcare record(e-HCR) is to combine it with advanced machine learning software to improve clinical decision-making which promote citizens timely record processing. The clinical inferences, which are typically not applicable to other components of the electronic health record have been considered a prerequisite for addressing various health concerns in administering a specific patient situation in a clinically logical and thought-provoking manner. The predictive model utilizing e-HCR will both reduce wasteful spending and advance clinical knowledge in order to increase the quality of care. The clinical data, however, presents a variety of challenges for data science that prevent the successful deployment of predictive models, taking into consideration all challenges with data representation, temporal processing, and the impact of data bias(Ahmed, Xi, Hou, Shah, & Hameed, 2023).

In a similar development, (Jain, Panesar, Talwar, & Sah, 2021) confirmed that IoT wireless connectivity and repository of electronically preserved data through artificial intelligence software, sensor devices and actuators have revolutionized intelligent medical diagnosis and therapy. As a result, the healthcare systems have been able to benefit from globalization for quick and efficient on-site or remote diagnosis and monitoring of different health related developments. By simultaneously transmitting and interpreting large data stored in the clinical data warehouse system, this improves effectiveness and lowers costs. IoT devices can be used to track the real-time location of medical devices and the location of clinical diagnoses thanks to a network of wireless connections and a repository of electronically maintained data, which highlighted the development of related technologies and tactics. However, (Radhakrishnan et al., 2023) noted that precision medicine, which is crucial for clinical data warehousing is swiftly developing novel treatments for diseases that are specific to individual patients based on their unique genetics, lifestyles, societal health determinants, and medical histories. The creation of targeted pharmaceuticals is more dependent on comprehensive patient information that goes beyond well-organized electronic health records and can only be obtained through a wide-ranging clinical repository. The authors emphasized that in-depth descriptions of a patient's medical history, family history, lifestyle, illness development, treatment plans, doctor's comments, and prognoses are all included in free-text clinical notes. Although not typically found in organized EHR data, these details are essential for the research on individualized disease therapy. Clinical notes are a tremendous gold mine of data on a patient's illness course, medical history, and therapy options stored in guarded databases only available for study following rigorous ethics review. Clinical notes and reports from ordinary patient care can provide a wealth of data that is clinically relevant and useful for research, including specific treatment plans, over-the-counter pharmaceutical use, dietary and physical activity habits, and precise diagnoses and prognoses. Even though access is limited due to the personal identifying and protected health information content, patient-level data are essential to use for research benefits(Zhuang, Shyu, Hong, Li, & Zhang, 2023).

Healthcare data mining is the process of sorting through enormous amounts of raw medical data and or well-organized health records in order to find and investigate any correlations and associations between facts and data parameters in order to derive valuable insights, evidences, scientific takeaways, and conclusions that can improve medical practice and or knowledge(Mbatha et al., 2023). Methods for mining and analyzing healthcare data have been around for a while, but due to several format obstacles and practical difficulties, they were only available to a small group of medical statisticians, clinical scientists, and healthcare professionals. Data mining is a part of larger procedure known as knowledge discovery from database theory, which involved a technological technique of identifying and understanding patterns from enormous and complicated databases. Through the adoption of artificial intelligence alongside machine learning on the data warehouse repository, the data mining techniques can help to manage information retrieval and pattern identification(Bharadiya, 2023). With the help of the clinical data warehouse technology, queries can be implemented quickly and patient-level reporting can be done speedily. Finding particular patient who meet the criteria for research studies and assisting in the discovery of novel connections between the causes and effects of diseases are two uses for it. The development of healthcare data warehouses has sparked a cognitive computing revolution that will help doctors treat patients' illnesses more effectively and result in better patient outcomes(Onyebuchi et al., 2024). To quickly respond to specific requests and generate tailored, intelligent recommendations, the cognitive computing system immediately analyses massive amounts of data that could be used to get around some obstacles. This have offered a thorough grasp of present applications of artificial intelligence in medicine as well as its potential in the future clinical information retrieval system(Matthew et al., 2024).

5. 5G SPECTRUM INFRASTRUCTURE FOR E-HEALTHCARE SYSTEM

A growing variety of devices and technology are being used in the healthcare industry to provide better, more effective services, turning medical facilities into smart hospitals(Matthew, Kazaure, & Okochi, 2022). The fifth generation network 5G offers continuous connectivity, making it unnecessary to switch between mobile and in-building Wi-Fi networks. It also makes it possible to combine many IoT radio networks that are incompatible into a single network. Numerous options exist with cloud computing to deliver high-quality, high-bandwidth, and reliable access to computing resources that may be quickly supplied or released when needed. Regarding the types of cloud computing, public, private, or hybrid there are variations in terms of service levels and deployment methods. The business requirements, including the levels of performance, security, and resilience, will determine which model is best. One of the most important technology for the digital transformation of current society is 5G technology, which is also necessary for smart healthcare since everything in smart healthcare system is expected to be connected(Javaid, Haleem, Singh, & Suman, 2023). 5G smart healthcare implementation and promotion can accelerate medical improvements and lessen inconsistent resource allocation. In addition to serving as the basis for cutting-edge communication services, 5G networks are also developing as the industrial digital transformation engine and the infrastructure underlying socioeconomic developmental catalyst(Matthew et al., 2022). The success of 5G is largely dependent on frequency band and regulations, which guarantee the spectrum's timely availability under the right circumstances to enable the wireless industry to meet demand for service improvement from consumers and businesses.

There are two types of 5G network infrastructure: non-standalone (NSA) infrastructures that still rely on some 4G Long Term Evolution (LTE) equipment, and standalone(SA) 5G infrastructures that have their own cloud-native network core connecting to 5G New Radio (NR) technologies(Matthew & Kazaure, 2021). The

NSA strategy leverages a combination of 5G Radio Access Network (RAN), 5G NR interface, and existing LTE infrastructure and core network to give a 5G-like experience until network carriers are able to build out the independent infrastructure needed for 5G(Shetty & Shetty, 2021). User equipment, such as the RAN and NR interface, and the 5G core network, which uses a service-based architecture framework with virtualized network services, make up a standalone 5G deployment. Typically hardware-based network operations are virtualized and executed as software. In order to maintain high sector throughput and let more users to connect to the network concurrently, 5G macro cells use multiple input, multiple output (MIMO) antennas, which are widely deployed(Bisht et al., 2023). Together with a large number of subterranean fiber networks, 5G wireless mobile networks make use of tiny cells with more distributed equipment, lower network congestion, and less population density, the 5G RAN element works well in these scenarios(Sufyan, Khan, Khashan, Mir, & Mir, 2023). The rationale behind this is that 5G RAN concentrates on lower-band radio frequencies, which have a greater coverage area but can transport less data. Redesigned to effectively interface with cloud-based 5G services and the IoT, the 5G Core Network infrastructure has dispersed servers around the network to minimize latency(Matthew et al., 2023). It also controls all mobile phone, data, and internet connections with the following key achievement.

Low Latency: Significantly reduced latency is a feature of 5G technology, which enhances the real-time data processing and retrieval capabilities of cloud data warehousing systems while also raising system efficiency(Prasad, Tanwar, & Bhavsar, 2021).

High Bandwidth: Cloud data warehouses can send and receive massive volumes of data rapidly and effectively because to 5G's high bandwidth capabilities, which optimizes data processing and analytics activities(P. K. Aggarwal et al., 2021).

Improved Connectivity: The use of 5G networks guarantees dependable and fast internet access, facilitating smooth communication among cloud data warehouse constituents and augmenting system efficiency(Sefati & Halunga, 2023).

Enhanced Data Security: In order to provide secure data transmission and storage in cloud data warehouses while maintaining data integrity and confidentiality, 5G's sophisticated security capabilities, such as network slicing and encryption, are utilized(Ayub, Mahmood, Kumari, & Sangaiah, 2021).

Scalability: The scalability needs of cloud data warehousing systems are supported by 5G technology, which makes it possible to expand infrastructure and resources effectively in order to keep up with demand for data processing(Khujamatov, Khasanov, Reypnazarov, & Akhmedov, 2021).

6. METHODOLOGY

In e-healthcare cloud IoT framework, the primary players have complete control over the data kept in the healthcare data warehouse repository through the cloud servers. The 5G spectrum and corporate software platforms as a service provide the enabling digital platform infrastructure refer **toFigure 1**. Infrastructures as a service (IaaS) refers to the suggested hardware, storage facility, software and physical devices of an IoT configuration that represent a brand-new way to provide cloud computing services(Nair & Tyagi, 2023). The software as a service (SaaS) environment suggested software tools that make up the intermediary layer, involving the amalgamation of the two infrastructures that gave rise to the platform as a service (PaaS), with functionalities of software libraries, tools, services, and implementable object-oriented programming codes that were authorized by the software supplier(Ugochukwu O Matthew et al., 2021). As IoT cloud database management technology advances which provides the resources required for an enterprise business model, the current study focused on the implementation of enterprise data warehouse for e-healthcare business operation. The paper addressed the fundamental components of an enterprise cloud data warehouse required for the implementation of e-healthcare within the scope of an e-healthcare management information system. The healthcare organizations genuinely trusted cloud infrastructure implementation; on the other hand, observations indicated that several other e-healthcare partners remain more skeptical over enterprise cloud security vulnerabilities(Alshamrani, 2022).

The enterprise cloud data warehouse, as seen through the lens of IT, is a top-down administrative business information system that project organizations as capable, knowledgeable, and cognizant of their business implementation objectives(Gagalova, Elizalde, Portales-Casamar, & Görges, 2020). Healthcare organizations will have access to servers and software services that provide scalability, maintainability, and massive data processing through the cloud data warehousing infrastructure via third-party cloud migration. The front-end framework provides the gateway protocol to the cloud database server that links the platform through remote client applications, consisting of the interfaces and software mechanisms that are required for service delivery. Integrating security into each service component, administrative tier, and application is essential for maintaining the integrity of the IoT solution and reducing the risk of cyberattacks when an organization deploys and leverages connected technologies to drive its business(Aslan, Aktuğ, Ozkan-Okay, Yilmaz, & Akin, 2023). For organizations to attain strong cybersecurity standards, IoT technology needs a wide range of capabilities which include access control, secure network protocols, data encryption, and other built-in security features which IoT platforms offer(Okafor, Ingle, Matthew, Saunders, & Delaney, 2024). For effective data warehouse information processing, the current study used ANNs in conjunction with deep learning pattern recognition that supported data mining techniques to analyze the transaction from the IoT cloud data warehouse system that necessitated e-healthcare smart system bimodal sensors.

An ANN is made up of nodes of weighted signals, which are networks of interconnected artificial neurons that may speak with one another to initiate a chain of commands(Nwanakwaugwu et al., 2023). The signal from each connection is added together to produce an integer value, and the output of each neuron is obtained as a non-linear function of the sum of its inputs. The ANNs are useful as bimodal data processing techniques because they can computably manipulate a wide range of input variables, infer complex and non-linear relationships between hidden input and output parameters, and express these relationships in existential nomenclature(Lyons & Göçmen, 2021). ANNs play a crucial role in character and picture identification because they continuously route signals from the input layer to the output layer, uncovering hidden patterns. It can be applied widely to cybersecurity data warehouse fraud detection as well as national security assessments, providing timely, actionable intelligence to complement data collection and identify and warn against potential threats to businesses and their clients(Jimmy, 2024). The foundation of the deep learning computing framework is Deep Neural Networks (DNNs) which also become the result of scientific advances in ANN research. The DNNs have enabled the integration of cutting-edge data mining methods with other revolutionary developments in computer vision, speech recognition, and natural language processing, among other computational applications, into the IoT cloud data warehousing business ecosystem(Ahmad, Shakeel, Mehfuz, & Ahmad, 2023).

In order to provide a machine with human recognition intelligence, pattern recognition is used in computer vision applications such as biological sequencing, biomedical imaging, biometric authentication, and image processing for cybersecurity validation, refer to **Figure 2**. This makes it possible for the computer to retrieve crucial data from image databases (datasets). When learning object is not sequential or time-dependent, a FFN that has been appropriately and proportionately trained to support grade realization on the pattern recognition task is applicable (Nath, Bharath, Dsouza, & Subramanian, 2024). With its revolutionary transformation and increased proficiency in tasks like object identification, picture classification, and restoration, FFN application in image processing has gained great significance. The ability of FFNs to extract complex properties from photographs and make intelligent decisions demonstrates the significance of these networks for automating image-related tasks. In natural language processing (NLP) tasks, FFN are employed to enhance the ability to derive significant insights from vast volumes of textual data. NLP finds practical applications in email spam filters, chatbots that converse in natural language, and information retrieval systems. The versatility of FFN in addressing complex NLP and image recognition challenges is exemplified by their practical applications(Ding, Abdel-Basset, Alrashdi, & Hawash, 2024).

Figure 2. Utilizing the ANN computational model for pattern identification (Abiodun et al., 2019)

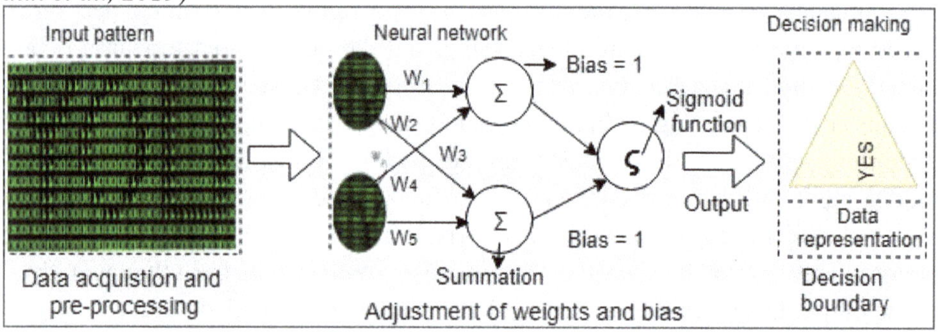

Figure 3. ANN-informed image processing for cloud IoT fingerprint recognition (Abiodun et al., 2019)

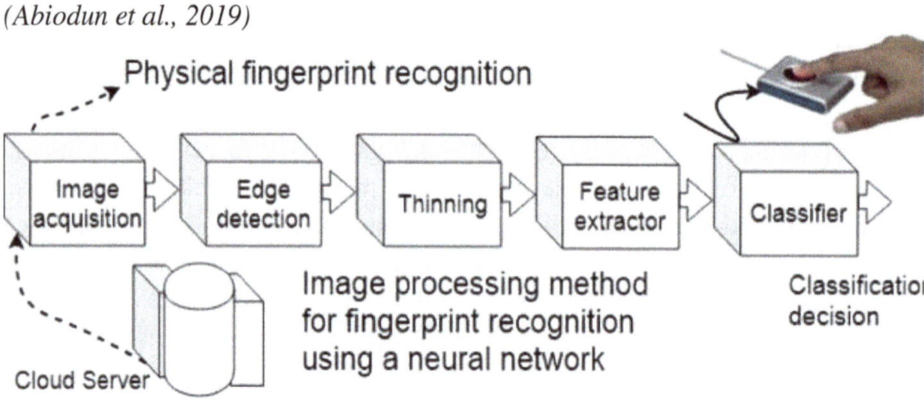

As seen in Figure 3, the ANN is built for pattern recognition (PR) and signal direction in a complex information gathering architecture within the IoT cloud data warehouse business information system. It accomplishes this by understanding patterns and relationships in the data and learning from experience, rather than by programming events. Neural network behaviors in autonomous system designs are affected by the architecture, the learning rule, and the transfer functions of the network's neurons, particularly when cloud data synchronization application is required. The hundreds of separate components that make up the layers of the neural structure also referred to as artificial neurons or processing elements are connected by coefficients, or weights(Worden, Tsialiamanis, Cross, & Rogers, 2023). The unitary neural structure that is arranged in layers is comprised of these neurons, each of which, when activated, produces a single neuronal output that is determined by the sum of its weighed inputs. Just like the FFNN, an ANN model gains knowledge about input-to-output design by determining the correlation between independent variables, or the inputs of the network, and dependent variables, or its outputs. Whereas category descriptors such as the existence or absence of organic functional groups in molecules are typical instances of output variables, observable variables such as spectral intensities at specific wavelengths are often used as input factors in the context of infrared spectra. When a network receives a set of training set samples, it learns by counting the number of occurrences in a dataset that fit into a specific category and spectrum. This is known as the machine learning approach.

Thereafter, changes are made to the network weights to reduce the discrepancies between the outputs of the network and the known true outputs. By using training set samples to modify the weights, the network can be used to deduce from a sample's spectrum whether it belongs to a class that is unknown. Several small processing units, like neurons, are layered in a classification technique called FFNs, which draws inspiration from biology. Each layer is connected to all earlier levels for flexibility. The output that the network produces from a given pattern is actually only tangentially related to the input pattern that it has learned. Figure 3 illustrates a novel approach to image processing for fingerprint recognition and biometric authentication for a cloud-based Internet of Things architecture. Using this method, you rub your finger across a smooth surface to feel its ridges and valleys. To create a range of computer-controllable integers, the minutiae a collection of unique points where the ridges and valleys converge are then subjected to NLP for identity authentication. Edge recognition and thinning are two pre-processing techniques used to reduce noise, make necessary adjustments to the image, and split it into segments(Abdulateef & Salman, 2021). Convolutional neural networks, or ConvNet ANN models, are a well-liked ANN model for the PR challenge. The incredible machines learning known as deep feedforward artificial neural networks, or convolutional neural networks (CNNs), are capable of handling speech, spoken language, video, object detection, and classification(Dargan, Kumar, Ayyagari, & Kumar, 2020).

It is challenging to predict how biometric identity technologies will perform in the broader technological context in the future because they are constantly evolving. Regarding the use of device and platform authentication, there are two main biometric trends to be mindful of: multimodal biometric authentication, which uses multiple biometric technologies at once instead of just one, and the use of a personal device as a biometric access token. Users can access all authorized IT resources and infrastructure systems with a single, distinct identity when biometric single sign-on technology is implemented(Farid, Elkhodr, Sabrina, Ahamed, & Gide, 2021). As opposed to the currently used face and fingerprint biometric recognition techniques, the finger-vein biometric identification approach uses internal vein patterns that are almost impossible to recreate. Compared to more traditional methods, finger-vein biometrics could offer a more secure method of vein recognition. Finger vein biometrics are sufficiently safe that they cannot be tampered with, compromised, or utilized fraudulently(Ali, Qiu, & Schmeelk, 2023). Complex image processing is required to eliminate the noise, retrieve the features, and then enhance them in standard finger-vein recognition approaches. This allows for the classification of images and attains highly accurate performance levels.

Figure 4. Demonstrating pattern recognition in face emotions using CNNs, with convoluted layers represented by L0 through L9 (Abiodun et al., 2019)

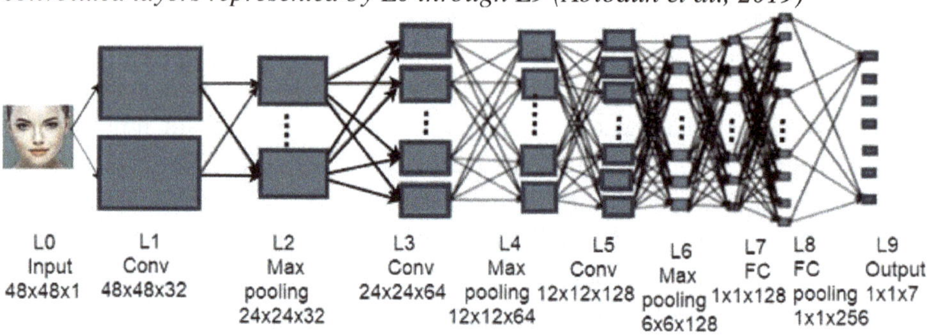

A standard CNN or deep learning-based neural network can decrease feature resolution in order to obtain picture properties and understand modal image data, as shown in Figure 4. CNN has recently demonstrated remarkable performance in several computer vision and image processing competitions, as demonstrated by the experimental and empirical PR implementation. Because Deep CNN uses many feature extraction methods, each of which is capable of independently learning representations from the input, it is able to learn with remarkable power. There has been a greater focus on studying CNNs because to the wealth of empirical data and the latest developments in hardware technology; intriguing deep CNN architectures have been proposed as a way to enhance computer vision and image processing(Mumuni & Mumuni, 2021). A number of innovative ideas that have been researched to advance CNN technology include regularization, parameter optimization, the use of different activation and loss functions, and architectural enhancements to improve accuracies and precisions(Amsaad et al., 2023). Furthermore, the most notable differences amongst CNNs are their convolution layer's common weights, receptive fields, and local connections, which ensure CNNs' superior performance in feature extraction and computation. By enabling CNN to distinguish between several images during feature extraction, it decreases the training parameters of the network and enhances the overall performance of feature extraction. By highlighting the important characteristics in the image, the layer significantly lessens the computational load on the model.

As a result of the local properties in the image being linked to the CNN layer, the training phase exhibits a noticeable increase in the matching rate. To build a system that can manage massive amounts of digital data, PR chooses analysis models such as preprocessing, scheme, and post-processing or decision-making models to accomplish generalization. It's also crucial to learn from a trained set of PR and the desired PR output when using ANN precisions. Integrating ANN into the distributed IoT systems and related infrastructures can successfully address the issues of criminal detection, cybercrime prevention, and cyber theft mitigation through PR(AL-Dosari, Fetais, & Kucukvar, 2024). The growth of the IoT and networked computers have enabled cybercrime to function globally. In the digital age, having a thorough awareness of cybersecurity procedures, whether internal or external, and being able to identify irregularities in information validation can be highly beneficial. Figure 4 provides a realistic demonstration of the various components of an ANN-based pattern recognition system, such as data collecting, feature extraction, classification, post-processing, and decision-making. By identifying features in photos, ANN pattern recognition is widely utilized to track cybersecurity developments in IoT critical infrastructures(Awotunde & Misra, 2022). In this case, a computer vision system has been trained to recognize particular patterns in photographs and can recognize images that include those patterns and block out any attempt suspected to be an intrusion.

7. MACHINE LEARNING DESIGN

Data and application protection is the main goal of cybersecurity studies which preserves sensitive information on the IoT data warehouse repository from attack, deletion, or illegal access(Mathew, Rodriguez, Rosa, Ayub, & Adasme, 2024). Given the demanding nature of e-healthcare digital ecosystem and the sensitive patient data handled by the systems, cybersecurity becomes imperative. By enabling algorithms to be trained collaboratively without disclosing the actual data, federated machine learning seeks to address the privacy and data governance concerns(M. Aggarwal, Khullar, & Goyal, 2024). Federated learning uses machine learning models to solve these problems and offer a privacy-preserving solution for the patient database system. A federated learning solution based on blockchain was developed within the context of distributed healthcare technology to preserve sensitive patient data(Naithani, Raiwani, Tiwari, & Chauhan, 2024). AI has been useful in the world of cybersecurity studies since it has been extensively implemented along with machine learning in response to user and machine log behavior. AI programs dynamically create algorithmic security solution and monitor behavioral trends in advancement of medical information system for effective healthcare delivery and privacy protection(Imoize, Balas, Solanki, Lee, & Obaidat, 2023).

Figure 5. Approach to ANN machine learning for data training techniques (Madhiarasan & Louzazni, 2022)

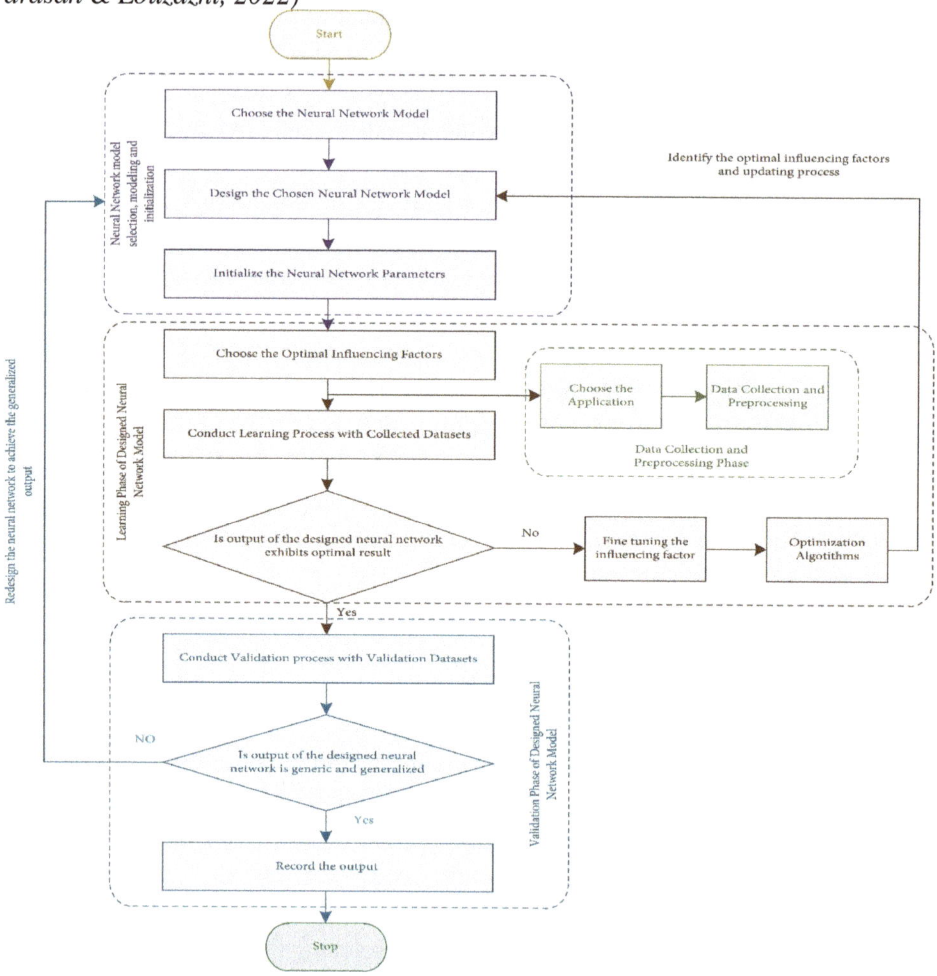

A step-by-step procedure for completing tasks is shown in Figure 5, which provides the generalization of ANN algorithmic design for data training to identify infiltration within the IoT cloud data warehouse e-healthcare business ecosystem.

First Action: The selection of an appropriate artificial neural network model, a feedforward, hybrid, or special neural network is the first stage in the neural network design process.

Second Action: When a neural network design is selected, the recommended model specifies the number of hidden layers, hidden neurons, input parameters, and other components.

Third Action: Set the initialization of the recommended model after completing the network design procedure.

Fourth Action: After the application has finished starting up, collect the data set and perform data normalization to eliminate inconsistent and missing data and improve output accuracy. Divide the collected data set's training and testing phases in the interim.

Fifth Action: Train the proposed neural network by adhering to the data collection and normalization protocols using a training data set.

Sixth Action: Verify whether the lead error is small and the performance is enough by looking at the output of the suggested neural network. The testing stage should be initiated if the suggested neural network model performs well and generates few errors during training. In the event that Step 2/Second Action is repeated, the performance was subpar. The procedure keeps going till the desired outcome is achieved.

Seventh Action: Upon completion of the training phase, apply the testing data sets the unseen raw data defined during the training phase, to the testing procedure of the proposed neural network model.

Eight Action: After testing, ascertain whether the proposed neural network model can function in a generic and well-generalized way. If not, carry on reframing the neural network until the desired generalized outcome is obtained (that is, until the least amount of error in the ideal result is produced during both the training and testing stages). The proposed neural network model ought to produce output that is significantly more broadly applicable.

Ninth Action: Stop the process.

8. DISCUSSION OF RESEARCH FINDING

Any ecosystem for AI development should be regulated by predetermined standards, norms, laws, and guidelines. All AI development projects must incorporate these into their introduction training as well as their ongoing assessments and evaluations(D. O. Oyekunle et al., 2025). It is important to continuously monitor all development and deployment activities and projects at all levels in order to identify deviations from these norms, standards, rules, and regulations. In the deployment of cloud-based enterprise e-healthcare data warehouse services, it is imperative to give serious thought to data privacy concerns and encryption regulations. A few instances of this are attribute-based encryption, identity-based encryption, public-key encryption, data encryption, and non-actor access denial. In order to ensure cybersecurity and controlled identity access via IoT cloud data warehouse federation, a structured approach such as pattern recognition and ANN multi-modal authentication should also be employed(Ebong et al., 2024). The stakes in cybersecurity are very high, thus being quick is crucial. Advancements in artificial intelligence and machine learning have revolutionized decision-making processes and enabled real-time cloud environment monitoring to thwart potential cybersecurity encroachments (Matthew et al., 2024). A critical intersection for database record protection in the field of healthcare technology development is the combination of AI and cybersecurity. As data warehouse technology advances medicine, it also presents cybersecurity issues that need to be handled carefully. At the vanguard of this crucial intersection are up-and-coming leaders who must foster innovation while protecting patient data and system resilience. These future healthcare executives will have a variety of duties to perform. By teaching people on the intricacies of cybersecurity and artificial intelligence, they create the groundwork for a conscientious ecosystem. In order to provide strong solutions, cooperation between medical doctors, tech specialists, and legislators becomes crucial.

This study starts a thorough investigation of the complex interrelationship between cybersecurity and artificial intelligence in healthcare. Through assessing the rapidly changing technological environment, exploring the subtleties of AI's influence on healthcare procedures, and analyzing the difficulties presented by cybersecurity risks, this research attempts to offer a comprehensive grasp of the interactions between these two crucial components. By detecting weaknesses and suggesting practical methods for reducing cyber threats, this study aims to help build a safe and robust healthcare system that leverages AI's benefits while protecting patient information and upholding the confidence of both people and organizations. Having an operational disaster recovery data center in a different location with minimal exposure to public platforms and the internet is the one surefire way to protect the company and guarantee business continuity. These technologies have many advantages, and the future lies in concentrating more on cybersecurity while investigating new technological application areas. These factors have been drawn to the current digital technology automation, especially in the healthcare industry, which puts healthcare organizations at serious risk for cybersecurity breaches. Because of the importance and sensitivity of healthcare data, these threats are more significant. Future studies on the development of cybersecurity (D. O. T. Oyekunle, Okwudili Matthew, Preston, & Boohene, 2024)prevention and protection mechanisms are therefore advised.

Figure 6. Semantic sensor-based e-health system application (Onyebuchi, Matthew, Kazaure, Okafor, et al., 2022)

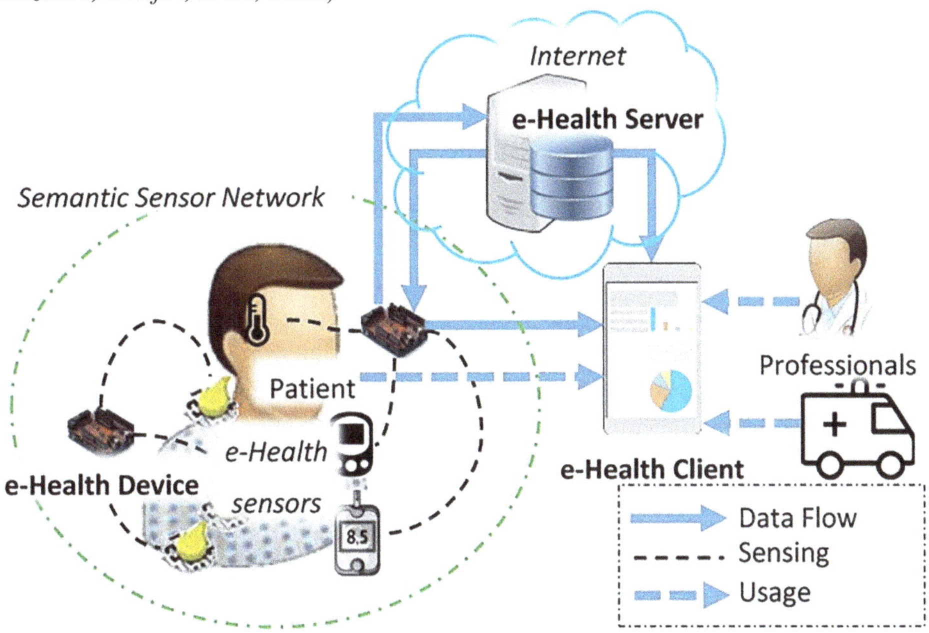

Figure **6** illustrates the components of the suggested electronic healthcare system, which includes IoT computing that has made it possible for the healthcare system to be automated through mobile client deliveries to access user-specific health information and operate any necessary e-Healthcare equipment for data collection. In light of this, the computer network of different e-Healthcare smart sensors might provide the mobile client with private and customized healthcare services, either as a distributed data warehouse system or a centralized database store(Gupta, Sharma, & Kalra, 2024). The power of cutting-edge technology is combined in this ground-breaking way to improve sensor data acquisition, clinical decision-making, advance medical research, and improve patient care(Haghayegh et al., 2024). EHR integration with AI is a significant advancement in the healthcare industry because of its ability to optimize results and personalize care. The EHR system is widely used in healthcare settings with the goal of improving the quality of patient care and streamlining medical record-keeping. The effectiveness of conventional EHR systems is, however, restricted by cyber-attacks, which include denial of service attacks (DoS), distributed denial of service attacks (DDoS), fake data injection, phishing, man in the middle attack and laborious data entry processes. By utilizing machine learning and human-computer interaction, AI-powered EHR systems can overcome these constraints and develop intelligent user interfaces. AI-driven medication discovery and individualized care also depend on the use of massive medical data, particularly EHR data(Rahman, Hossan, Uddin, & Hossain, 2024). AI systems are able to evaluate the unique characteristics of each patient and forecast the onset of a disease or suggest customized treatment regimens. To improve the effectiveness of AI research using EHR data, data standardization and improvement are necessary. The combination of several data modalities, including structured, semi-structured, and unstructured data, has potential for offering important insights into disease diagnosis and prognosis, notwithstanding the difficulties involved in maintaining EHR data(Z. Liu et al., 2022). The combination of these several data modalities can provide multimodal insights in healthcare through AI technologies, especially machine learning. One of the most important steps toward precision medicine and better clinical decision-making is the integration of AI with EHR. Healthcare providers can gain a more thorough understanding of patients' health and improve treatment results by utilizing cutting-edge technologies. Additionally, this integration has important ramifications for medical research since it gives scientists access to rich, diverse data that might propel healthcare innovations. The integration of multimodal data especially EHR and medical imaging data becomes even more crucial as the healthcare sector continues to embrace digitalization and artificial intelligence(Chen et al., 2024). This integration may open up new avenues for clinical research and customized healthcare, leading to ground-breaking developments in the area.

9. FUTURE RESEARCH FOCUS:WAY FORWARD FOR AI AND CYBERSECURITY

The development of privacy-preserving AI systems that support collaborative healthcare research is now being impeded by cybersecurity threats resulting from compromised sensitive data. Given that there are obvious benefits to employing AI to evaluate cybersecurity data, there are also significant privacy concerns. The wider range of privacy-preserving AI methods, such as secure multiparty computing, blockchain, federated learning, encryption, and suggested hybrid systems that combine aspects of the existing methods to prevent data breaches, will be the focus of future study. Federated learning, either alone or in conjunction with differential privacy, is the most promising technique to be implemented, in accordance to a study that examined the effectiveness, accuracy, and privacy of the various e-healthcare technology options. The healthcare sector can profit greatly from the deployment of EHR systems to enable better patient information access, better care coordination, fewer mistakes, more efficient diagnosis and treatment, and lower costs are a few of them. Healthcare professionals may optimize time, resources, and results while delivering better, patient-centered care by utilizing EHR technology as future adoption evolves.

10. CONCLUSION

Since cybercrime is a major risk to business and personal infrastructures, effective strategies must eventually be put into place to limit its impact. From the current study, using an ANN computer algorithm for bimodal sensor access can identify standard operating environment and potential users in the smart e-healthcare digital ecosystem. The paper described the IoT cloud data warehouse technology platform as a component of the ongoing investigation into the administration, processing, and analysis of a vast amount of data from the health grid ecosystem that functions as an e-health system and a national investment in healthcare. In order to analyze the transaction from the IoT cloud data warehousing system, the authors introduced ANN bimodal sensor around the e-healthcare smart system for end user authentication. This strategy makes sure that hackers are unable to access the data warehouse repository. By allowing digital devices to handle massive data transfer volumes, the 5G spectrum infrastructure would enable them become more self-sufficient in providing healthcare services. It will also contribute to the development of a more customized health ecosystem by facilitating instantaneous social networks of linked IoT medical equipment and secure communication.

This study established that the current model can be applied to risk management, fraud detection, identity authentication, and checkmate cybersecurity issues in smart e-healthcare services. In order to perform data integration tasks, bimodal sensor access was introduced by means of an ANN computer algorithm. Future scholars will benefit from this work's thorough explanations and analysis as they broaden their knowledge of image recognition and data mining in the vast e-healthcare cloud data warehouse. Lastly, the study problem statement were addressed, as the paper recommended collaboration with cybersecurity experts to maintain a high degree of attention as the quantity of cyber threats increases in order to stay one step ahead of cybercriminals. They can mitigate the impact of cybercrime and protect individuals and organizations from its detrimental impacts by implementing innovative methods and tactics around digital infrastructures.

REFERENCES

Abdulateef, S. K., & Salman, M. D. (2021). A Comprehensive Review of Image Segmentation Techniques. *Iraqi Journal for Electrical & Electronic Engineering*, 17(2), 166–175. DOI: 10.37917/ijeee.17.2.18

Abiodun, O. I., Jantan, A., Omolara, A. E., Dada, K. V., Umar, A. M., Linus, O. U., & Kiru, M. U. (2019). Comprehensive review of artificial neural network applications to pattern recognition. *IEEE Access : Practical Innovations, Open Solutions*, 7, 158820–158846. DOI: 10.1109/ACCESS.2019.2945545

Aceto, G., Persico, V., & Pescapé, A. (2020). Industry 4.0 and health: Internet of things, big data, and cloud computing for healthcare 4.0. *Journal of Industrial Information Integration*, 18, 100129. DOI: 10.1016/j.jii.2020.100129

Aggarwal, M., Khullar, V., & Goyal, N. (2024). A comprehensive review of federated learning: Methods, applications, and challenges in privacy-preserving collaborative model training. *Applied Data Science and Smart Systems*, 570-575.

Aggarwal, P. K., Jain, P., Mehta, J., Garg, R., Makar, K., & Chaudhary, P. (2021). Machine learning, data mining, and big data analytics for 5G-enabled IoT. *Blockchain for 5G-Enabled IoT: The new wave for Industrial Automation*, 351-375.

Ahanger, T. A., Aljumah, A., & Atiquzzaman, M. (2022). State-of-the-art survey of artificial intelligent techniques for IoT security. *Computer Networks*, 206, 108771. DOI: 10.1016/j.comnet.2022.108771

Ahmad, S., Shakeel, I., Mehfuz, S., & Ahmad, J. (2023). Deep learning models for cloud, edge, fog, and IoT computing paradigms: Survey, recent advances, and future directions. *Computer Science Review*, 49, 100568. DOI: 10.1016/j.cosrev.2023.100568

Ahmed, A., Xi, R., Hou, M., Shah, S. A., & Hameed, S. (2023). Harnessing big data analytics for healthcare: A comprehensive review of frameworks, implications, applications, and impacts. *IEEE Access : Practical Innovations, Open Solutions*, 11, 112891–112928. DOI: 10.1109/ACCESS.2023.3323574

AL-Dosari, K., Fetais, N., & Kucukvar, M.AL-Dosari. (2024). Artificial intelligence and cyber defense system for banking industry: A qualitative study of AI applications and challenges. *Cybernetics and Systems*, 55(2), 302–330. DOI: 10.1080/01969722.2022.2112539

Al Hamid, H. A., Rahman, S. M. M., Hossain, M. S., Almogren, A., & Alamri, A. (2017). A security model for preserving the privacy of medical big data in a healthcare cloud using a fog computing facility with pairing-based cryptography. *IEEE Access : Practical Innovations, Open Solutions*, 5, 22313–22328. DOI: 10.1109/ACCESS.2017.2757844

Al-Issa, Y., Ottom, M. A., & Tamrawi, A. (2019). eHealth cloud security challenges: A survey. *Journal of Healthcare Engineering*, •••, 2019. PMID: 31565209

Alam, S., Shuaib, M., Ahmad, S., Jayakody, D. N. K., Muthanna, A., Bharany, S., & Elgendy, I. A. (2022). Blockchain-based solutions supporting reliable healthcare for fog computing and Internet of medical things (IoMT) integration. *Sustainability (Basel)*, 14(22), 15312. DOI: 10.3390/su142215312

Aldhaheri, A., Alwahedi, F., Ferrag, M. A., & Battah, A. (2023). Deep learning for cyber threat detection in IoT networks: A review. *Internet of Things and Cyber-Physical Systems*.

Alghofaili, Y., Albattah, A., Alrajeh, N., Rassam, M. A., & Al-Rimy, B. A. S. (2021). Secure cloud infrastructure: A survey on issues, current solutions, and open challenges. *Applied Sciences (Basel, Switzerland)*, 11(19), 9005. DOI: 10.3390/app11199005

Ali, M. L., Qiu, M., & Schmeelk, S. (2023). *Access Control, Biometrics, and the Future.* Paper presented at the Proceedings of the 2023 5th International Conference on Image, Video and Signal Processing. DOI: 10.1145/3591156.3591158

Alshamrani, M. (2022). IoT and artificial intelligence implementations for remote healthcare monitoring systems: A survey. *Journal of King Saud University. Computer and Information Sciences*, 34(8), 4687–4701. DOI: 10.1016/j.jksuci.2021.06.005

Amiri, Z., Heidari, A., Navimipour, N. J., Unal, M., & Mousavi, A. (2024). Adventures in data analysis: A systematic review of Deep Learning techniques for pattern recognition in cyber-physical-social systems. *Multimedia Tools and Applications*, 83(8), 22909–22973. DOI: 10.1007/s11042-023-16382-x

Amsaad, F., Prasanna, P., Pravallika, T., Mamatha, G., Raviteja, B., Lakshmi, M., . . . Tashtoush, Y. (2023). *Toward Secure and Efficient CNN Recognition with Different Activation and Optimization Functions.* Paper presented at the International Conference on Advances in Computing Research. DOI: 10.1007/978-3-031-33743-7_45

Argaw, S. T., Troncoso-Pastoriza, J. R., Lacey, D., Florin, M.-V., Calcavecchia, F., Anderson, D., & Eshaya-Chauvin, B. (2020). Cybersecurity of Hospitals: Discussing the challenges and working towards mitigating the risks. *BMC Medical Informatics and Decision Making*, 20(1), 1–10. DOI: 10.1186/s12911-020-01161-7 PMID: 32620167

Aslan, Ö., Aktuğ, S. S., Ozkan-Okay, M., Yilmaz, A. A., & Akin, E. (2023). A comprehensive review of cyber security vulnerabilities, threats, attacks, and solutions. *Electronics (Basel)*, 12(6), 1333. DOI: 10.3390/electronics12061333

Awotunde, J. B., & Misra, S. (2022). *Feature extraction and artificial intelligence-based intrusion detection model for a secure internet of things networks Illumination of artificial intelligence in cybersecurity and forensics*. Springer.

Ayub, M. F., Mahmood, K., Kumari, S., & Sangaiah, A. K. (2021). Lightweight authentication protocol for e-health clouds in IoT-based applications through 5G technology. *Digital Communications and Networks*, 7(2), 235–244. DOI: 10.1016/j.dcan.2020.06.003

Bharadiya, J. P. (2023). A Comparative Study of Business Intelligence and Artificial Intelligence with Big Data Analytics. *American Journal of Artificial Intelligence*, 7(1), 24.

Bisht, N., Malik, P. K., Das, S., Islam, T., Asha, S., & Alathbah, M. (2023). Design of a Modified MIMO Antenna Based on Tweaked Spherical Fractal Geometry for 5G New Radio (NR) Band N258 (24.25–27.25 GHz) Applications. *Fractal and Fractional*, 7(10), 718. DOI: 10.3390/fractalfract7100718

Chelliah, B. J. (2022). *An Efficient Storage Solution for Healthcare Management Systems Using Cloud.* Paper presented at the 2022 Third International Conference on Smart Technologies in Computing, Electrical and Electronics (ICSTCEE).

Chen, X., Xie, H., Tao, X., Wang, F. L., Leng, M., & Lei, B. (2024). Artificial intelligence and multimodal data fusion for smart healthcare: Topic modeling and bibliometrics. *Artificial Intelligence Review*, 57(4), 91. DOI: 10.1007/s10462-024-10712-7

Dargan, S., Kumar, M., Ayyagari, M. R., & Kumar, G. (2020). A survey of deep learning and its applications: A new paradigm to machine learning. *Archives of Computational Methods in Engineering*, 27(4), 1071–1092. DOI: 10.1007/s11831-019-09344-w

Ding, W., Abdel-Basset, M., Alrashdi, I., & Hawash, H. (2024). Next generation of computer vision for plant disease monitoring in precision agriculture: A contemporary survey, taxonomy, experiments, and future direction. *Information Sciences*, 665, 120338. DOI: 10.1016/j.ins.2024.120338

Ebong, G. N., Matthew, U. O., Olofin, B., Andrew-Vitalis, N., Fatai, L. O., Waliu, A. O., & Oladipupo, M. A. (2024). *Multimedia Cloud Data Warehouse Design for Knowledge Sharing in the University Environment: A Proposed Digital Solution Implementing Interactive Learning Strategies in Higher Education.* IGI Global. DOI: 10.4018/979-8-3693-3559-8.ch010

Farid, F., Elkhodr, M., Sabrina, F., Ahamed, F., & Gide, E. (2021). A smart biometric identity management framework for personalised IoT and cloud computing-based healthcare services. *Sensors (Basel)*, 21(2), 552. DOI: 10.3390/s21020552 PMID: 33466730

Gagalova, K. K., Elizalde, M. A. L., Portales-Casamar, E., & Görges, M. (2020). What you need to know before implementing a clinical research data warehouse: Comparative review of integrated data repositories in health care institutions. *JMIR Formative Research*, 4(8), e17687. DOI: 10.2196/17687 PMID: 32852280

Gupta, M., Sharma, P., & Kalra, R. (2024). *Federated learning and artificial intelligence in e-healthcare Federated Learning and AI for Healthcare 5.0.* IGI Global.

Haghayegh, F., Norouziazad, A., Haghani, E., Feygin, A. A., Rahimi, R. H., Ghavamabadi, H. A., & Felfeli, T. (2024). Revolutionary Point-of-Care Wearable Diagnostics for Early Disease Detection and Biomarker Discovery through Intelligent Technologies. *Advancement of Science*, 11(36), 2400595. DOI: 10.1002/advs.202400595 PMID: 38958517

Heart, T., Ben-Assuli, O., & Shabtai, I. (2017). A review of PHR, EMR and EHR integration: A more personalized healthcare and public health policy. *Health Policy and Technology*, 6(1), 20–25. DOI: 10.1016/j.hlpt.2016.08.002

Hon, K. (2024). *Artificial neural networks Technology and Security for Lawyers and Other Professionals*. Edward Elgar Publishing.

Imoize, A. L., Balas, V. E., Solanki, V. K., Lee, C.-C., & Obaidat, M. S. (2023). *Handbook of Security and Privacy of AI-Enabled Healthcare Systems and Internet of Medical Things*. CRC Press.

Jain, P., Panesar, S. F., Talwar, B. F., & Sah, M. K. (2021). IoT-Based Solutions for Smart Healthcare. *Emerging Technologies for Healthcare: Internet of Things and Deep Learning Models*, 25-67.

Javaid, M., Haleem, A., Singh, R. P., & Suman, R. (2023). *5G technology for healthcare: Features, serviceable pillars, and applications*. Intelligent Pharmacy.

Jimmy, F. (2024). Cyber security Vulnerabilities and Remediation Through Cloud Security Tools. *Journal of Artificial Intelligence General science (JAIGS) ISSN: 3006-4023, 2*(1), 129-171.

Khujamatov, K., Khasanov, D., Reypnazarov, E., & Akhmedov, N. (2021). Existing technologies and solutions in 5G-enabled IoT for industrial automation. *Blockchain for 5G-Enabled IoT: The new wave for Industrial Automation*, 181-221.

Kumaresan, M., Gopal, R., Mathivanan, M., & Poongodi, T. (2022). *Amalgamation of blockchain, IoT, and 5G to improve security and privacy of smart healthcare systems Blockchain Applications for Healthcare Informatics*. Elsevier.

Lacity, M. C., Khan, S. A., & Yan, A. (2017). *Review of the empirical business services sourcing literature: an update and future directions Outsourcing and offshoring business services*. Springer.

Li, X., Lu, Y., Fu, X., & Qi, Y. (2021). Building the Internet of Things platform for smart maternal healthcare services with wearable devices and cloud computing. *Future Generation Computer Systems*, 118, 282–296. DOI: 10.1016/j.future.2021.01.016

Liu, H., Crespo, R. G., & Martínez, O. S. (2020). *Enhancing privacy and data security across healthcare applications using blockchain and distributed ledger concepts.* Paper presented at the Healthcare. DOI: 10.3390/healthcare8030243

Liu, Z., Zhang, J., Hou, Y., Zhang, X., Li, G., & Xiang, Y. (2022). *Machine learning for multimodal electronic health records-based research: Challenges and perspectives.* Paper presented at the China Health Information Processing Conference.

Lyons, J. T., & Göçmen, T. (2021). Applied machine learning techniques for performance analysis in large wind farms. *Energies*, 14(13), 3756. DOI: 10.3390/en14133756

Madhiarasan, M., & Louzazni, M. (2022). Analysis of artificial neural network: Architecture, types, and forecasting applications. *Journal of Electrical and Computer Engineering*, 2022, 2022. DOI: 10.1155/2022/5416722

Mathew, U. O., Rodriguez, D. Z., Rosa, R. L., Ayub, M. S., & Adasme, P. (2024). *Advancing Healthcare 5.0 through Federated Learning: Opportunity for Security Enforcement using Blockchain.* Paper presented at the 2024 International Conference on Software, Telecommunications and Computer Networks (SoftCOM). DOI: 10.23919/SoftCOM62040.2024.10722012

Matthew, U. O., Aderinola, M., Shuaibu, I., Kazaure, J. S., Ohabuiro, J., Daniel, O. O., & Nwamouh, U. C. (2023). Device to Device Communication Using Optimized Frequency Spectrum Reuse (OFSR) in Multi-Layered Cellular Network. *HAFED POLY Journal of Science. Management and Technology*, 5(2), 172–191.

Matthew, U. O., & Kazaure, J. S. (2021). Chemical polarization effects of electromagnetic field radiation from the novel 5G network deployment at ultra high frequency. *Health and Technology*, 11(2), 305–317. DOI: 10.1007/s12553-020-00501-x PMID: 33527067

Matthew, U. O., Kazaure, J. S., John, O., & Haruna, K. (2021). Telecommunication Business Information System and Investment Ecosystem in a Growing Economy: A Review of Telecom Investment in Nigeria. [IJICTHD]. *International Journal of Information Communication Technologies and Human Development*, 13(2), 1–20. DOI: 10.4018/IJICTHD.2021040101

Matthew, U. O., Kazaure, J. S., & Okafor, N. U. (2021). Contemporary development in E-Learning education, cloud computing technology & internet of things. *EAI Endorsed Transactions on Cloud Systems*, 7(20), e3–e3.

Matthew, U. O., Kazaure, J. S., & Okochi, P. I. (2022). 5G Mid-Range Electromagnetic Spectrum Implementation for Critical Infrastructure Development: Electromagnetic Spectrum Sustainability. [IJITN]. *International Journal of Interdisciplinary Telecommunications and Networking*, 14(1), 1–26. DOI: 10.4018/IJITN.307103

Matthew, U. O., Onumaku, V. C., Fatai, L. O., Adekunle, T. S., Waliu, A. O., Ndukwu, C. C., & Ebong, G. N. (2024). *E-Healthcare Data Warehouse Design and Data Mining Using ML Approach Reshaping Healthcare with Cutting-Edge Biomedical Advancements*. IGI Global.

Mazhar, T., Irfan, H. M., Haq, I., Ullah, I., Ashraf, M., Shloul, T. A., Ghadi, Y. Y., Imran, , & Elkamchouchi, D. H. (2023). Analysis of Challenges and Solutions of IoT in Smart Grids Using AI and Machine Learning Techniques: A Review. *Electronics (Basel)*, 12(1), 242. DOI: 10.3390/electronics12010242

Mbatha, S. Z., Mulaudzi, T. V., Mbita, Z., Adeola, H. A., Batra, J., Blenman, K. R., & Dlamini, Z. (2023). *Artificial Intelligence–Enhanced Drug Discovery and the Achievement of Next-Generation Human-Centered Health System Society 5.0 and Next Generation Healthcare: Patient-Focused and Technology-Assisted Precision Therapies*. Springer.

Mishra, V., Gupta, K., Saxena, D., & Singh, A. K. (2024). A Global Medical Data Security and Privacy Preserving Standards Identification Framework for Electronic Healthcare Consumers. *IEEE Transactions on Consumer Electronics*, 70(1), 4379–4387. DOI: 10.1109/TCE.2024.3373912

Mumuni, A., & Mumuni, F. (2021). CNN architectures for geometric transformation-invariant feature representation in computer vision: A review. *SN Computer Science*, 2(5), 340. DOI: 10.1007/s42979-021-00735-0

Nair, M. M., & Tyagi, A. K. (2023). *AI, IoT, blockchain, and cloud computing: The necessity of the future Distributed Computing to Blockchain*. Elsevier.

Naithani, K., Raiwani, Y., Tiwari, S., & Chauhan, A. S. (2024). *Artificial Intelligence Techniques Based on Federated Learning in Smart Healthcare Federated Learning for Smart Communication using IoT Application*. Chapman and Hall/CRC.

Nath, V. G., Bharath, S. P., Dsouza, A., & Subramanian, A. (2024). Machine Learning Algorithms for Smart Gas Sensor Arrays. *Nanostructured Materials for Electronic Nose*, 185-225.

Nifakos, S., Chandramouli, K., Nikolaou, C. K., Papachristou, P., Koch, S., Panaousis, E., & Bonacina, S. (2021). Influence of human factors on cyber security within healthcare organisations: A systematic review. *Sensors (Basel)*, 21(15), 5119. DOI: 10.3390/s21155119 PMID: 34372354

Nwanakwaugwu, A. C., Matthew, U. O., Kazaure, A. A., & Haruna, K. (2023). *Data Mining Business Intelligence Applications in Retail Services Using Artificial Neural Networks Handbook of Research on Cybersecurity Risk in Contemporary Business Systems*. IGI Global.

Okafor, N., Ingle, R., Matthew, U., Saunders, M., & Delaney, D. (2024). Assessing and Improving IoT Sensor Data Quality in Environmental Monitoring Networks: A Focus on Peatlands. *IEEE Internet of Things Journal*, 11(24), 40727–40742. DOI: 10.1109/JIOT.2024.3454241

Onyebuchi, A., Matthew, U. O., Kazaure, J. S., Ebong, G. N., Ndukwu, C. C., Nwanakwaugwu, A. C., & Okey, O. D. (2024). *Cloud-Based IoT Data Warehousing Technology for E-Healthcare: A Comprehensive Guide to E-Health Grids Pioneering Smart Healthcare 5.0 with IoT, Federated Learning, and Cloud Security*. IGI Global.

Onyebuchi, A., Matthew, U. O., Kazaure, J. S., Nwanagwaugwu, A. C., Nwamouh, U. C., & Adamu, U. A. (2022). Cloud based IoT Electronic Healthcare Data Warehouse Integration in emerging 5G Health Grid Ecosystem.

Onyebuchi, A., Matthew, U. O., Kazaure, J. S., Okafor, N. U., Okey, O. D., Okochi, P. I., Taiwo, J. F., & Matthew, A. O. (2022). Business demand for a cloud enterprise data warehouse in electronic healthcare computing: Issues and developments in e-healthcare cloud computing. [IJCAC]. *International Journal of Cloud Applications and Computing*, 12(1), 1–22. DOI: 10.4018/IJCAC.297098

Oyekunle, D. O., Esseme, A. C. B., Oladipupo, M. A., Oseni, V. E., Adebola, N. T., Nwaiku, M., & Matthew, U. O. (2025). *Artificial Neural Network Algorithm in Nutritional Assessment: Implication for Machine Learning Prediction in Nutritional Assessments Precision Health in the Digital Age: Harnessing AI for Personalized Care*. IGI Global Scientific Publishing.

Oyekunle, D. O. T., Okwudili Matthew, U., Preston, D., & Boohene, D. (2024). Trust beyond technology algorithms: A theoretical exploration of consumer trust and behavior in technological consumption and AI projects. *Journal of Computer and Communications, 12*(06), 10.4236.

Panimalar, S., & Gunasundari, S. (2023). *A survey based on privacy-preserving over health care data analysis.* Paper presented at the International Conference on Emerging Trends in Expert Applications & Security. DOI: 10.1007/978-981-99-1946-8_40

Patil, R. Y., Patil, Y. H., & Bannore, A. (2024). *Cybersecurity in medical Internet of Things: Issues, challenges, and future directions Security Implementation in Internet of Medical Things*. CRC Press.

Prasad, V. K., Tanwar, S., & Bhavsar, M. D. (2021). Advance cloud data analytics for 5G enabled IoT. *Blockchain for 5G-Enabled IoT: The new wave for Industrial Automation*, 159-180.

Radhakrishnan, L., Schenk, G., Muenzen, K., Oskotsky, B., Ashouri Choshali, H., Plunkett, T., Israni, S., & Butte, A. J. (2023). A certified de-identification system for all clinical text documents for information extraction at scale. *JAMIA Open*, 6(3), ooad045. DOI: 10.1093/jamiaopen/ooad045 PMID: 37416449

Shrimali, R. (2020). How IoT is transforming the healthcare industry. Embedded Computing Design, Volansys LLC (accessed May 5, 2021) available at: https:// www. embeddedcomputing. com/application/healthcare/telehealth-healthcare-iot/ how-iot-is-transforming-the-healthcare-industry

Rahman, M. H., Hossan, K. M. R., Uddin, M. K. S., & Hossain, M. D. (2024). Improving Collaborative Interactions Between Humans and Artificial Intelligence to Achieve Optimal Patient Outcomes in the Healthcare Industry. *Available atSSRN* 5029975. DOI: 10.2139/ssrn.5029975

Rani, S., & Srivastava, G. (2024). Secure hierarchical fog computing-based architecture for industry 5.0 using an attribute-based encryption scheme. *Expert Systems with Applications*, 235, 121180. DOI: 10.1016/j.eswa.2023.121180

Raul, A. C. (2021). *The privacy, data protection and cybersecurity law review*. Law Business Research Limited.

Saba Raoof, S., & Durai, M. (2022). A comprehensive review on smart health care: Applications, paradigms, and challenges with case studies. *Contrast Media & Molecular Imaging*, 2022(1), 2022. DOI: 10.1155/2022/4822235 PMID: 36247859

Sadhu, P. K., Yanambaka, V. P., & Abdelgawad, A. (2022). Internet of things: Security and solutions survey. *Sensors (Basel)*, 22(19), 7433. DOI: 10.3390/s22197433 PMID: 36236531

Sardi, A., Rizzi, A., Sorano, E., & Guerrieri, A. (2020). Cyber risk in health facilities: A systematic literature review. *Sustainability (Basel)*, 12(17), 7002. DOI: 10.3390/su12177002

Sefati, S. S., & Halunga, S. (2023). Ultra-reliability and low-latency communications on the internet of things based on 5G network: Literature review, classification, and future research view. *Transactions on Emerging Telecommunications Technologies*, 34(6), e4770. DOI: 10.1002/ett.4770

Sengan, S., Kamalam, G., Vellingiri, J., Gopal, J., Velayutham, P., & Subramaniyaswamy, V. (2020). Medical information retrieval systems for e-Health care records using fuzzy based machine learning model. *Microprocessors and Microsystems*, •••, 103344.

Shetty, R. S., & Shetty, R. S. (2021). 5G NSA Design and Deployment Strategy. *5G Mobile Core Network: Design, Deployment, Automation, and Testing Strategies*, 103-165.

Shrivastava, V., & Chaturvedi, A. K. (2024). A review on intrusion detection system for distributed network based on Machine Learning. *Journal of Integrated Science and Technology*, 12(2), 739–739.

Soni, D., & Kumar, N. (2022). Machine learning techniques in emerging cloud computing integrated paradigms: A survey and taxonomy. *Journal of Network and Computer Applications*, 205, 103419. DOI: 10.1016/j.jnca.2022.103419

Sufyan, A., Khan, K. B., Khashan, O. A., Mir, T., & Mir, U. (2023). From 5G to beyond 5G: A comprehensive survey of Wireless network evolution, challenges, and promising technologies. *Electronics (Basel)*, 12(10), 2200. DOI: 10.3390/electronics12102200

Szalados, J. E. (2021). Medical Records and Confidentiality: Evolving Liability Issues Inherent in the Electronic Health Record, HIPAA, and Cybersecurity. *The Medical-Legal Aspects of Acute Care Medicine: A Resource for Clinicians, Administrators, and Risk Managers*, 315-342.

Tange, K., De Donno, M., Fafoutis, X., & Dragoni, N. (2020). A systematic survey of industrial Internet of Things security: Requirements and fog computing opportunities. *IEEE Communications Surveys and Tutorials*, 22(4), 2489–2520. DOI: 10.1109/COMST.2020.3011208

Vellela, S. S., Reddy, B. V., Chaitanya, K. K., & Rao, M. V. (2023). *An Integrated Approach to Improve E-Healthcare System using Dynamic Cloud Computing Platform.* Paper presented at the 2023 5th International Conference on Smart Systems and Inventive Technology (ICSSIT). DOI: 10.1109/ICSSIT55814.2023.10060945

Venkatachalam, K., Yang, Z., Trojovský, P., Bacanin, N., Deveci, M., & Ding, W. (2023). Bimodal HAR-An efficient approach to human activity analysis and recognition using bimodal hybrid classifiers. *Information Sciences*, 628, 542–557. DOI: 10.1016/j.ins.2023.01.121

Vilakazi, K., & Adebesin, F. (2023). A Systematic Literature Review on Cybersecurity Threats to Healthcare Data and Mitigation Strategies. *EPiC Series in Computing*, 93, 240–251. DOI: 10.29007/hf15

Worden, K., Tsialiamanis, G., Cross, E., & Rogers, T. (2023). *Artificial neural networks Machine Learning in Modeling and Simulation: Methods and Applications*. Springer.

Zala, K., Thakkar, H. K., Dholakia, N., Shukla, M., & Thumar, D. (2024). Designing an Attribute-Based Encryption Scheme with an Enhanced Anonymity Model for Privacy Protection in E-Health. *SN Computer Science*, 5(2), 203. DOI: 10.1007/s42979-023-02541-2

Zhuang, Y., Shyu, C.-R., Hong, S., Li, P., & Zhang, L. (2023). Self-sovereign identity empowered non-fungible patient tokenization for health information exchange using blockchain technology. *Computers in Biology and Medicine*, 157, 106778. DOI: 10.1016/j.compbiomed.2023.106778 PMID: 36934533

Chapter 5
Cybersecurity Issues on E-Healthcare Cloud Data Warehouse System:
Blockchain-Based Federated Learning Approach

Ogheneruona Maria Esegbona-Isikeh
https://orcid.org/0009-0005-6073-9442
Birmingham City University, UK

Morgan Nwaiku
https://orcid.org/0009-0001-8984-8387
Teesside University, UK

Victor Nosakhare Oriakhi
https://orcid.org/0009-0005-2005-8378
University of Salford, UK

Chukwuka Michael Oforgu
https://orcid.org/0009-0005-1216-1957
University of the West of England, UK

Oluwatosin Samuel Falebita
https://orcid.org/0009-0006-6750-482X
Colorado State University, USA

Ugochukwu Okwudili Matthew
https://orcid.org/0000-0003-0828-9710
Federal University of Lavras, Brazil

Alain Claude Bah Esseme
https://orcid.org/0009-0005-8086-4566
Nexus Cloud Technologies, UK

Victor Onuchi Onyenagubom
https://orcid.org/0009-0001-1084-9193
Teesside University, UK

ABSTRACT

In order to detect denial-of-service (DoS) and distributed denial of service (DDoS) intrusions on the organization's e-healthcare data warehouse infrastructure, the authors of this study proposed a computing framework that combines a federated learning system based on blockchain technology. A Message Queuing Telemetry Transport (MQTT) broker gathers data from an IoT node and sends it to the computing platform for analysis. As a platform for the creation of several new technologies and

DOI: 10.4018/979-8-3373-2827-0.ch005

applications, IoT has created new opportunities in the age of cloud communication. Due to the increasing use of cloud data warehouse technologies, computer networks have had serious security concerns, and there are security vulnerabilities in the IoT as well. DoS and DDoS attacks on IoT e-healthcare servers may compromise general stability, efficacy of the services, and real-time information federation. This study provided an efficient MQTT broker approach to secure servers from cyberattacks and presented state-of-the-art defenses against DoS/DDoS attacks in the IoT digital healthcare ecosystem.

INTRODUCTION

Healthcare providers throughout the world can leverage cloud computing to increase return on investment and improve service quality by utilizing artificial intelligence (AI), machine learning, big data analytics and the Internet of Things (IoT) to effect precision medicine(Sahu, Gupta, Ambasta, & Kumar, 2022),(Matthew, Onumaku, et al., 2024),(Onyebuchi, Matthew, Kazaure, Okafor, et al., 2022). Healthcare industry has undergone changes because of the combination of cloud computing and AI, which offers strong platforms and solutions that improve patient care, expedite processes, and promote personalized medicine(Aminizadeh et al., 2024). These technologies have the potential to solve some of the most important problems facing healthcare as they develop further, creating a more effective, efficient, and universally transformed healthcare future. Cloud computing has become an important innovation in today's advanced healthcare environment, altering the way business organization acquire, manage, and exchange medical data(Onyebuchi et al., 2024). They are also streamlining their processes and creating cutting-edge telehealth solutions along with significant reduction of costs, enhancing the efficacy and efficiency of healthcare services. Healthcare is expected to change significantly as a result of cloud computing, with a projected global market value of over $89 billion by 2027, coupled with exponential growth in infrastructure as a service (IaaS), software as a service(SaaS) and platform as a service(PaaS)(Wong, Vengusamy, & Bastrygina, 2024),(Matthew, Asuni, & Fatai, 2024).

Healthcare providers can improve patient outcomes, provide better treatment, and spur industry innovation by adopting cloud computing, creating major positive impact on patient outcomes and operational efficiency for healthcare service organizations. The electronic health record (HER) systems' customizability and flexibility are increased by the use of cloud computing in the healthcare industry(Mandarino, Pappalardo, & Tramontana, 2024). In the past, customized solutions required a high level of information technology (IT) and programming experience but with the development of AI and its connection with cloud computing, large-scale dataset analysis can assist in creating customized care plans that are tailored to each patient's specific need. The effectiveness of electronic healthcare (e-healthcare) workflows is further enhanced by this flexibility. In the context of healthcare, cloud computing refers to the availability of data centers to consumers over the internet, dispersed from central servers over multiple locations(Dang, Piran, Han, Min, & Moon, 2019). Healthcare stakeholders now have a flexible way to remotely access servers that safely manage large amounts of data, regardless of their physical location. IoT integrates a wide range of industries and professions, such as traffic management, energy management, environmental monitoring, smart grid management, critical infrastructure surveillance, and healthcare management(Tabaa, Monteiro, Bensag, & Dandache, 2020). These days, the modern society is seeing new innovations in these domains that aim to simplify infrastructure and give customers reliable solutions. Because IoT technologies have so many different features, critical application of healthcare systems require extra care to guarantee timely and cloud computing for safe conveyance of their data. Many businesses throughout the world are currently using IoT to combine different hospitals and improve patient health monitoring and record federation by using real-time information system monitoring. Patients are also benefiting from this technology because it allows them to obtain continuous monitoring without constantly visiting hospitals. Currently, e-healthcare services are provided to patients by many hospitals, and doctors are always keeping an eye on the progress of these patients(Matthew, Kazaure, Amaonwu, et al., 2021).

With regard to providing necessary services through cloud IoT infrastructure, these hospitals and the patients have legal agreements. Protecting patient data, confidentiality is essential to demonstrating the system's dependability and intelligence sharing within digital health ecosystem. In e-healthcare systems, servers play a vital role since they provide real-time patient monitoring and administration of clinical procedures(Padmaja & Seshadri, 2021). Patient health monitoring may be at risk if these servers are unavailable for a brief period of time or more due to service disruptions arising from network vulnerability. Network vulnerabilities have grown as a result of IoT network expansion and skilled hackers have begun to undertake sophisticated attacks on vital resources(Mallick & Nath, 2024). Sensitive patient records may become extremely difficult to access in the crucial and demanding field of e-health if there is a significant attack on the network, such as a denial-of-service (DoS) and distributed denial-of-service attack(Sari & Sopuru, 2021). Given that blockchain technology's intrinsic qualities make it appropriate for tracking and storing medical data, it presents potential for advancement and can address a number of issues facing the present healthcare systems(Yaqoob, Salah, Jayaraman, & Al-Hammadi, 2022). In order to mitigate the effects of attacks, both enterprise IT organizations and service providers must continue to protect their own cloud critical infrastructures where blockchain technology is used to establish a decentralized network of nodes that exchange information and computational resources(Kharche, Badholia, & Upadhyay, 2024). These nodes can then use this unchangeable ledger to protect the confidentiality of data kept in their ethereal domains, guaranteeing that integrity will always be preserved even in the face of technological upheaval. Several networking layers must be functional in the languages that devices use to guarantee strong security, intelligent routing, and analytics operations. Comprehending these protocols in the network allows traffic to be prioritized, safeguarded, and routed appropriately. As opposed to conventional systems, blockchains decentralized architecture improves security against hacks and data loss while guaranteeing resilience against single points of failure(Falayi, Wang, Liao, & Yu, 2023).

Due to size restrictions and storage costs, blockchain cannot be utilized to store all the data in EHR records; however, it can be used to index the data using hashing methods of federated learning(Guduri, Chakraborty, Maheswari, & Margala, 2023). With the use of a central server and a number of clients acting as nodes to carry out local training using their local data, federated learning is a distributed machine-learning technique for DoS ad DDoS intrusion detection(S. Agrawal et al., 2022). A standard global model is initially sent to a group of clients by the central server, while the local models are then returned to the server by clients, who used the local data to train the global model(Ye et al., 2024). An additional training cycle is initiated by the server after combining the local models into a new global model. It is possible to repeat this process multiple times until a threshold is met or the global model converges. Fundamentally speaking, federated learning is a cooperative machine learning method that uses local data samples from several devices or servers to train and device an algorithm without ever transferring the actual data(Supriya & Gadekallu, 2023). In situations when access rights, security and data privacy present serious obstacles, this idea is revolutionary. In a similar development, AI models will allow hospitals to work together to improve patient outcomes without exchanging sensitive patient data, or where digital devices can learn from user behavior to improve features without sacrificing privacy, there are many possibilities and scenarios that federated learning is bringing to e-healthcare system. No matter how it is stored, sensitive information including genetic health records and demographic data is subject to strict protection requirements under privacy laws like the General Data Protection Regulation (GDPR) in Europe and the Health Insurance Portability and Accountability Act (HIPAA) in the United States(Rahnasto, 2023). To tackle these obstacles, novel approaches that leverage the advantages of the blockchain are required, including data integrity, decentralization for security and resilience, and robust authorization. It is necessary to include other features like upholding privacy regulations, being economical, providing accessibility to all pertinent parties, offering scalable storage options for large amounts of data, and optimizing efficiency while utilizing smart commissions.

Figure 1. Enterprise healthcare cloud data warehouse system supporting clinical transactions (Knosp, Craven, Dorr, Bernstam, & Campion Jr, 2022)

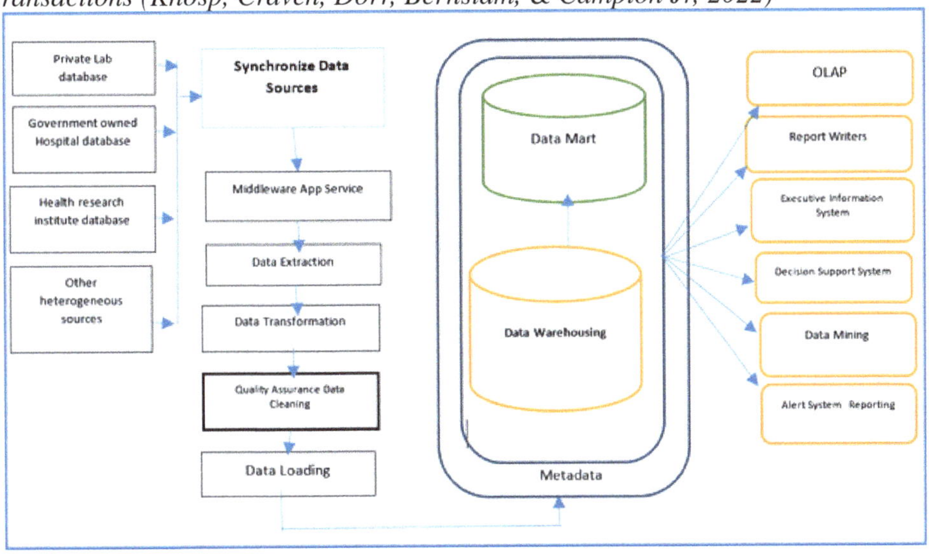

In **Figure 1** above, the e-healthcare enterprise data warehouse is a database, or group of databases, that unifies data from various heterogeneous sources and applications for a business organization and makes it accessible for analysis and utilization throughout the organization while being integrated across various IoT operational platforms. Enterprise data warehouses help organizations to find hidden patterns, trends, and correlations among enormous, complex datasets stored on the IoT cloud repositories (Dhatterwal, Kaswan, Baliyan, & Jain, 2022). Database synchronization helps with hybrid integration, which involves storing data on-premise servers and in cloud services like Google Cloud platforms, Microsoft Azure, and AWS cloud data warehouse repositories(Mathur, 2024). It also ensures data integrity between databases and automatically replicates changes back and forth. Prior to being sent and stored, processes such as AWS data synchronization or Azure data sync manage data enrichment, filtration, transformation, and aggregation, and vice versa. Without interfering with business activities, this happens in real-time while preserving data consistency and correctness. Data mining allows businesses to segment their customer bases, find cross-selling opportunities, detect fraud, and estimate demand, all of which contribute to a competitive advantage in the marketplace as key component of organizational business intelligence activities(Javaid, 2024),(Nwanakwaugwu, Matthew, Kazaure, & Haruna, 2023). Furthermore, data mining allows for the extraction of useful insight from huge, complicated data sets, resulting in a thorough understanding of an organization's operations and market dynamics. Strategic data mining integration within a strong data warehouse infrastructure enables businesses to make data-driven decisions, capitalize on new opportunities, and navigate an increasingly competitive landscape with confidence and clarity(J. Ranjan & Foropon, 2021).

Medical personnel can access a wide variety of patient data through cloud computing, share it with important parties, and provide prompt protocols. The enterprise data warehouse is the biggest and most computationally demanding business application systems, made up of enormous databases that store historical data on volumes ranging from gigabytes to terabytes of stored information(Ebong et al., 2024). These databases are confronted with two challenges related to the system's workload: first, they have rapidly rising data volumes and application workloads; second, there are more users utilizing the system at once due to its distributed nature(Zhang, Martin, Powley, & Chen, 2017). The enterprise data warehouse systems are implemented on large-scale parallel computers, such as symmetric multiprocessor system environments, clusters, massively parallel processing systems, and parallel database software, in order to meet the performance requirements. Healthcare practitioners may enhance patient care throughout the entire digital ecosystem supply, boost cooperation, and streamline communications by utilizing cloud computing(Onyebuchi, Matthew, Kazaure, Nwanagwaugwu, et al., 2022). Cloud computing in healthcare systems can assist providers improve patient engagement by enabling remote access to prescriptions, test results, and medical information. Patients are better able to participate in their care since they can access and control their medical records from anywhere at any time, which has distinguished federated learning as unique cloud-based machine learning paradigms due to its modest yet significant data processing and model training(Nadella et al., 2024). The potential of privacy violations and improper use of data under conventional data handling procedures has increased as we continue to produce enormous volumes of data through our digital activities. This has necessitated network security intrusions that have spread throughout the observed networked IoT cloud databases and how they affect organizational business security goals over time.

When deploying distributed cloud data warehouse systems, federated learning (FL) leverages blockchain technology to enhance security and privacy in perceptive data transportation systems(X. Li et al., 2024). Data integrity and security are enhanced by blockchain and IoT integration, particularly in FL for data internetworking operations. By exchanging just model updates and storing data locally, this approach enhances privacy. Effective IoT collaboration is made possible by blockchains transparency, which is crucial for data warehouse accountability. Its consensus algorithms further ensure network integrity by verifying updates and transactions across devices, preventing attacks, and encouraging a collaborative information sharing environment(W. Li, Tan, & Wang, 2020). It is anticipated that federated learning will serve as the foundation for the upcoming generation of artificial intelligence collaboration networks. Studies on cloud data warehouse knowledge-based technology have shown that advanced concept technology can implement the real network security scenario, and that contemporary technology has significantly more accurate concept of the security problem than traditional technology. This study significantly advanced the analysis of cybersecurity attacks on cloud data warehouse-protected communication and threat intelligence related to e-healthcare. This research's main contribution will be the threat intelligence pertaining to e-healthcare, which ensures that e-healthcare organizations can be safeguarded against DoS and DDoS attacks on critical infrastructure and provides information about possible phony data injections. The paper is structured into introduction, background of the study, research contribution, theoretical framework, and proposed model, discussion of research findings, future research work and conclusion.

BACKGROUND OF THE STUDY

Cloud data warehouse systems enable healthcare providers to effectively manage the growing volume of digital health data while upholding security and legal compliances. This comprises medical images, test results, patient data, and electronic health records. Protecting sensitive patient medical data is a top priority for healthcare professionals. Healthcare data regulations like GDPR and HIPAA imposes legal duties on the healthcare administrators to safeguard patient data and notify patients of any breaches(Isibor, 2024). Due to the severe consequences for noncompliance, stringent data collecting, privacy protection, and cybersecurity enforcement are required to stop breaches. The privacy of health data is still a major problem in the digital age of the twenty-first century. This paper assesses the efficacy of HIPAA more precisely in a manner to adequately handle present-day cybersecurity risks, as provided by the general data protection regulation. This paper makes the case that the healthcare organizations around the world should take on the challenge of updating data privacy legislation to reflect the present-day cybersecurity globalization trend. In addition, this paper suggests that healthcare providers use the new methods to improve security and consistency in risk analysis. In light of the sharp increase in data breach events inside the healthcare system, revisions to healthcare laws are necessary to enact strict patient protections. In order to preserve the confidentiality, integrity, and security of electronically stored protected health information, healthcare administrators are required by the HIPAA Security Rule to employ the appropriate administrative, technical, and physical safeguards(Szalados, 2021). The enforcement of the privacy and security rules with DoS/DDoS cybersecurity attack defense mechanisms will be a major emphasis of this study.

RESEARCH CONTRIBUTION

This study implemented e-healthcare cloud data warehouse IoT federated learning system, built IDS system using Message Queuing Telemetry Transport (MQTT) broker to mitigate cybersecurity false data injection which prevented DoS and DDoS attack scenario. Understanding MQTT, blockchain, and federated learning, all of which were discussed in relation to the topic of cybersecurity in this study. Combining these technologies improved the security, scalability, and efficiency of cloud data warehouse IoT connectivity for security and privacy regulations in electronic healthcare systems.

THEORETICAL FRAMEWORK

Data and technology play a crucial role in the global health industry as health institutions deal with mounting pressure to provide innovative and seamless services that are accessible to every citizens(Pappas & Frisch, 2022). Digital technology has the potential to enhance public health and health financing, fortify health systems, and expand access to the marginalized communities(Forslund et al., 2024). It is anticipated that future healthcare will be data-connected and technology-integrated due to potentials available in artificial intelligence and data analytics(Ratta & Sharma, 2024). The infrastructure and resources required by healthcare businesses to create, implement, and oversee their own healthcare applications growth are made available by IoT cloud platforms(Onyebuchi, Matthew, Kazaure, Okafor, et al., 2022). Healthcare providers may now concentrate on innovation and application development rather than worrying about underlying infrastructure management provided by platform as service(PaaS) which provides them operational leverages(Matthew, Kazaure, & Okafor, 2021). Healthcare businesses can access virtualized computing resources, such as servers, storage, and networking capabilities, through cloud infrastructure delivery. Infrastructure as service (IaaS) enables healthcare organizations to manage growing workloads, quickly expand their communications, and allocate resources as efficiently as possible(Molo et al., 2021). The original purpose of PaaS was to facilitate code authoring by having the PaaS provider handle the operations and infrastructure. Alongside the initial public cloud platform for all PaaS, private and hybrid PaaS options administered by corporate IT departments were created because many firms opted not to have everything in the public cloud.

In PaaS, the client is given the ability to handle applications and data since the provider in public PaaS or the IT department in private PaaS control the runtime, middleware, operating system, virtualization, servers, storage, and networking(Mathur, 2024). PaaS comes in a variety of forms, including privately configured cloud delivery, hybrid, and public. Applications on public cloud services were the initial target of PaaS, but it later expanded to encompass private and hybrid solutions. Software as service (SaaS) is the root of public PaaS, which lies in the cloud computing space between SaaS and IaaS(Mathur, 2024). IaaS offers virtual hardware from a supplier with scalable virtualization options, in contrast to PaaS, where server maintenance is handled by the provider, IaaS requires the user to continue managing the server. Benefits from the cloud infrastructure strategy include increased scalability, reduced cost of ownership, and better flexibility of cyber threat intelligence. Cyber threat intelligence is an adaptable, dynamic system that blocks and neutralizes cyberattacks on the target network by gathering and analyzing data from threat histories(Lanza, Lahmadi, & François, 2024). The threat intelligence is not a hardware-dependent solution in itself, rather encompasses methods, strategies, and processes and is an essential part of a company's comprehensive security framework. A cybersecurity system relies on threat intelligence and analysis to make sure it detects as many attacks as possible since threats change and grow over time. Gaining understanding through threat intelligence enable the organization to stop or lessen network threats(Saeed, Suayyid, Al-Ghamdi, Al-Muhaisen, & Almuhaideb, 2023). Cyber intelligence and analysis have advantages that go beyond what the IT staff, analysts, and administrators can reap. A comprehensive and action-oriented cyber threat intelligence system can benefit the entire company business infrastructure(Möller, 2023). Cybersecurity system administrators can create the most effective plan to safeguard their network by using the insights that cyber threat intelligence offers.

Figure 2. Cloud Infrastructure delivery and IoT platform for e-healthcare (Gupta, 2023)

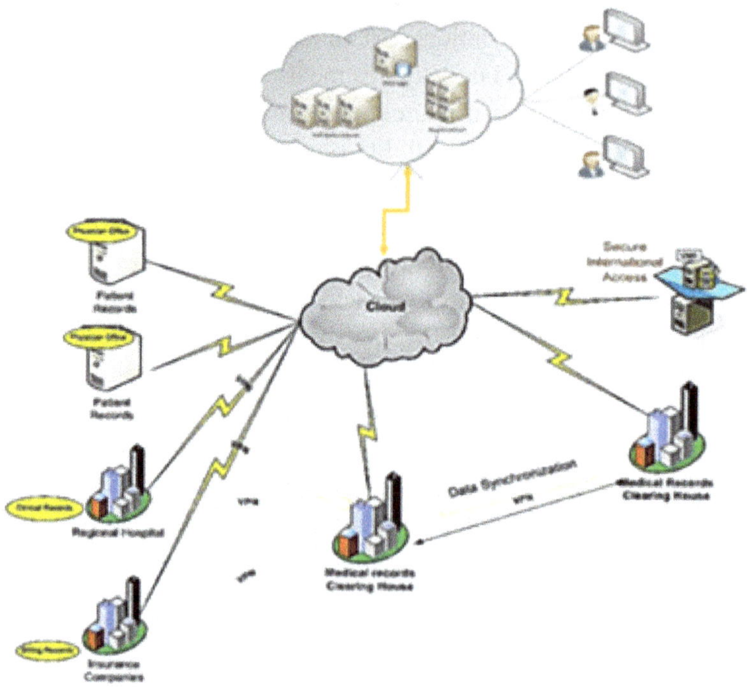

In Figure 2 above, the IoT cloud technology for e-healthcare used utility computing concepts to provide metrics for service improvement needed for the national health grid ecosystem implementation, thereby meeting the need for ubiquitous health data mining operation needed for citizen healthcare management. In order to ensure the sustainability of e-healthcare, cloud IoT computing has attempted to maintain the quality of service (QoS) and reliability issues of other grid computing models(Nair & Tyagi, 2023). The global market for IoT and cloud computing have expanded quickly over the years, analysts predict that this growth will continue, particularly for companies that deal with big data in e-healthcare and IoT-connected medical intelligence(Gandhi & Kumar, 2024). Adding real-time communications services voice, video, and messaging to applications without having to design back-end infrastructure and interfaces is made possible by communications platforms as a service (CPaaS), a cloud-based platform(Kelaidonis et al., 2017). SaaS systems are generally multi-tenant, while they normally achieve more efficiency by sharing some resources across clients, fully segregated environments are frequently made available for a premium(Rimal & Choi, 2012). IaaS is the most fundamental type of cloud computing, in which users lease infrastructure resources like physical computers from cloud providers rather than owning them. Utilizing the infrastructure, which consists of operating systems, applications and middleware are included in PaaS, however, applications from SaaS providers are usually run on PaaS or IaaS platforms(Malallah, Qashi, Abdulrahman, Omer, & Yazdeen, 2023). Making a SaaS solution scalable for a fluctuating number of users while maintaining the constant and instantaneous availability that users demand would be very challenging without IaaS. In a cloud computing setting, where resources are shared by numerous users, DoS and DDoS attack pose serious security challenges(Uddin, Kumar, & Chamola, 2024). The DoS/DoS aims to make resources or services inaccessible by overloading system channels with excessively high volumes of fictitious traffic. Attackers using DoS and DDoS aim to overload resources like memory, CPU processing power, or network bandwidth by obstructing network traffic or preventing users from accessing services(Al-Tamimi, Almoamari, Nehme, & Basurra, 2024). Since it can be challenging to differentiate between genuine user requests and DoS/DDoS attacks, even when the former originate from a large number of distant IoT workstations, dealing with DDoS attacks at all stages in cloud systems is a huge concern(Heidari & Jabraeil Jamali, 2023).

DOS AND DDOS ATTACKS ON CLOUD INFRASTRUCTURE

Healthcare providers place a high priority on the security and confidentiality of sensitive medical data along IaaS, PaaS and SaaS cloud system layers; yet, these platforms are vulnerable to DoS/DDoS attacks, which can originate from within the business organization ecosystem or from outside the organization business world(Sequeiros, Chimuco, Samaila, Freire, & Inácio, 2020). The availability of services are impacted by this kind of attack at the SaaS and PaaS levels, which are most vulnerable to external DDoS attacks(Shaar & Efe, 2018). A DoS attack is a type of cyberattack used in IoT cloud computing, such as distributed data warehouse infrastructure, where the attacker aims to prevent authorized users from accessing a machine or network resource by temporarily or permanently interrupting the host's functions(Snehi & Bhandari, 2021). Within the cloud system, mostly in the PaaS and IaaS tiers, an internal cloud-based DDoS attack might take many different forms. For instance, the trial periods of some providers' cloud services could be exploited by cybercriminals. Consequently, a DoS attack on the victim's internal computer can be initiated by an authorized user inside the cloud environment(Kumari & Jain, 2023). DDoS attacks can take many different forms(Nafea et al., 2024), notwithstanding healthcare organizations can use cloud computing to drive innovation, enhance patient care, and maximize operational efficiency if they plan ahead, implement strong security measures, and carefully choose their cloud service vendors(R. Ranjan & Ch, 2024). DDoS attacks are divided into two groups according to (Bala & Behal, 2024), which include flooding and logical or software attacks. According to (Shukla, Krishna, & Patil, 2024),SYN flooding, ICMP flooding, and User Datagram Protocol(UDP) flooding have been noted as examples of flooding attacks; ping of death, teardrop attack, and land attack have been described as logical attacks. A DDoS attack, sometimes referred to as a TCP SYN flood, is a sort of DoS attack in which a server is bombarded with an excessive amount of SYN requests in an attempt to overwhelm it with open connections(Aslam, Srivastava, & Gore, 2022). To effectively combat DDoS attacks, firewalls can be configured to reject internet protocols(IP) addresses, and router ports from initiating attacks (Saharan & Gupta, 2024). Several DoS/DDoS attacks on networks, such as the ping of death, SYN flood, ICMP/PING flood, and UDP flood, were described in the paper(Bindra & Sood, 2019). Similarly, (M. M. Aslam et al., 2022) established the circumstances in which attacks like jamming and kill command are considered DoS attacks. To thwart eavesdropping and jamming attempts,(Ahmad et al., 2024) proposed cycle duty spread spectrum, and priority message involving network collisions avoidance.

Figure 3. Synchronized DDoS attack on a cloud server infrastructure (Khairuddin, Isa, Shukran, Ismail, & Maskat, 2024)

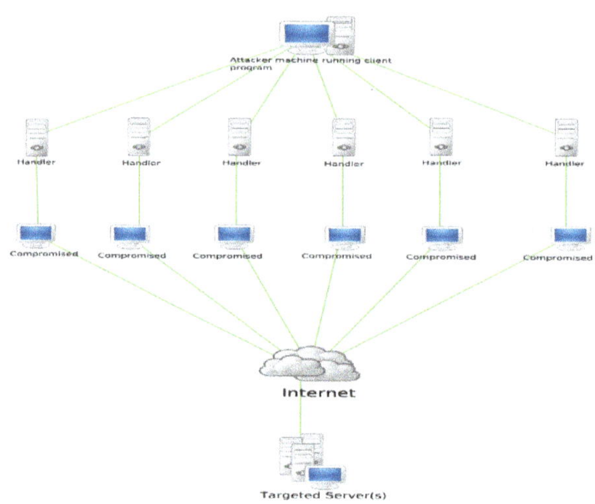

A number of DDoS defense strategies have been identified by(ul Sami, Ahmad, Asif, & Ullah, 2018), including implementation of IDS systems, filtering off attack packets, and single/multi-source attacks which is a mechanism that can change its defense in response to the intensity of the attack. The vector machine classifier can analyze any attack pattern on the application layer based on the entropy of each HTTP GET request made from the source IP address which is grounded in information theory and leverages user browsing behavior(Praseed & Thilagam, 2022), helping suspicious requests detection base on entropy. Attacks can take many different forms as they can involve sending millions of requests to a server in an attempt to slow it down, flooding it with a large volume of incorrect data, or sending requests from an unauthorized IP address(Shukla et al., 2024), **refer toFigure 3**. The incoming traffic flooding, the target in a DDoS attack comes from a variety of sources which require more advanced tactics to counter; trying to stop one source of the attack is not enough because there are several sources. A DoS/DDoS attack can be likened to a swarm of individuals barging through a store's front entrance, making it difficult for consumers to get in and disrupting business operations(Möller, 2023). DoS attack perpetrators frequently target websites or services, such credit card payment gateways or data warehouse repository, that are stockpiled on the well-known web servers. These attacks may be motivated by hacktivism, blackmail, or retaliation(Brooks, Yu, Ozcelik, Oakley, & Tusing, 2021). Proposing countermeasures depends on the degree of congestion which requires security protocols in collaborative environments(Rai, Badrinath, Kamath, Kumar, & Gatti, 2024). However, some researchers have also experimented with blockchain, federated learning, and machine learning techniques to understand the various models for DoS/DDoS attack detection. This suggests that several coordinated efforts are required to safeguard cloud data warehouse IoT networked resources against these attacks, and that traditional network analysis approaches alone are insufficient(Jamil, Schelén, Monrat, & Andersson, 2024).

FEDERATED LEARNING METHOD BASED ON BLOCKCHAIN

Federated learning is a new distributed AI technique that allows machine learning models to be trained collaboratively without exchanging patient data(Sheller et al., 2020). A real-time distributed networking system based on the MQTT protocol is proposed in this research, which also delves into the examination of several federated learning techniques. Federated learning aims to solve the privacy and data governance issues by allowing algorithms to be trained jointly without sharing the actual data(Bharati, Mondal, Podder, & Prasath, 2022). Concerns about patient privacy and data security are seriously jeopardized by the common practice of centralizing data from many institutions. The technology that can train machine learning models at scale across several medical institutions without transferring the data is essential to resolving this issue. IoT-derived sensitive data, such as patient health records and sensitive financial information, is used by federated learning to train and evaluate machine learning models(Rauniyar et al., 2023). Federated learning is therefore the path to developing learning models while protecting privacy. In conventionally federated learning, mobile devices use on-device data samples to calculate their local model update, which they then transmit to a central server. The global model is updated by the central server, which compiles the local model updates from various devices. Mobile devices retrieve the most recent global model in order to calculate their subsequent local model revision. Until the central server reaches the required precision, the cycle keeps going. The disadvantage of this strategy is its whole reliance on the dependability of a central server for global model update computation and storage. Malicious activity results in a faulty global model update, which affects the precision of later local model updates and makes the federated learning process as a whole incorrect. In an unsecured setting, it is a good way to replace the central server that is vulnerable to attacks. Blockchain technology can be used with federated learning to lessen the security risks associated with a central server information data warehousing(Ali, Li, & Yousafzai, 2024). Information security and privacy can be maintained by the adaptation of blockchain technology between the client and server nodes. Blockchain provides decentralization, incentive mechanisms, and cyberattack resistance, while federated learning enables the collaborative integration of data aggregation and machine learning models in a remote environment(Ali et al., 2024). Federated learning provided by blockchain speeds up member verification and selection. Cognitive computing may improve accuracy, resistance to data injection cyberattacks, and incentive systems for the healthcare sector by incorporating blockchain into federated learning(Khan et al., 2024).

Figure 4. Blockchain-based network federated learning system (Majeed & Hong, 2019)

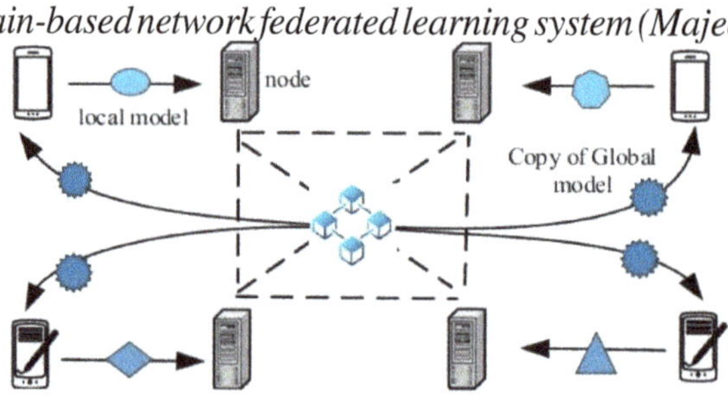

By offering an incredibly feasible plan for the training of reliable decentralized learning models, the combination of blockchain and federated learning guarantees the privacy of user data(Jiang et al., 2024). The parameters of the trained model can be safely and irrevocably stored on the blockchain, offering impenetrable defense against malevolent activity and unwanted access. To assure the security of the sharing process, (Lu, Huang, Dai, Maharjan, & Zhang, 2020) proposed a safe data sharing architecture that has been validated by the blockchain. This design distributes and maintains the federated learning model and parameter transfer process on the blockchain. A multi-weight subjective logic model was used to create an effective reputation computation technique based on the interaction history of task publishers and proposed reputation records. A blockchain-based federated learning approach was proposed by(Kim, Park, Bennis, & Kim, 2019), for the device verification and consensus, the local gradients of each iteration are recorded in blocks, and the end-to-end latency and optimal block production rate are examined. In order to select nodes, integrate the learned model into the blockchain, and carry out two-stage validation, (Lu, Huang, Zhang, Maharjan, & Zhang, 2020) introduced a hybrid blockchain architecture-based federated learning model that consists of a permissioned blockchain and a local directed acyclic graph. In addition to maintaining the security and reliability of the blockchain, (Lu, Huang, Zhang, et al., 2020) combined blockchain with federated learning to give the system the optimal decision-making power of artificial intelligence, enabling blockchain's efficiency and communication to improve its functionality.

PROPOSED FRAMEWORK

In order to analyze the attack pattern, the current paper proposed a method comparable to the time-to-live (TTL) value of the arriving packet and the packet buffer utilization rate of the server with predefined values. These packets may be the result of botnet activity or subnets employing different DoS/DDoS attack methods. Within the digital ecosystem, the IoT network of physical objects, including e-healthcare data warehouse system, cars, buildings, and other items that are all assigned unique identifiers that enable them to communicate with one another without the need for human intervention, permit communication and exchange messages through popular machine-to-machine connection MQTT protocol. When using a MQTT setup, clients publish messages, which are then parsed by the BIG-IP system. BIG-IP is a group of software and hardware platforms that offer services with an emphasis on security, dependability, and performance, operating in virtualized environments and have hardware implementation functionality on public clouds and other managed infrastructures where rack space is a vital resource(Mukhopadhyay, Bose, & Roy, 2020). The BIG-IP system's ability to route various protocol and application traffic types to the right target server is one of its main uses. This is made possible by the system's Local Traffic Manager(LTM) module, which has the ability to transmit traffic either directly to a pool of load balancing servers, or to a next-hop router, a pool of routers, or a specific network node(Mukhopadhyay et al., 2020). Important features including implementing security policies to network traffic, quickening

HTTP connections, and enhancing connections throughout a wide-area network are offered by additional modules on the BIG-IP system. Based on the parsed messages, the BIG-IP system triggers any defined MQTT-specific iRule events and loads the MQTT messages to a pool of message brokers based on connection. Message brokers then forward and carry the messages to servers that have subscribed. When clients publish messages to a MQTT configuration, the BIG-IP system analyzes those messages, triggers any defined MQTT-specific iRule events, and loads balances the MQTT messages to a pool of message brokers based on connectivity. Sending the messages to servers that have subscribed is done by the message brokers.

Figure 5. MQTT federated learning architecture based on blockchain for cloud IoT data warehouse

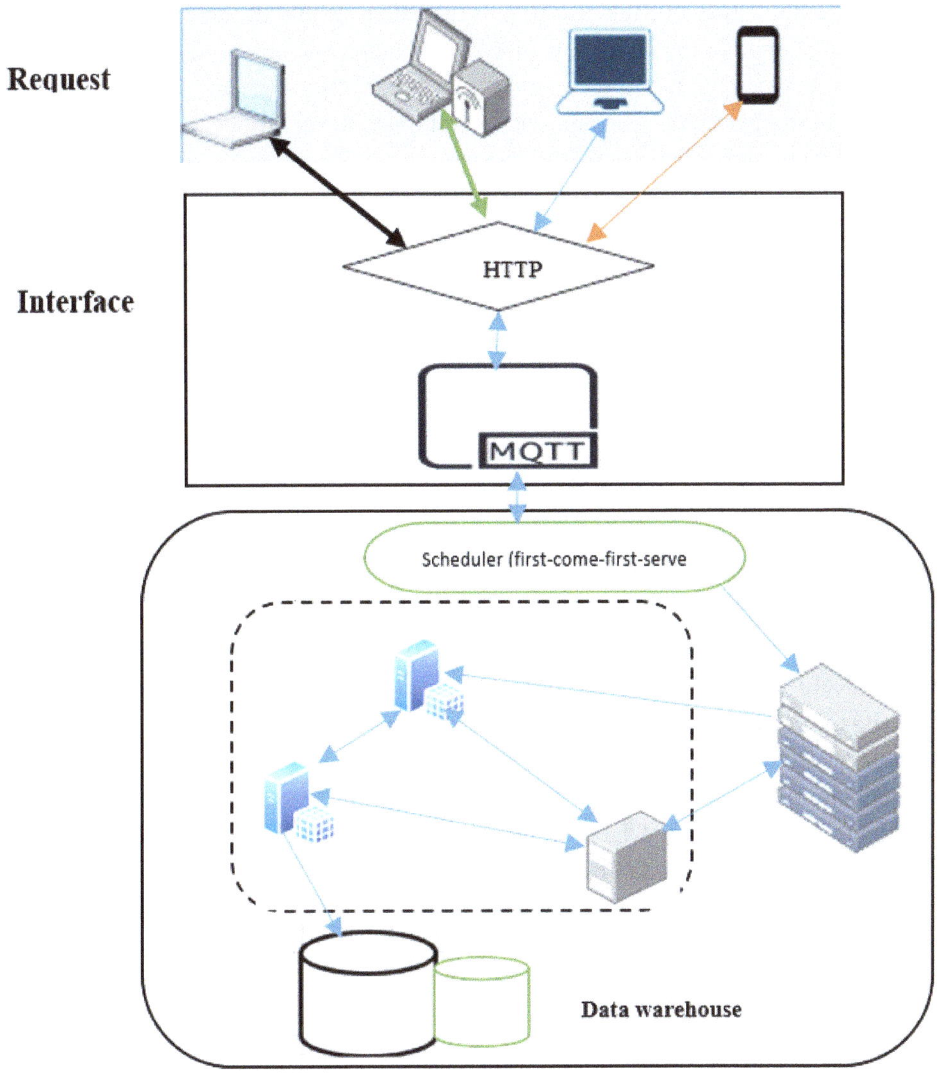

The main system design of the MQTT federated learning blockchain IoT framework was mostly made up of numerous pieces that were combined in a coordinated method, as illustrated in Figure 4. The cloud cluster program in charge of sensing device response is first installed on the IoT node and updated as needed(Mavromatis et al., 2019). In order to conduct scenario analysis, data is gathered from an IoT node by a MQTT broker and sent to the computing platform. A MQTT broker uses the publish/subscribe method to operate multiple subscribers, each of whom is subscribed to a particular topic, and forwards the data as it is received. Thirdly, the cloud platform employed in this study coupled the MQTT and the intrusion detection system that notifies security mechanism protocols. The whole thing is comprised of an IoT cloud with several MQTT clients and nodes, as Figure 5 shows. Any customer can send and receive data by logging into the IoT cloud platform. MQTT and the federated learning data warehouse server comprise the bulk of the IoT cloud node. Apart from rapid data transport, the MQTT component is a protocol subscriber and broker that allows several activities after obtaining the data. This study uses federated learning supervision to provide specific data to a verifiable receiver in service compliance with HIPAA regulation, following data collection from a component for reliable data transfer and storage.

On account that BIG-IP natively supports the MQTT protocol and offers industry-leading secure sockets layer (SSL) speed and visibility for both incoming and outbound traffic, offering opportunity to encrypt everything from the client to the server to affordably safeguard the whole user experience. Additionally, it guards against DoS and DDoS attacks that could be fatal and offers internet content adaptation protocol (ICAP) services for integration with virus and data loss prevention(N. Agrawal & Tapaswi, 2019). An extensible transparent proxy server is made possible by the ICAP, a lightweight request-response protocol similar to HTTP(Pathan & Buyya, 2007). In addition to standardizing the implementation of new features, this frees up resources. BIG-IP is an originator and endpoint of the MQTT protocol due to its comprehensive proxy design. Using their in-depth knowledge of the protocol, iRules are able to intelligently parse the MQTT protocol and decide on traffic at various events (certain points in a network connection's session flow, like MQTT_CLIENT_INGRESS and MQTT_SERVER_INGRESS). Utilizing software-defined networking (SDN), cloud computing, and mobility, the information bellow provides examples of common BIG-IP MQTT configuration applications that drive innovation and profitability for corporate businesses(Shafiq, Rahman, Shaon, Mahmud, & Hosen, 2024).

DISCUSSION OF RESEARCH FINDINGS

MQTT uses a publish-subscribe approach in which clients connect with brokers in the capacity of publishers or subscribers. By delivering messages from publishers to interested subscribers who have registered for particular topics, the broker oversees topics and subscriptions. Through the MQTT protocol, BIG-IP LTM facilitates the support of IoT clients by publishing helpful data to MQTT Brokers (servers). Following that, information is sent by the MQTT brokers to each and every subscriber base on blockchain paradigm. BIG-IP LTM is able to use MQTT traffic load balancing for its IoT clients thanks to MQTT support. Encrypting everything from the client to the server allows you to reasonably safeguard the whole user experience. BIG-IP LTM provides industry-leading SSL performance and visibility for both inbound and outgoing traffic. Operating at the application layer via transmission control protocol (TCP) or other specialized circumstances like user datagram protocol (UDP), MQTT is a messaging protocol designed for devices with limited resources. It serves as a substitute for HTTP in low-bandwidth settings in IoT networks. Together with offering ICAP services for integration with virus and data loss protection, it also fights against potentially devastating DoS/DDoS attacks. To generate system model based BIG-IP system operation, the paper adopted use case to stop MQTT DoS/DDoS attacks:

Model #1: Preventing MQTT DoS and DDoS attacks based on blockchain federated learning subject, the application delivery components in the BIG-IP system provide enhanced performance, security, high availability, and access management preventing DoS/DDoS intrusion. Supervising the publishing message's subject, and if it doesn't meet the validation requirements, terminate the connection. By doing this, messages with false subject won't be delivered to the message brokers, which aid in stopping subject-based MQTT DoS/DDoS assaults.

Model #2: Blockchain federated learning MQTT publish message length validation along BIG-IP supervisory mechanism. The amount of data being transferred is usually known to application parties. A publishing message's duration can be confirmed using such information; if it turns out to be shorter than expected, the connection should be closed. By doing this, message brokers will not be overloaded with large communications that fail to get through.

Model#3: Load balancing and pool selection using usernames as unique identifiers where BIG-IP system approved computing clients based on blockchain federated learning modality. Utilizing the username as a distinctive means of directing traffic towards a message broker and assigning a device or end user to a load balancer pool, this allows stickiness between an end user and a message broker. When a device has to reconnect to the message broker that is hosting the active client session, the mapping comes in handy since it allows the device to leverage the message broker's status information to influence decisions.

Model#4: Client certificate authentication over transport layer security (TLS) based on blockchain federated learning. After BIG-IP terminates SSL/TLS encrypted MQTT messages, the unencrypted traffic can be sent to the backend broker. For the reason that all SSL/TLS functionality and settings can be offloaded to the BIG-IP, this enables the broker to scale. The BIG-IP can use iRules to carry out Client Certificate Authentication in addition to ending SSL/TLS. In order to facilitate back-end Broker authentication, the BIG-IP can incorporate the username and the client's name from the client certificate into the backend connection.

FUTURE RESEARCH FOCUS

Information security and privacy can be maintained by the adaptation of blockchain technology between the client and server nodes. Blockchain provides decentralization, incentive mechanisms, and cyberattack resistance, while federated learning enables the collaborative integration of data aggregation and machine learning models in a remote environment. Federated learning provided by blockchain speeds up member verification and selection. Cognitive computing may improve accuracy, resistance to data injection cyberattacks, and incentive systems for the healthcare sector by incorporating blockchain into federated learning. Future research should incorporate blockchain technology and machine learning to improve the system's resistance to DoS and DDoS attacks and experiment with any limitation of the implementation. The system's daily record will be used to train the current model, which will allow for the prompt observation of attack behavior and the efficient application of adaptive defense mechanisms based on training instances and report every shortcoming.

CONCLUSION

A paradigm shift in the healthcare sector has been brought about by the incorporation of cloud computing, which has opened up new opportunities for better patient care, operational effectiveness, and data management. Healthcare companies may provide more patient-centered, accessible, and collaborative services as they take advantage of cloud computing. Organizations can collaborate with cloud service providers, IT outsourcing firms that specialize in offering specialized cloud computing solutions for the healthcare sector, to fully utilize the potential of cloud computing in the healthcare sector. A pivotal data warehouse federation will arise from embracing the transformative potential of cloud computing and setting off on a path towards a more effective, safe, and patient-centered healthcare ecosystem. The strategy put out in the current research concentrated on improving the server's capacity to recognize attack patterns and implement proactive defenses against DoS/DDoS intrusions. In order to reduce cybersecurity fake data injections and prevent DoS and DDoS scenario activities, the study established an IoT federated learning architecture for e-healthcare cloud data warehouses and built an intrusion detection system utilizing MQTT brokers. With our suggested method, attack packets can be quickly recognized and dropped before the attack reaches its peak point, and intrusions can be distinguished by their pre-calculated TTL values.

REFERENCES

Agrawal, N., & Tapaswi, S. (2019). Defense mechanisms against DDoS attacks in a cloud computing environment: State-of-the-art and research challenges. *IEEE Communications Surveys and Tutorials*, 21(4), 3769–3795. DOI: 10.1109/COMST.2019.2934468

Agrawal, S., Sarkar, S., Aouedi, O., Yenduri, G., Piamrat, K., Alazab, M., Bhattacharya, S., Maddikunta, P. K. R., & Gadekallu, T. R. (2022). Federated learning for intrusion detection system: Concepts, challenges and future directions. *Computer Communications*, 195, 346–361. DOI: 10.1016/j.comcom.2022.09.012

Ahmad, I., Rodriguez, F., Kumar, T., Suomalainen, J., Jagatheesaperumal, S. K., Walter, S., . . . Ylianttila, M. (2024). Communications security in Industry X: A survey. *IEEE Open Journal of the Communications Society.*

Al-Tamimi, B. N., Almoamari, H., Nehme, A., & Basurra, S. (2024). *Cybersecurity Challenges and Implications for the Adoption of Cloud Computing and IoT: DDoS Attacks as an Example Decision Making and Security Risk Management for IoT Environments*. Springer.

Ali, S., Li, Q., & Yousafzai, A. (2024). Blockchain and federated learning-based intrusion detection approaches for edge-enabled industrial IoT networks: A survey. *Ad Hoc Networks*, 152, 103320. DOI: 10.1016/j.adhoc.2023.103320

Aminizadeh, S., Heidari, A., Dehghan, M., Toumaj, S., Rezaei, M., Navimipour, N. J., & Unal, M. (2024). Opportunities and challenges of artificial intelligence and distributed systems to improve the quality of healthcare service. *Artificial Intelligence in Medicine*, 149, 102779. DOI: 10.1016/j.artmed.2024.102779 PMID: 38462281

Aslam, M. M., Ahmed, Z., Du, L., Hassan, M. Z., Ali, S., & Nasir, M. (2022). An Overview of Recent Advances of Resilient Consensus for Multiagent Systems under Attacks. *Computational Intelligence and Neuroscience*, 2022(1), 6732343. DOI: 10.1155/2022/6732343 PMID: 39411550

Aslam, N., Srivastava, S., & Gore, M. (2022). ONOS flood defender: An intelligent approach to mitigate DDoS attack in SDN. *Transactions on Emerging Telecommunications Technologies*, 33(9), e4534. DOI: 10.1002/ett.4534

Bala, B., & Behal, S. (2024). AI techniques for IoT-based DDoS attack detection: Taxonomies, comprehensive review and research challenges. *Computer Science Review*, 52, 100631. DOI: 10.1016/j.cosrev.2024.100631

Bharati, S., Mondal, M., Podder, P., & Prasath, V. (2022). Federated learning: Applications, challenges and future directions. *International Journal of Hybrid Intelligent Systems*, 18(1-2), 19–35. DOI: 10.3233/HIS-220006

Bindra, N., & Sood, M. (2019). Detecting DDoS attacks using machine learning techniques and contemporary intrusion detection dataset. *Automatic Control and Computer Sciences*, 53(5), 419–428. DOI: 10.3103/S0146411619050043

Brooks, R. R., Yu, L., Ozcelik, I., Oakley, J., & Tusing, N. (2021). Distributed denial of service (DDoS): A history. *IEEE Annals of the History of Computing*, 44(2), 44–54. DOI: 10.1109/MAHC.2021.3072582

Dang, L. M., Piran, M. J., Han, D., Min, K., & Moon, H. (2019). A survey on internet of things and cloud computing for healthcare. *Electronics (Basel)*, 8(7), 768. DOI: 10.3390/electronics8070768

Dhatterwal, J. S., Kaswan, K. S., Baliyan, A., & Jain, V. (2022). *Integration of cloud and IoT for smart e-healthcare Connected e-health: Integrated IoT and cloud computing*. Springer.

Ebong, G. N., Matthew, U. O., Olofin, B., Andrew-Vitalis, N., Fatai, L. O., Waliu, A. O., & Oladipupo, M. A. (2024). *Multimedia Cloud Data Warehouse Design for Knowledge Sharing in the University Environment: A Proposed Digital Solution Implementing Interactive Learning Strategies in Higher Education*. IGI Global. DOI: 10.4018/979-8-3693-3559-8.ch010

Falayi, A., Wang, Q., Liao, W., & Yu, W. (2023). Survey of distributed and decentralized IoT securities: Approaches using deep learning and blockchain technology. *Future Internet*, 15(5), 178. DOI: 10.3390/fi15050178

Forslund, M., Mathieson, K., Djibo, Y., Mbindyo, C., Lugangira, N., & Balasubramaniam, P. (2024). Strengthening the evidence base on the use of digital health technologies to accelerate progress towards universal health coverage. *Oxford Open Digital Health*, 2, oqae033. DOI: 10.1093/oodh/oqae033

Gandhi, P., & Kumar, R. (2024). Artificial Intelligence of Things (AIoT) for Intelligent Data Design. *Reshaping Intelligent Business and Industry: Convergence of AI and IoT at the Cutting Edge*, 507-517.

Guduri, M., Chakraborty, C., Maheswari, U., & Margala, M. (2023). Blockchain-based federated learning technique for privacy preservation and security of smart electronic health records. *IEEE Transactions on Consumer Electronics*, 70(1), 2608–2617. DOI: 10.1109/TCE.2023.3315415

Gupta, M. (2023). *A novel scheme to manage the e-healthcare system using cloud computing and the internet of things Computational Intelligence in Healthcare*. CRC Press.

Heidari, A., & Jabraeil Jamali, M. A. (2023). Internet of Things intrusion detection systems: A comprehensive review and future directions. *Cluster Computing*, 26(6), 3753–3780. DOI: 10.1007/s10586-022-03776-z

Isibor, E. (2024). Regulation of Healthcare Data Security: Legal Obligations in A Digital Age. *Available atSSRN* 4957244. DOI: 10.2139/ssrn.4957244

Jamil, M. N., Schelén, O., Monrat, A. A., & Andersson, K. (2024). Enabling Industrial Internet of Things by Leveraging Distributed Edge-to-Cloud Computing: Challenges and Opportunities. *IEEE Access : Practical Innovations, Open Solutions*, 12, 127294–127308. DOI: 10.1109/ACCESS.2024.3454812

Javaid, H. A. (2024). Improving Fraud Detection and Risk Assessment in Financial Service using Predictive Analytics and Data Mining. *Integrated Journal of Science and Technology, 1*(8).

Jiang, Y., Ma, B., Wang, X., Yu, G., Yu, P., Wang, Z., Ni, W., & Liu, R. P. (2024). Blockchained federated learning for internet of things: A comprehensive survey. *ACM Computing Surveys*, 56(10), 1–37. DOI: 10.1145/3659099

Kelaidonis, D., Vlacheas, P., Stavroulaki, V., Georgoulas, S., Moessner, K., Hashi, Y., . . . Demestichas, P. (2017). Cloud internet of things framework for enabling services in smart cities. *Designing, Developing, and Facilitating Smart Cities: Urban Design to IoT Solutions*, 163-191.

Khairuddin, M. A., Isa, M. R. M., Shukran, M. A. M., Ismail, M. N., & Maskat, K. (2024). Detecting Distributed Denial-of-Service (DDoS) Attacks Through the Log Consolidation Processing (LCP) Framework. *JOIV: International Journal on Informatics Visualization*, 8(3), 1064. DOI: 10.62527/joiv.8.3.2184

Khan, I. A., Razzak, I., Pi, D., Khan, N., Hussain, Y., Li, B., & Kousar, T. (2024). Fed-inforce-fusion: A federated reinforcement-based fusion model for security and privacy protection of IoMT networks against cyber-attacks. *Information Fusion*, 101, 102002. DOI: 10.1016/j.inffus.2023.102002

Kharche, A., Badholia, S., & Upadhyay, R. K. (2024). Implementation of blockchain technology in integrated IoT networks for constructing scalable ITS systems in India. *Blockchain: Research and Applications*, 100188.

Kim, H., Park, J., Bennis, M., & Kim, S.-L. (2019). Blockchained on-device federated learning. *IEEE Communications Letters*, 24(6), 1279–1283. DOI: 10.1109/LCOMM.2019.2921755

Knosp, B. M., Craven, C. K., Dorr, D. A., Bernstam, E. V., & Campion, T. R.Jr. (2022). Understanding enterprise data warehouses to support clinical and translational research: Enterprise information technology relationships, data governance, workforce, and cloud computing. *Journal of the American Medical Informatics Association : JAMIA*, 29(4), 671–676. DOI: 10.1093/jamia/ocab256 PMID: 35289370

Kumari, P., & Jain, A. K. (2023). A comprehensive study of DDoS attacks over IoT network and their countermeasures. *Computers & Security*, 127, 103096. DOI: 10.1016/j.cose.2023.103096

Lanza, C., Lahmadi, A., & François, J. (2024). *Ransomware Analysis: Knowledge Extraction and Classification for Advanced Cyber Threat Intelligence*. CRC Press. DOI: 10.1201/9781003528999

Li, W., Tan, J., & Wang, Y. (2020). *A framework of blockchain-based collaborative intrusion detection in software defined networking*. Paper presented at the Network and System Security: 14th International Conference, NSS 2020, Melbourne, VIC, Australia, November 25–27, 2020, Proceedings 14. DOI: 10.1007/978-3-030-65745-1_15

Li, X., Hu, Y., Zeng, L., An, Y., Yang, J., & Xiao, X. (2024). Blockchain-based federated learning approaches in internet of things applications. *Security and Privacy*, 7(6), 435. DOI: 10.1002/spy2.435

Lu, Y., Huang, X., Dai, Y., Maharjan, S., & Zhang, Y. (2020). Federated learning for data privacy preservation in vehicular cyber-physical systems. *IEEE Network*, 34(3), 50–56. DOI: 10.1109/MNET.011.1900317

Lu, Y., Huang, X., Zhang, K., Maharjan, S., & Zhang, Y. (2020). Blockchain empowered asynchronous federated learning for secure data sharing in internet of vehicles. *IEEE Transactions on Vehicular Technology*, 69(4), 4298–4311. DOI: 10.1109/TVT.2020.2973651

Majeed, U., & Hong, C. S. (2019). *FLchain: Federated learning via MEC-enabled blockchain network*. Paper presented at the 2019 20th Asia-Pacific Network Operations and Management Symposium (APNOMS).

Malallah, H. S., Qashi, R., Abdulrahman, L. M., Omer, M. A., & Yazdeen, A. A. (2023). Performance analysis of enterprise cloud computing: a review. *Journal of Applied Science and Technology Trends, 4*(01), 01-12.

Mallick, M. A. I., & Nath, R. (2024). Navigating the Cyber security Landscape: A Comprehensive Review of Cyber-Attacks, Emerging Trends, and Recent Developments. *World Scientific News*, 190(1), 1–69.

Mandarino, V., Pappalardo, G., & Tramontana, E. (2024). A Blockchain-Based Electronic Health Record (EHR) System for Edge Computing Enhancing Security and Cost Efficiency. *Computers*, 13(6), 132. DOI: 10.3390/computers13060132

Mathur, P. (2024). Cloud computing infrastructure, platforms, and software for scientific research. *High Performance Computing in Biomimetics: Modeling, Architecture and Applications*, 89-127.

Matthew, U. O., Asuni, O., & Fatai, L. O. (2024). *Green Software Engineering Development Paradigm: An Approach to a Sustainable Renewable Energy Future Advancing Software Engineering Through AI, Federated Learning, and Large Language Models*. IGI Global. DOI: 10.4018/979-8-3693-3502-4.ch018

Matthew, U. O., Kazaure, J. S., Amaonwu, O., Adamu, U. A., Hassan, I. M., Kazaure, A. A., & Ubochi, C. N. (2021). *Role of internet of health things (IoHTs) and innovative internet of 5G medical robotic things (IIo-5GMRTs) in COVID-19 global health risk management and logistics planning Intelligent Data Analysis for COVID-19 Pandemic*. Springer.

Matthew, U. O., Kazaure, J. S., & Okafor, N. U. (2021). Contemporary development in E-Learning education, cloud computing technology & internet of things. *EAI Endorsed Transactions on Cloud Systems*, 7(20), e3–e3.

Matthew, U. O., Onumaku, V. C., Fatai, L. O., Adekunle, T. S., Waliu, A. O., Ndukwu, C. C., & Ebong, G. N. (2024). *E-Healthcare Data Warehouse Design and Data Mining Using ML Approach Reshaping Healthcare with Cutting-Edge Biomedical Advancements*. IGI Global.

Mavromatis, A., Colman-Meixner, C., Silva, A. P., Vasilakos, X., Nejabati, R., & Simeonidou, D. (2019). A software-defined IoT device management framework for edge and cloud computing. *IEEE Internet of Things Journal*, 7(3), 1718–1735. DOI: 10.1109/JIOT.2019.2949629

Möller, D. P. (2023). *Threats and threat intelligence Guide to Cybersecurity in Digital Transformation: Trends, Methods, Technologies, Applications and Best Practices*. Springer.

Molo, M. J., Badejo, J. A., Adetiba, E., Nzanzu, V. P., Noma-Osaghae, E., Oguntosin, V., Baraka, M. O., Takenga, C., Suraju, S., & Adebiyi, E. F. (2021). A Review of Evolutionary Trends in Cloud Computing and Applications to the Healthcare Ecosystem. *Applied Computational Intelligence and Soft Computing*, 2021(1), 1843671. DOI: 10.1155/2021/1843671

Mukhopadhyay, B., Bose, R., & Roy, S. (2020). A novel approach to load balancing and cloud computing security using SSL in IaaS environment. *International Journal (Toronto, Ont.)*, 9(2).

Nadella, G. S., Meduri, K., Gonaygunta, H., Addula, S. R., Satish, S., Harish, M., & Maturi, S. (2024). Advancing Edge Computing with Federated Deep Learning: Strategies and Challenges. *International Journal for Research in Applied Science and Engineering Technology*, 12(4), 3422–3434. DOI: 10.22214/ijraset.2024.60602

Nafea, A. A., Hamdi, M. M., saad Abdulhakeem, B., Shakir, A. T., Alsumaidaie, M. S. I., & Shaban, A. M. 2024, April. Detection Systems for Distributed Denial-of-Service DDoS Attack Based on Time Series: Review, A. In 2024 21st International Multi-Conference on Systems, Signals & Devices (SSD) (pp. 43-48). IEEE.

Nair, M. M., & Tyagi, A. K. (2023). *AI, IoT, blockchain, and cloud computing: The necessity of the future Distributed Computing to Blockchain*. Elsevier.

Nwanakwaugwu, A. C., Matthew, U. O., Kazaure, A. A., & Haruna, K. (2023). *Data Mining Business Intelligence Applications in Retail Services Using Artificial Neural Networks Handbook of Research on Cybersecurity Risk in Contemporary Business Systems*. IGI Global.

Onyebuchi, A., Matthew, U. O., Kazaure, J. S., Ebong, G. N., Ndukwu, C. C., Nwanakwaugwu, A. C., & Okey, O. D. (2024). *Cloud-Based IoT Data Warehousing Technology for E-Healthcare: A Comprehensive Guide to E-Health Grids Pioneering Smart Healthcare 5.0 with IoT, Federated Learning, and Cloud Security*. IGI Global.

Onyebuchi, A., Matthew, U. O., Kazaure, J. S., Nwanagwaugwu, A. C., Nwamouh, U. C., & Adamu, U. A. (2022). Cloud based IoT Electronic Healthcare Data Warehouse Integration in emerging 5G Health Grid Ecosystem.

Onyebuchi, A., Matthew, U. O., Kazaure, J. S., Okafor, N. U., Okey, O. D., Okochi, P. I., Taiwo, J. F., & Matthew, A. O. (2022). Business demand for a cloud enterprise data warehouse in electronic healthcare computing: Issues and developments in e-healthcare cloud computing. [IJCAC]. *International Journal of Cloud Applications and Computing*, 12(1), 1–22. DOI: 10.4018/IJCAC.297098

Padmaja, K., & Seshadri, R. (2021). A real-time secure medical device authentication for personal E-Healthcare services on cloud computing. *International Journal of System Assurance Engineering and Management*, •••, 1–11. DOI: 10.1007/s13198-021-01148-1

Pappas, H., & Frisch, P. (2022). *Leveraging technology as a response to the COVID pandemic: Adapting diverse technologies, workflow, and processes to optimize integrated clinical management*. CRC Press.

Pathan, A.-M. K., & Buyya, R. (2007). A taxonomy and survey of content delivery networks. *Grid computing and distributed systems laboratory, University of Melbourne. Technical Report*, 4, 70.

Praseed, A., & Thilagam, P. S. (2022). HTTP request pattern based signatures for early application layer DDoS detection: A firewall agnostic approach. *Journal of Information Security and Applications*, 65, 103090. DOI: 10.1016/j.jisa.2021.103090

Rahnasto, J. (2023). Genetic data are not always personal—Disaggregating the identifiability and sensitivity of genetic data. *Journal of Law and the Biosciences*, 10(2), lsad029. DOI: 10.1093/jlb/lsad029 PMID: 38023689

Rai, N., Badrinath, A., Kamath, A., Kumar, V. A., & Gatti, R. R. (2024). *Security Challenges of IoT-Enabled Vehicular Communications and Their Countermeasures Communication Technologies and Security Challenges in IoT: Present and Future*. Springer.

Ranjan, J., & Foropon, C. (2021). Big data analytics in building the competitive intelligence of organizations. *International Journal of Information Management*, 56, 102231. DOI: 10.1016/j.ijinfomgt.2020.102231

Ranjan, R., & Ch, B. (2024). A comprehensive roadmap for transforming healthcare from hospital-centric to patient-centric through healthcare internet of things (IoT). *Engineering and Science*, 30, 1175. DOI: 10.30919/es1175

Ratta, P., & Sharma, S. (2024). A blockchain-machine learning ecosystem for IoT-Based remote health monitoring of diabetic patients. *Healthcare Analytics*, 5, 100338. DOI: 10.1016/j.health.2024.100338

Rauniyar, A., Hagos, D. H., Jha, D., Håkegård, J. E., Bagci, U., Rawat, D. B., & Vlassov, V. (2023). Federated learning for medical applications: A taxonomy, current trends, challenges, and future research directions. *IEEE Internet of Things Journal*.

Rimal, B. P., & Choi, E. (2012). A service-oriented taxonomical spectrum, cloudy challenges and opportunities of cloud computing. *International Journal of Communication Systems*, 25(6), 796–819. DOI: 10.1002/dac.1279

Saeed, S., Suayyid, S. A., Al-Ghamdi, M. S., Al-Muhaisen, H., & Almuhaideb, A. M. (2023). A systematic literature review on cyber threat intelligence for organizational cybersecurity resilience. *Sensors (Basel)*, 23(16), 7273. DOI: 10.3390/s23167273 PMID: 37631808

Saharan, S., & Gupta, V. (2024). Prevention of DDoS attacks: a comprehensive review and future directions. *Information Security Journal: A Global Perspective*, 1-33.

Sahu, M., Gupta, R., Ambasta, R. K., & Kumar, P. (2022). Artificial intelligence and machine learning in precision medicine: A paradigm shift in big data analysis. *Progress in Molecular Biology and Translational Science*, 190(1), 57–100. DOI: 10.1016/bs.pmbts.2022.03.002 PMID: 36008002

Sari, A., & Sopuru, J. (2021). E-Health Threat Intelligence Within Cyber-Defence Framework for E-Health Organizations. *Smart Systems for E-Health: WBAN Technologies, Security and Applications*, 161-179.

Sequeiros, J. B., Chimuco, F. T., Samaila, M. G., Freire, M. M., & Inácio, P. R. (2020). Attack and system modeling applied to IoT, cloud, and mobile ecosystems: Embedding security by design. *ACM Computing Surveys*, 53(2), 1–32. DOI: 10.1145/3376123

Shaar, F., & Efe, A. (2018). DDoS attacks and impacts on various cloud computing components. *International Journal of Information Security Science*, 7(1), 26–48.

Shafiq, S., Rahman, M. S., Shaon, S. A., Mahmud, I., & Hosen, A. S. (2024). A Review on Software-Defined Networking for Internet of Things Inclusive of Distributed Computing, Blockchain, and Mobile Network Technology: Basics, Trends, Challenges, and Future Research Potentials. *International Journal of Distributed Sensor Networks*, 2024(1), 9006405. DOI: 10.1155/2024/9006405

Sheller, M. J., Edwards, B., Reina, G. A., Martin, J., Pati, S., Kotrotsou, A., & Colen, R. R. (2020). Federated learning in medicine: Facilitating multi-institutional collaborations without sharing patient data. *Scientific Reports*, 10(1), 12598. DOI: 10.1038/s41598-020-69250-1 PMID: 32724046

Shukla, P., Krishna, C. R., & Patil, N. V. (2024). Iot traffic-based DDoS attacks detection mechanisms: A comprehensive review. *The Journal of Supercomputing*, 80(7), 9986–10043. DOI: 10.1007/s11227-023-05843-7

Snehi, M., & Bhandari, A. (2021). Vulnerability retrospection of security solutions for software-defined Cyber–Physical System against DDoS and IoT-DDoS attacks. *Computer Science Review*, 40, 100371. DOI: 10.1016/j.cosrev.2021.100371

Supriya, Y., & Gadekallu, T. R. (2023). A survey on soft computing techniques for federated learning-applications, challenges and future directions. *ACM Journal of Data and Information Quality*, 15(2), 1–28. DOI: 10.1145/3575810

Szalados, J. E. (2021). Medical Records and Confidentiality: Evolving Liability Issues Inherent in the Electronic Health Record, HIPAA, and Cybersecurity. *The Medical-Legal Aspects of Acute Care Medicine: A Resource for Clinicians, Administrators, and Risk Managers*, 315-342.

Tabaa, M., Monteiro, F., Bensag, H., & Dandache, A. (2020). Green Industrial Internet of Things from a smart industry perspectives. *Energy Reports*, 6, 430–446. DOI: 10.1016/j.egyr.2020.09.022

Uddin, R., Kumar, S. A., & Chamola, V. (2024). Denial of service attacks in edge computing layers: Taxonomy, vulnerabilities, threats and solutions. *Ad Hoc Networks, 152*, 103322. ul Sami, I., Ahmad, M. B., Asif, M., & Ullah, R. (2018). DoS/DDoS detection for E-Healthcare in internet of things. *International Journal of Advanced Computer Science and Applications*, 9(1).

Wong, B. K. M., Vengusamy, S., & Bastrygina, T. (2024). *Healthcare digital transformation through the adoption of artificial intelligence Artificial Intelligence, big data, blockchain and 5G for the digital transformation of the healthcare industry.* Elsevier.

Yaqoob, I., Salah, K., Jayaraman, R., & Al-Hammadi, Y. (2022). Blockchain for healthcare data management: Opportunities, challenges, and future recommendations. *Neural Computing & Applications*, 34(14), 1–16. DOI: 10.1007/s00521-020-05519-w

Ye, R., Wang, W., Chai, J., Li, D., Li, Z., Xu, Y., . . . Chen, S. (2024). *Openfedllm: Training large language models on decentralized private data via federated learning.* Paper presented at the Proceedings of the 30th ACM SIGKDD Conference on Knowledge Discovery and Data Mining. DOI: 10.1145/3637528.3671582

Zhang, M., Martin, P., Powley, W., & Chen, J. (2017). Workload management in database management systems: A taxonomy. *IEEE Transactions on Knowledge and Data Engineering*, 30(7), 1386–1402. DOI: 10.1109/TKDE.2017.2767044

Chapter 6
Federated Learning for Secure and Privacy-Preserving Medical Diagnostics

Gaurav Gupta
https://orcid.org/0000-0002-5192-4428
Shoolini University, India

Ravi Kant
https://orcid.org/0000-0002-7924-239X
Shoolini University, India

Abdulahi Mahammed Adem
https://orcid.org/0009-0001-2866-0698
Shoolini University, India

ABSTRACT

Federated learning is an emerging powerful approach for training ML models across decentralized data sources, such as in healthcare, without actually transferring the sensitive data to a central server. Although FL naturally reduces the risks of privacy since data are confined to local devices, it still can be highly vulnerable to sophisticated attacks such as model inversion, data poisoning, and inference attacks. Advanced privacy-preserving techniques that are nowadays studied for addressing the privacy and security concerns of this paper include differential privacy, homomorphic encryption, and secure aggregation. These, therefore, open the room for FL to be adopted as a solution in some of the privacy-sensitive domains. This paper conducts a thorough review of the techniques discussed and outlines a

DOI: 10.4018/979-8-3373-2827-0.ch006

customized security framework for healthcare applications that allow patient data to be safeguarded without detrimental effects on model performance and accuracy. Conclusion:

INTRODUCTION

Artificial intelligence is surely transforming the health diagnostics landscape: more precision, speed, and expansiveness in medical decision-making frameworks. Increased availability of comprehensive health information, coupled with advances in ML, has facilitated the successful implementation of AI in a varied domain of diagnostics, from medical imaging and genomics to health monitoring technologies that individuals wear (Sahu et al. 2022). Thus, artificial intelligence models can look at complex patterns in X-rays, MRI, and CT scans and highlight serious health conditions such as cancer, heart diseases, and neurological conditions to the attention of radiologists (Piorkowski, Obuchowicz, and Najjar 2023). On the other hand, advances in algorithms using artificial intelligence have also heavily pushed research forward in the area of genomics, making the identification of genetic markers affiliated with different diseases more effective, which is an essential part of personalized medicine (Rezayi, R Niakan Kalhori, and Saeedi 2022). Wearable health technologies are increasingly incorporating artificial intelligence in the process of monitoring physiological indicators in real-time, like heart rate, blood glucose level, and patterns of sleep, therefore allowing timely notifications about any potential health-related concerns (Nahavandi et al. 2022). By such contextual applications, it is easily comprehensible that artificial intelligence may also plays significant role in the identification of disorders that could affect human health.

In addition to such general progressions, several research studies have shed light on more specific aspects in the adoption of AI in health care. Some of these have included AI-based models in medical image diagnostics, such as the huge potential for identifying early signs of diseases like breast cancer and diabetic retinopathy that can bring better patient outcomes (Gulati, Guleria, and Goyal 2024). AI-driven predictive algorithms are now used for real-time patient monitoring with wearable devices that offer personalized health management solutions (Naithani et al. 2024). Additionally, the adoption of AI in genomic applications has increased the safe handling of genetic data, thereby facilitating precision medicine to be used to treat complex conditions like cancer and rare diseases (Naik et al. 2024). These developments have emphasized the adaptability and flexibility of AI technologies to address a wide range of healthcare challenges, which makes them indispensable in modern medical practice.

However, traditional centralized ML models-that require aggregating data to a single site for training create a host of challenges, more so in the healthcare sector (Abdulrahman et al. 2021). The sensitivity of medical data makes stringent privacy policies imperative, while traditional frameworks for centralized learning increase such risks of leakage and unauthorized access. Centralizing data also creates vulnerabilities in security due to the fact that attacks on a single server can lead to breaches involving highly sensitive patient data (Argaw et al. 2020). Additionally, health information scattered across various organizations makes the process of transfer and sharing quite complex while protecting privacy standards (Sheikh et al. 2021). With diagnostics increasingly using artificial intelligence, these issues in health care are essential to address security and confidentiality of patient information.

FL is a new approach overcoming those challenges with a decentralized ML model (Martinez Beltran et al. 2023). In FL, model is trained in multiple devices or organizations, but the data resides in its local environment (Martinez Beltran et al. 2023). On the contrary, each client in federated network is training model on their dataset locally and sending model updates to a host server. Such a server aggregates model updates into an improved global model. The decentralized approach has advantages regarding data security and patient privacy but concurrently enables the training of AI models on a lot of different datasets distributed across many locations (Rahman et al. 2022). FL facilitates the retention of data at its original source, preserving individual privacy, minimizing security threats, and creating opportunities for cooperative endeavors among various healthcare organizations while ensuring data confidentiality is upheld.

Recent studies have presented transformative impact of FL in healthcare. (Nazir and Kaleem 2023) showed that FL enhances the accuracy of diagnostic systems without violating data privacy through its application in medical images. (H. Wang et al. 2023) studied the use of FL in genomics further, which may allow it to securely analyze genetic information across institutions. These developments highlight FL's capability to combat key challenges in health information management while preserving confidentiality and scalability. Moreover, (Singh and Singh 2023) explored the role that FL plays in the success of multi-hospital alliances for the early diagnosis of diabetic retinopathy: it showed a marked accuracy improvement in diagnostics. (Khan and Abaoud 2023) applied FL with numerous datasets gathered from wearable health instruments in real-time patient monitoring systems to raise alerts about the progression of critical conditions in a timely manner. Such applications depict the flexibility of FL for providing secure data sharing and promoting clinical decision-making. In addition, recent new findings, like differential privacy techniques and homomorphic encryption, are reinforcing the framework of FL to make the former more resilient to some potential breaches (Xie et al. 2024). These breakthroughs present FL as a cornerstone on which future advancement in AI health systems is based-to ensure scalability, privacy, and collaborative possibilities across world institutions. Figure 1 shows the working of FL in such a system, the central server maintains a global model with initial parameters, and participants-in this system, also referred to as clients or nodes-retain their local datasets secure, not sharing them with any external party.

Figure 1. FL

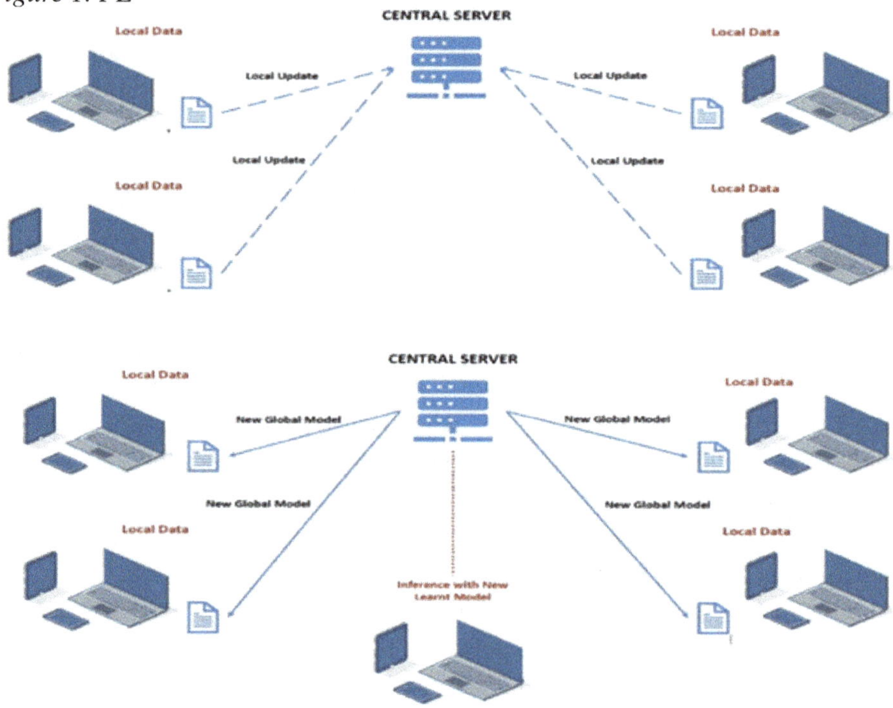

1.1. Objective

This paper aims to study security and privacy aspects of FL, especially within the sensitive healthcare diagnostics domain. Taking advantage of state-of-the-art cryptographic techniques, such as differential privacy, homomorphic encryption, and secure aggregation, this research will mitigate some fundamental threats related to data leakage, unofficial access to specific datasets, and compliance with privacy regulations, including GDPR. The ultimate goal should be that the collaborative learning models of health care ensure maximum security with no reduced utility in the model.

1.2. Motivation

This motivation stems from the growing reliance on AI/ML in healthcare, where sharing and aggregation of large-scale data are very crucial in building a robust model. Traditional centralized learning systems raise many serious concerns with regard to data privacy and accordance with frameworks such as GDPR and HIPAA. FL offers decentralized method that maintains the privacy of data localization, but even this approach is not threat-proof against model inversion, data poisoning, and inference attacks. Healthcare data, whether in the form of imaging, genomics, or in real-time monitoring using wearable, is sensitive; hence, FL systems should include the deployment of additional layers of security. This is the motivation toward the exploration and application of state-of-the-art security techniques that ensure protection of patient data with preserved privacy without any compromises on performance and accuracy of the models.

The paper is structured as: Section 1 background of FL and its relevance in healthcare. Section 2 explaining the detailed descriptions of the foundational concepts in FL based on how FL works and why it matters for decentralized, privacy-preserving ML in sensitive domains like health. Section 3 delves into the health-related applications of FL. Section 4 Identifies and discusses privacy and security issues specific to FL. Section 5 Describes the central techniques for improving FL security: differential privacy, homomorphic encryption, and secure aggregation. Section 6 captures challenges and difficulties in deploying the proposed techniques. Section 7 is the conclusion of the paper summarizing key takeaways for the application in health.

2. CORE CONCEPTS OF FL

FL is state-of-the-art ML technique that overcomes shortcomings of centralized models by incorporating a decentralized model in learning (Ogundokun et al. 2022). Instead of all data needing to be transmitted to some host server, FL allows local model training on data autonomously by individual devices or institutions such as hospitals and research centers. That reflects that any participant in a federated network owns full control over his datasets and shares only the learned parameters with the centralized server, such as model weights or gradients.

The essence of FL itself is collaborative yet secure, first, global model is initialized on central server (Hu et al. 2021). Each participant downloads the global model to train it locally on their specific dataset. After training, the local updates basically, the model's learned parameters are forwarded to the central server. Importantly, no raw data is transmitted, just the model updates. It is the main server that consequently updates these models to arrive at a more robust and globally generalizable improved model. This is done multiple times, thereby enabling model to learn from different heterogeneous data that are geographically distributed while maintaining data privacy. The central server may employ techniques such as secure aggregation to ensure that local updates are aggregated in a manner that prevents leaking sensitive information. This architecture represents a fundamental paradigm shift from previous centralized learning mechanisms, whereby all information is collected and processed at one single source, toward a more privacy-sensitive, safer, and scalable infrastructure, which is befitting the health data sources' characteristics of decentralization.

2.1. Key Advantages of FL in Healthcare

FL provides a lot of value in the healthcare space, especially mitigating some of the key weaknesses of traditional ML approaches. Its core advantage lies in being intrinsically able to guarantee data privacy (Coelho et al. 2023). Due to the fact that FL keeps patient data within the local environments of their originating institutions or devices, this makes sure sensitive medical information stays at the point of origin, thereby reducing risks due to data breaches. This aspect is highly crucial in the healthcare sector, as the privacy policies, such as GDPR and HIPAA, demand very strict measures when it comes to handling patient data (Rauniyar et al. 2024). Aside from privacy protection, FL makes it possible to have decentralized computation and, therefore, is very useful in clinical settings where data normally resides in a disaggregated manner among institutions (Taha et al. 2023). Medical facilities, outpatient centers, and research organizations can contribute to FL without losing confidentiality in their data and hence enable wide collaboration (Taha et al. 2023). This collaborative methodology, besides improving the dataset available for training AI models, increases the generalizability of the resultant models by training on a broader range of datasets. This approach is particularly significant in the area of medical diagnostics, where differences in patient demographics, devices, and procedural norms can make a centralized model less effective (Rieke et al. 2020). Another important benefit of FL in healthcare is its scalability (Sáinz-Pardo Díaz and López García 2023). As number of participants increases, it will keep on learning from a varied data source without having to transfer data, which could be costly and time-consuming. This again makes FL appropriate for scaling AI-powered diagnostics across large healthcare networks or even across borders. Furthermore, FL enables real-time updates, keeping the models adaptive and responsive in the face of new medical insights, which is particularly important in fields like oncology, where timely and accurate diagnostics have a disproportionate impact on patient outcomes (Prasad et al. 2022).

3. FL IN MEDICAL DIAGNOSTICS

FL is increasingly recognized as an effective mechanism in the field of medical diagnostics because it allows health organizations, research institutions, and IoMT devices to collaborate on common interests while protecting patient confidentiality. This distributed framework is a game-changer for various aspects of medical diagnostics, including medical imaging, genomics, and wearable health monitoring (Sáinz-Pardo Díaz and López García 2023). By allowing AI models to improve diagnostic accuracy without the need to pool data into centralized location. FL addresses significant challenges in healthcare, especially within data privacy, security, and collaboration across institutions (Coelho et al. 2023). It trains models without sharing raw data, hence increasing the possibility of more personalized and real-time diagnostics.

3.1. Applications in Medical Imaging

Medical imaging is the richest data areas in health, and it needs some deep AI techniques for image analysis, including MRI, CT scans, X-rays, and histopathology slides. FL enjoys a unique advantage wherein healthcare institutions collaborate on training an AI model with no exchange of patient data for collaboration, conquering the data fragmentation seen across hospitals, clinics, and research institutions (Taha et al. 2023).

MRI and CT scans: In MRI and CT scans, FL can allow various hospitals and diagnostic centers to train AI models on their local data by focusing on a single disease or condition. This can be done by a model being trained across hospitals for the detection of tumors in MRI scans (Taha et al. 2023). By doing so, it enhances robustness as a result of learning from a more diverse data set without any sensitive imaging data leaving the premises. Each of these updates, such as the weights learned from a local model in each hospital, are aggregated back at a central server, where these updates are aggregated to improve the global model. In this manner, the combined model benefits from an array of imaging data from different regions, ethnicities, and equipment, which leads to enhanced diagnostic accuracy.

FL also plays an important role in surmounting device-specific biases (Abreha, Hayajneh, and Serhani 2022). That is, not all hospitals will be using the same imaging machines for diagnosing the ailment, and such machines may have various resolutions and capabilities. As a result of such differences, inconsistencies may arise if some centralized model is trained on the pooled data. With FL, each institution's model will learn from its own data, taking into account the specificities of that particular imaging technology, hence making the global model more adaptive and generalizable. This is of great importance in specific areas, like oncology, where subtlety in images may provide a huge difference in diagnosis and treatment planning.

X-rays and Histopathology: In applications like X-rays and histopathology, where high-resolution images provide the backbone for diagnosis on minute details related to fractures, abnormalities within the lung, or cancerous cells, FL enables knowledge sharing for model development across various pathology labs and radiology departments (Nazir and Kaleem 2023). Histopathology deals with the study of tissues and requires the identification of abnormalities at the cellular level, which often changes with demographics and stages of diseases (van der Laak, Litjens, and Ciompi 2021). FL allows for the combination of model updates from multiple labs, hence generalization across different patient cohorts as well as different staining techniques being used in various laboratories.

One such practical application of FL in this domain involves the detection of lung diseases like pneumonia or tuberculosis from chest X-rays (Malik and Anees 2024). FL allows radiology departments across different hospitals to create more accurate AI models to find these conditions in diverse populations without necessarily sharing sensitive patient images. Moreover, FL would speed up diagnosis and allow hospitals to deploy models that were trained with numerous different datasets; thus, these models can detect conditions even earlier and more reliably than single-institution training.

3.2. Genomics and Personalized Medicine

Genomics create very large datasets that comprise extremely sensitive genetic information (Byrd et al. 2020). In this regard, data privacy becomes paramount. FL proposes to provide a solution that can enable hospitals and research institutions to collaborate on training AI models that analyze genetic data without transferring the actual genomic sequences across the networks (Cremonesi et al. 2023).

FL in Genomic Research: Other genomic research involves the investigation of the patterns and various mutations in DNA sequences related to different cancers, neurological disorders, and other genetic rare conditions (Pfeifer and Jin 2024). Because of the sensitivity of genomic data, institutes are very reluctant to share their data; this often makes the process of research rather slow. FL enables researchers to collaboratively build models analyzing large-scale variations in genetic diversity across diverse populations without compromising privacy (Cremonesi et al. 2023).

For instance, in cancer genomics, FL enables various research institutions to train models to learn from datasets residing across multiple institutions and identify those mutations that are associated with specific types of cancers. For example, a model that has been trained through FL might develop patterns that suggest a higher risk for certain cancers or predict how a patient responds to different levels of treatments while ensuring patient confidentiality as per regulations like GDPR or HIPAA (Rauniyar et al. 2024), (Rieke et al. 2020).

Recent studies have pointed towards FL potential in genomic analysis; recently, (Kumar Singh, Khanna, and singh 2023) showed FL to get used for identification of biomarkers with respect to breast cancer, integrating multi-institutional genomic data. Similarly, (Zhou et al. 2024) demonstrated FL towards the study of rare neurological conditions where data sparsity would have further inhibited classical methodology. Such applications indicate the potential of FL to speed up genomic research without compromising on protecting privacy. For instance, FL research has been directed to understand inherited cardiac diseases for which multi-institutional collaborative research was able to be preserved with patient confidential data (Issac and Kumar 2024).

Personalized Medicine and FL: FL has great importance in personalized medicine for allowing individualized treatment per the patient's genetic makeup (Rauniyar et al. 2024). Diseases that involve conditions such as cancer, diabetes, or cardiovascular conditions have thus sought answers in personalized medicine, which provides treatment that caters to unique genetic characteristics defining an individual patient (Rieke et al. 2020). Developing AI models for such a task is possible only with big diverse data representative of different populations and genetic backgrounds.

With FL, a variety of hospitals and research institutions can collaborate in building AI models capable of predicting how different patients react to certain treatments based on their genetic markers without necessarily sharing their datasets (Sahu et al. 2022). This will make sure that the treatment plans can be more precisely tailored to each patient's genetic composition and, therefore, better outcomes of the treatment are ensured while reducing the possibility of adverse reactions. Besides, models of FL are more likely to detect rare genetic conditions when they have been trained on data from different institutions, rather than on more homogeneous datasets.

3.3. Wearable Devices and Real-time Diagnostics

Wearable devices play crucial role in healthcare through real-time monitoring: smartwatches, continuous glucose monitors, and fitness trackers (Mansour, Saeed Darweesh, and Soltan 2024). As a rule, these are part of the so-called broader Internet of Medical Things ecosystem that continuously follows heart rate, glucose levels, sleep patterns, and many more. The approach, however, encompasses a volume of data emanating from the process that is also difficult to handle in real time and does raise serious privacy concerns, making the deployment of centralized AI solutions very difficult.

FL in Wearable Health Monitoring: This is where FL tries to address the problem by enabling on-device AI training, meaning every wearable device trains a model locally on the user's data (Arikumar et al. 2022). That device then sends updates to a central server for combination, where raw data-like an individual's heart rate or glucose levels-is never transmitted over the network. Because such systems adopt this kind of decentralized approach, they preserve privacy for users while offering diagnostics in real-time, thanks to the data they collect in natural environments such as homes or during daily activities.

For instance, continuous glucose monitors collect data on blood sugar levels when managing diabetes. With FL, these can develop personalized models that predict glucose fluctuations depending on diet, physical activity, and medication (H. Y. Lu et al. 2024). This will enable real-time interventions-for example, recommending changes in insulin doses or food intake-without sensitive health data being exposed to third parties.

Chronic Disease Monitoring and Early Intervention: To this effect, hypertension, heart diseases, and respiratory conditions will need not only to be continuously monitored, but timely interventions will also be required, to avoid complications (El-Rashidy et al. 2021). Wearable devices with FL capabilities will build predictive models that flag off early warning signals such as abnormal heartbeats, high blood pressure, or an unusual pattern of breathing heralding an imminent serious complication (Gayathri et al. 2024).

FL improves the accuracy of prediction by these models, since they are trained on data from diverse populations (Banabilah et al. 2022). The more varied health profiles the models learn from, the better. This is particularly important for wearable devices because these are prone to biases, a large part of which comes from training on small datasets. This means that with more federated devices, the global model improves, benefiting its users through more reliable and personalized diagnostics. Application of FL in the medical diagnosis is summarized in Table 1.

Table 1. Summary of applications of FL in healthcare

Category	Description	Key Applications	Benefits	Related Works
Medical Diagnostics	✓ Enables collaboration without sharing data. ✓ Ensures privacy in training AI models.	✓ Medical Imaging ✓ Genomics ✓ Wearable Devices	✓ Preserves data privacy. ✓ Enhances diagnostic accuracy. ✓ Supports real-time, personalized solutions.	(Xu et al. 2021)
Applications in Medical Imaging	✓ Allows local training on imaging data. ✓ Reduces the need for central data pooling.	✓ MRI for tumor detection ✓ CT scans for diagnosis	✓ Reduces device-specific biases. ✓ Improves model robustness. ✓ Enhances diagnostic precision.	(Adnan et al. 2022)
X-rays and Histopathology	✓ Facilitates collaboration for disease diagnosis. ✓ Combines insights without sharing raw images.	✓ Chest X-rays for lung diseases ✓ Histopathology for cancer detection	✓ Speeds up diagnosis. ✓ Generalizes models across institutions. ✓ Protects patient confidentiality.	(Nazir and Kaleem 2023).
Genomics and Personalized Medicine	✓ Enables collaboration on genomic analysis. ✓ Maintains privacy of genetic data.	✓ Genomic research ✓ Personalized medicine for cancer and rare genetic conditions	✓ Supports personalized treatment. ✓ Enhances research on genetic mutations. ✓ Ensures data security.	(Cremonesi et al. 2023).
Devices and Real-time Diagnostics	✓ Local training on user data. ✓ Enables real-time health monitoring.	✓ Continuous glucose monitors ✓ Fitness trackers for heart rate and blood pressure	✓ Provides real-time intervention. ✓ Preserves user privacy. ✓ Improves chronic disease monitoring.	(H. Y. Lu et al. 2024).

4. PRIVACY AND SECURITY IN FL

Rising use of FL in healthcare diagnostics heralds a need for increased emphasis on data security and privacy (Rauniyar et al. 2024). When patient data is this sensitive and highly regulated, it must be safeguarded by provisions that are nothing short of robust security and privacy mechanisms. While FL reduces privacy risks significantly by keeping data local, a number of challenges still need to be addressed to maintain data confidentiality and cope with system vulnerabilities (Aouedi et al. 2023). This section discusses key considerations in healthcare privacy, major techniques for preserving privacy in FL, and security challenges that arise within this form of distributed learning.

4.1. Data Privacy in Healthcare

Data breaches in the healthcare industry form a wide segment, from sensitive information about medical history to genetic information and diagnostic records (Churi et al. 2021). Confidentiality is at once an ethical obligation and a binding duty under strict regulations in different countries of the world, such as the General Data Protection Regulation, Europe (Gefenas et al. 2022), and the Health Insurance Portability and Accountability Act in the United States (Rauniyar et al. 2024). These regulations put strict restrictions on the use, accommodation, and release of patient information, and the prime focus of this legislation has been the privacy security of individuals. These would be processed on a central server in the traditional form of a centralized learning system, where patient data is collected from several institutions. Of course, this places a great risk on data privacy. Any breach in such a centralized system can result in the leakage of a lot of patient data, leading to possible identity theft, financial fraud. Secondly, even if the centralized systems are secure, transferring data across different institutions has its own chances of interception or unauthorized access.

FL handles these issues by ensuring that no raw patient data is required to leave the local confines of a particular healthcare institution. Instead, it is only the updates regarding the learned model of weights or gradients that are transmitted to the central server for aggregation (Aouedi et al. 2023). This limits sensitive data exposure and thus mitigates the risk of breaches during data transfer. However, while FL solves many of the privacy issues inherent in centralized systems, it is by no means immune. Sometimes model updates can still leak some information about underlying data; thus, additional techniques to guarantee privacy preservation must be applied to make sure that patient confidentiality is fully maintained.

4.2. Privacy-Preserving Mechanisms in FL

Advanced privacy-preserving mechanisms that FL can employ include secure aggregation, homomorphic encryption, and differential privacy to further protect patient data both in training and aggregation. The techniques are designed to make sure no sensitive information is inadvertently leaked during collaborative model training and thus are crucial for compliance with regulations such as the GDPR and HIPAA (Rauniyar et al. 2024).

Differential Privacy: Differential privacy is the most used technique to provide privacy protection in FL (Ouadrhiri and Abdelhadi 2022). This involves injecting noise into the model updates that are sent from the local devices or institutions to the main server; hence, it is very difficult to trace specific details about the underlying data (Ni et al. 2021). It guarantees that no meaningful information about the patients could be inferred, even if an adversary intercepted model update (Ni et al. 2021). The principal benefit of differential privacy is that it does provide a mathematical guarantee of the privacy of individuals being protected, independent of how much data one shares. When implemented, for instance, in healthcare, differential privacy ensures that fine patient-specific details related to any disease or condition do not leak through the model updates (Ni et al. 2021). Consider a scenario in cancer detection where a hospital is training a FL model. In this regard, differential privacy will ensure that none of the attackers can infer which patients out of all the patients within the dataset have been diagnosed with cancer from the output of the models (Aouedi et al. 2023).

Secure Multiparty Computation (SMC): Another highly important approach to preserving privacy in FL is Secure Multi-Party Computation (Sotthiwat et al. 2021). SMC enables several parties jointly to check a function over their private inputs. In other words, each of the participants can make a contribution to model training in the FL process without leaking data locally. SMC ensures that sensitive information of participating institutions does not leak while updating the global model (Tran et al. 2021). For example, SMC allows multiple hospitals to jointly train an AI model for heart disease diagnosis in a FL scenario without sharing the raw ECG data (X. Wang et al. 2023). These updates are computed securely, and a central server can aggregate updates without learning anything about the data in each hospital. This technique becomes really important in environments where various institutions are not prepared to collaborate owing to various concerns arising out of data leakage.

Homomorphic Encryption: Homomorphic encryption is a more computationally intensive but highly secure technique, which lets computations be done directly on the encrypted data (B. Wang et al. 2023). The model updates during FL will be encrypted before sending to the central server. Aggregation is done over encrypted data. There is no need to decrypt the data for computation by the central server, which ensures sensitive information is kept safe through the process. Homomorphic encryption is also helpful in health care situations where the possibility of leakage in data is considered to be high-for example, in genomics (B. Wang et al. 2023). Thus, encrypting the updates of the model will protect the hospitals and research institutions from the scenario in which the attacker can retrieve meaningful information about the patients' genetic information, even though it might have reached the central server.

While homomorphic encryption is supposed to introduce computational overhead, its capability for secure computations on encrypted data makes it rather interesting and powerful in guaranteeing data privacy in the context of FL (Aziz et al. 2023).

4.3. Security Challenges in FL

Even with privacy-preserving techniques in use, FL would still be vulnerable to various types of security threats in the form of model inversion attacks, poisoning attacks, and inference attacks, all of which have a potential to compromise either the integrity of the learning process or the confidentiality of the data.

Model Inversion Attacks: In this attack, the adversary targets at recovering the original data from the model updates (Wen, Yiu, and Hui 2021). Although FL does not share raw data, model updates could carry information that may be leveraged, if analysed properly, to infer restricted information related to individual patients. For example, in case of a medical imaging-based application, an attacker might aim at recovering a blurry version of the MRI scan from the gradients of the model. Although the image might not be entirely clear, it would probably still contain enough detail to identify the patient from any tumor features (Geiping et al. 2020).

To alleviate model inversion attacks, FL systems should have the capability to inject different techniques of preserving privacy, such as differential privacy or leverage more secure protocols for aggregation that make it hard to derive sensitive information from these updates (Lyu et al. 2024). Also, frequent model updates can be averaged over time to obscure the contributions of individual data points, making it harder for the attackers to reverse-engineer the underlying data.

Poisoning Attacks: In poisoning attacks, malicious participants deliberately upload corrupted or misleading model updates to the central server with an aim of degrading performance of global model (Wang et al. 2022). This could be very hazardous in health diagnostics, where the results could lead to some very incorrect or harmful medical diagnosis (Wang et al. 2022). For instance, the global model may be less effective in detecting cancerous lesions in future patients if poisoned updates are submitted by one of the participating hospitals in cancer detection FL.

In poisoning attacks, FL systems should make use of a strong verification mechanism to detect and filter suspicious updates (Awan, Luo, and Li 2021). Anomaly detection algorithms flag those that are very different from the expected pattern (Ding et al. 2024). Encryption ensures that communication channels between participants and a central server can avoid any attempt by the attacker to tamper with the updates in transmission.

Inference Attacks: Inference attacks also involve trying to infer sensitive information about individual participants or their data by observation over model updates (Aouedi et al. 2023). This is even when no raw data is shared at times;

model behavior divulges something about the underlying dataset. For example, if the FL model suddenly becomes very good at diagnosing some very rare disease, an attacker might infer that one of the participants of the network has contributed data about that particular disease (A. Ali et al. 2023).

FL systems would therefore apply secure aggregation protocols such that updates by individuals are combined in a manner that any identifiable information is masked. Noise injection, such as in differential privacy, could further ensure that inference attacks do not reveal sensitive patterns from updates.

5. TECHNIQUES FOR ENHANCING SECURITY IN FL

Sound security of FL in its sensitive applications, like healthcare, is of utmost importance, as breaches of privacy and data breaches have higher consequences there compared to elsewhere. While FL eliminates the raw data exposure risk by preserving the data on local devices, further security mechanisms must be integrated into the model updates and the overall learning process. Concretely, it would be quite useful if one could offer some guarantee that sensitive information is not revealed due to enabling effective model training using different techniques such as differential privacy, and secure aggregation. These methods save data from leakage and make FL systems robust against sophisticated attacks like model inversion, poisoning, and inference attacks.

5.1. Differential Privacy Integration

Differential privacy probably represents the most important methodology adopted in order to enhance security in FL (M. Ali et al. 2023). It indeed guarantees that sensitive information about a given data record cannot be extracted, even in the presence of an adversary who may intercept model updates sent from local machine to the central server, by adding noise carefully calibrated to the model updates. It gives a mathematical guarantee that the contribution of an individual's data remains private; thus, it is highly effective to apply in very sensitive health sectors where patients' confidentiality is paramount (M. Ali et al. 2023).

How Differential Privacy Works in FL: In the context of FL, one may ensure differential privacy by adding random noise into the gradients or weights of the locally trained models before the process of transmission for aggregation (Baek et al. 2021). This noise will mask the contribution of any single data point, ensuring that the local model contribution to the global model doesn't leak any specific information about the underlying data. As an example, if a FL system is set up for the analysis of medical images, such as MRI, differential privacy guarantees that changes from each hospital or diagnostic center would be anonymized (Sandhu et al. 2023). In other words, even in the case of an attacker intercepting these updates, they could not reconstruct sensitive patient information, like identifying characteristics from MRI images. This added noise is sufficiently small to preserve the model's utility, hence the model learns useful patterns without compromising privacy.

Another critical advantage of differential privacy is that, in this way, FL can be made to conform with such regulations as General Data Protection Regulation, where individual data protection needs to be vigorous. Differential privacy contributes to fulfilling legal requirements on data protection in healthcare by not allowing sensitive information to be inferred from model updates (Ouadrhiri and Abdelhadi 2022).

5.2. Homomorphic Encryption

While differential privacy protects individual contributions by adding noise, homomorphic encryption gives additional security by enabling the performance of computations while data is encrypted. This means model updates can be encrypted in transmission to a central server and still be aggregated and processed at that server without requiring decryption. In that way, even if an attacker has access to the server or intercepts updates while sending, an attacker would not be able to decipher encrypted information.

How Homomorphic Encryption Works in FL: In a homomorphic encryption-based FL system, model updates are encrypted first by the local devices or institutions, then are forwarded to the central server (Lozi et al. 2022). In turn, this server would operate on those without ever decrypting them. Then it would send the encrypted model, updated in this way, back to the participants, who might decrypt it using their private keys. The beauty of homomorphic encryption is in a security feature enabling computations on encrypted data. Recalling the simple example of several hospitals collaboratively training a model that predicts disease outcomes from patient data, homomorphic encryption ensures that at every step the updates of every hospital are kept fully protected (Khalid et al. 2023). Not even an attacker who managed to breach the server could learn anything useful from the encrypted updates. Although homomorphic encryption offers security, the computational overhead is definitely present because data encryption and decryption might be computationally expensive, as well as operations over encrypted data. However, continuous improvement in cryptographic techniques is actually reducing this computational overhead. Therefore, homomorphic encryption turns to be a feasible approach toward secure FL in healthcare, particularly in those applications that contain highly sensitive information, like genetics or medical images (Abaoud, Almuqrin, and Khan 2023).

5.3. Secure Aggregation Techniques

Another fundamental technique that contributes to privacy and security in FL is Secure Aggregation. The goal of secure aggregation in FL is to ensure updates of an individual model should not be inspected, intercepted, or reverse-engineered while carrying out the aggregation (Fereidooni et al. 2021). This has critical implications within the domain of FL, where model updates are often communicated over networks that might be insecure, hence vulnerable to interception by adversaries.

How Secure Aggregation Works in FL: This is in a conventional FL setup: A hospital or IoMT device updates the model locally and forwards the updated model to a central server for aggregation (Gupta et al. 2023). Secure aggregation techniques ensure these updates are encrypted in such a way that the server can aggregate but not inspect individual updates (Song et al. 2023). It is usually provided, with the help of cryptographic protocols, namely SMC or secret sharing, which allows multiple participants to compute a task over their data while keeping the data itself hidden from one another and the central server. For example, in a FL model that focuses on monitoring chronic conditions like heart disease through wearable health devices, secure aggregation would guarantee that no one entity has access to the raw health data coming from individual devices (Bebortta et al. 2023). Devices encrypt their model updates, while the central server collects these encrypted updates without an ability to see the contribution of each device (Fereidooni et al. 2021). That ensures that even in the case of server compromise, the privacy of such patients who use these devices remains assured.

Advanced Secure Aggregation Methods: One such advanced method for secure aggregation includes threshold aggregation, where model updates from participants are aggregated only if the minimum required number of participants contribute their updates (Song et al. 2020). In other words, there is no disclosure of any information about an individual participant from the collective update. This will be very useful in medical applications, where even small datasets from various individual hospitals or clinics may possess highly sensitive information. Another approach consists of verifiable aggregation, which comes with the guarantee that the central server cannot tamper with or somehow alter the model updates during the process of aggregation (Xu et al. 2022). With this setup, participants can ensure the performed aggregation was correct without letting their data be revealed. This builds an additional layer of trust that maintains the integrity of the global model via the learning process.

6. CHALLENGES AND LIMITATIONS OF FL IN HEALTHCARE

While FL unlocks a plethora of benefits in healthcare diagnostics, significant challenges and constraints persist that must be addressed in order to realize its effectual deployment. These result from intrinsic complexities within healthcare data and system infrastructure and the pluralistic nature of the medical landscape. The main challenges include data heterogeneity and non-IID data, communication bottlenecks, and scalability for big-scale healthcare systems. Understanding these limitations is crucial for the best implementation of FL in real-world healthcare applications and also to realize its full promise of being privacy preserving and efficient in performing medical diagnostics.

6.1. Data Heterogeneity and Non-IID Data

One of the biggest challenges to applying FL in health care is data heterogeneity (Sachin, Annappa, and Ambesange 2024). Healthcare data, generally collected from different institutions, devices, and geographic regions, are non-independent and identically distributed, which means there is considerable variation between data from one source and another. Such heterogeneity arises for several reasons, including medical practices, diagnostic equipment, patient populations, and even local environmental factors, which can shape what type of data will be gathered and how those data are distributed. Non-IID data in a FL system may result in an imbalanced learning where the global model gets biased toward the data of certain institutions or regions (Z. Lu et al. 2024). For instance, there is great heterogeneity in medical imaging data. MRI scans may turn out quite different in resolution when taken from devices or under protocols employed at different hospitals (Sáinz-Pardo Díaz and López García 2023). Such heterogeneity of data gives skepticism to the fact that the global model will generalize well across different institutions. Non-IID data is even more sophisticated to handle (Z. Lu et al. 2024). A number of works propose personalization in FL where models are fine-tuned for certain institutions, or through advanced aggregation methods considering variability in data distributions.

6.2. Communication Bottlenecks and Latency

Another limitation with the application of FL in healthcare involves communication bottlenecks and latency between local devices and the central servers (Rahman et al. 2022). In a FL setup, local devices must send model updates periodically to the central server for aggregation into updates of the global model. The process involves participants and servers being in constant contact, which might be a little problematic when dealing with healthcare applications in real time.

In real-time patient monitoring, for example, updates coming from wearable devices are extremely important to be in a timely fashion. For instance, this would be of great help to note critical health conditions such as arrhythmias or sudden spikes in blood pressure. At the same time, if there is latency or bandwidth limitation in the communication network, these could lead to slower model training and diagnostics. Moreover, poor or no Internet infrastructure makes communication with the central server spasmodic or impossible in remote or poorly resourced areas.

The inefficiency in communication can be avoided by employing communication-efficient FL methods that either send updates less frequently or compress updates to save bandwidth (Almanifi et al. 2023). Edge computing can also be embedded in the FL system for local processing of model updates with minimum frequent communication with the central server, thereby alleviating part of the latency issue (Xia et al. 2021). These solutions involve some sort of trade-off in terms of slower global model convergence.

6.3. System Scalability and Computational Constraints

Another challenging problem is scaling up the FL systems across many hospitals, devices, or IoMT networks (Rani et al. 2023). Large-scale healthcare networks require FL support hundreds or thousands of participants that actively contribute to updating models. The more participants there are, the higher the computation pressure on the central server rises exponentially, whereas it is hard to manage the update aggregation in a timely manner (Zhang et al. 2021).

This is exacerbated by the computational capabilities that each participant has; they are different. The large hospitals may have high-level computing resources and therefore can process complex models quickly, while smaller clinics or IoMT devices may not have comparable computational powers to handle such models. Different means of computation can also cause imbalanced contributions in model training (Prasad et al. 2022).

For instance, in a FL system for radiological diagnostics, powerful servers of some participating hospitals may have the capability to train large deep learning models, whereas IoMT devices in home-care environments can only have limited processing power (Sachin et al. 2023). Another critical challenge of the design of such systems is guaranteeing that all participants will contribute efficiently to the global model without being overwhelmed by other participants who are resource-poor (Wen et al. 2022).

This challenge can partly be met through model compression, where the dimensions and complexity of models under training are reduced to make them more plausible for bounded resource devices (Imteaj et al. 2022). Other techniques, such as federated averaging, even help in efficient aggregation through a reduction in the number of communications or data transferred (Qi et al. 2024). Other ways include hierarchical FL: within such a setting, the local servers serve to intermediate devices and central servers that make a local aggregation of updates before forwarding to a central server, reducing load on central infrastructure (Lim et al. 2020).

However, even with these solutions, the scalability of FL remains a significant concern, mainly in healthcare, where the intricacy of models and variability in data can make it difficult to ensure that the system scales efficiently without sacrificing performance or accuracy.

6.4. Ethical Concerns in FL for Healthcare

Adoption of FL significantly raises ethical concerns; hence, its implementation should be judiciously made by careful consideration. Key areas of concerns are as follows:

Data Privacy and Security: Even though FL reduces the necessity of sharing data, it is important to have model updates secure and prevent any adversarial attacks. Research has recently identified vulnerabilities in FL systems, such as model inversion attacks, where a sensitive patient's information could be reconstructed(Gupta and Alam 2022).

Algorithmic Bias and Fairness: FL models must deal with the latent bias that can be built up from imbalanced or non-representative data sets. For example, if training models on skewed datasets biased toward certain demographics is allowed, it may allow disparities in diagnosis accuracy or prescription recommendation (Chen et al. 2023).

Informed Consent: The patients for whose data are indirectly put into FL systems need to be appropriately informed on the handling of their information, regardless of it remaining local. Communication that clearly portrays FL's purpose, benefits, and risks to establish trust is very necessary(Rahman et al. 2022).

Regulatory Compliance: This is an issue of adhering to the privacy regulation, such as GDPR and HIPAA. The mechanism in FL must include differential privacy and secure aggregation techniques, as stated by (Silva and Soto 2022).

Scalability and Resource Distribution: With FL, the computational requirements as well as communication may produce inequities among institutes that may have proper infrastructures. Equitable availability of the FL technology becomes important in developing collaborations with the globe for health-related matters (Bashir et al. 2023).

Addressing these ethical concerns will not only enhance FL's acceptance in the healthcare sector but also ensure that its deployment aligns with the principles of equity, transparency, and accountability.

7. FUTURE DIRECTIONS IN FL FOR MEDICAL DIAGNOSTICS

FL will be increasingly transformational in medical diagnostics, especially as the technology continues to evolve with other emerging technologies. While FL already offers a privacy-preserving approach to the collaboration of ML, future developments could decidedly upscale its scalability, security, and application in diverse healthcare settings. The cross-border collaboration of data contribution, integration with FL, and IoMT, along with ways that emerging technologies such as quantum computing and 5G networks may influence the future of FL in healthcare, are summarized in Table 2.

Table 2. Feature direction of FL in medical diagnosis

No	Key Area	Description	Potential Benefits
1	Cross-Border Data Collaboration	FL enables secure, global collaboration for diagnostics and research without sharing raw data.	Enhances diagnostic accuracy and pandemic preparedness globally.
2	Integration with IoMT and AI	FL allows real-time monitoring through IoMT devices while preserving privacy.	Enables real-time diagnostics and personalized treatment.
3	Emerging Technologies (Quantum, 5G)	Quantum computing accelerates FL training; 5G enables real-time data transmission between IoMT devices.	Faster diagnostics and improved communication across healthcare systems.
4	Personalized Medicine	FL aggregates patient data securely to enable individualized treatments.	Tailored treatments and improved patient outcomes.
5	Decentralized Clinical Trials	FL enables secure, multi-institution clinical trials without centralizing data.	Boosts trial diversity and efficiency.
6	Privacy-Enhancing Technologies (PETs)	PETs integrated with FL improve security in collaborative healthcare learning.	Enhances data privacy while allowing collaboration.
7	FL for Rare Diseases	FL helps in diagnosing rare diseases by pooling data from global institutions.	Increases accuracy in diagnosing rare conditions.
8	Real-Time Diagnostics & Telemedicine	FL provides continuous model updates for remote diagnostics and telemedicine.	Enhances care and decision-making in telemedicine.
9	Blockchain Integration with FL	Blockchain ensures secure and transparent FL model updates and data sharing in healthcare.	Increases security and trust in FL systems.

8. CONCLUSION

FL has emerged among the most essential enablers of secure, privacy-preserving medical diagnostics, solving many problems connected with centralized ML. FL enables the collaboration between institutions and devices in training AI models while avoiding sensitive patient data sharing; it enables privacy preservation and enhances data security by facilitating the use of AI across healthcare settings. In this study, we have seen the basic machinery of FL, applications on medical diagnostics, the used privacy and security techniques, and open challenges and limitations that need to be resolved. From medical imaging to genomics, wearables, FL bears tremendous potential in fostering a new generation of real-time diagnostics, facilitating collaboration between healthcare institutions, and distributed AI solutions that protect patient confidentiality. FL is not to be underestimated in the future scope of its impact in health. As AI technology adoptions continue across health, FL is a robust framework through which those innovations could be scaled across institutions, devices, and geographical regions without loss of privacy. FL enables collaboration in medical research and diagnostics on a truly global scale, having the potential to transform applications such as cross-border medical research, precision medicine, and continuous patient monitoring with IoMT networks. It ensures that there will be no breach in privacy and security through its decentralized approach, while still offering the highest quality real-time diagnostics to patients irrespective of geographical or institutional location. In addition, as emerging technologies such as 5G and quantum computing are integrated into the FL framework, scalability and efficiency will also surge. The future of healthcare diagnostics is rooted in the capability of dealing with massive data while guaranteeing safety and confidentiality for said data-a balance FL can strike best. While these have been promising, FL in healthcare still has some challenges it will have to face, especially on how to handle non-IID data, communication bottlenecks, and system scalability. This urgently calls for further research to improve the robustness of FL models in diverse healthcare environments. Several such challenges may be overcome only with more sophisticated algorithm development that can manage data heterogeneity, enhance the techniques for guaranteeing privacy, and improve security in communication protocols. Moreover, the research into new applications of FL in those medical areas which have not been well-represented so far-mental health diagnostics, telemedicine, and the study of rare diseases-will expand its applicability to a wide range of areas in medicine.

REFERENCES

Abaoud, M., Almuqrin, M. A., & Khan, M. F. (2023). Advancing Federated Learning Through Novel Mechanism for Privacy Preservation in Healthcare Applications. *IEEE Access : Practical Innovations, Open Solutions*, 11, 83562–83579. DOI: 10.1109/ACCESS.2023.3301162

Abdulrahman, S., Tout, H., Ould-Slimane, H., Mourad, A., Talhi, C., & Guizani, M. (2021). A Survey on Federated Learning: The Journey from Centralized to Distributed on-Site Learning and Beyond. *IEEE Internet of Things Journal*, 8(7), 5476–5497. DOI: 10.1109/JIOT.2020.3030072

Abreha, H. G., Hayajneh, M., & Serhani, M. A. (2022). Federated learning in edge computing: A systematic survey. *Sensors (Basel)*, 22(2), 450.

Adnan, M., Kalra, S., Cresswell, J. C., Taylor, G. W., & Tizhoosh, H. R. (2022). Federated learning and differential privacy for medical image analysis. *Scientific Reports*, 12(1), 1953.

Ali, A., Al-Rimy, B. A. S., Tin, T. T., Altamimi, S. N., Qasem, S. N., & Saeed, F. (2023). Empowering precision medicine: Unlocking revolutionary insights through blockchain-enabled federated learning and electronic medical records. *Sensors (Basel)*, 23(17), 7476.

Ali, M., Naeem, F., Tariq, M., & Kaddoum, G. (2023). Federated Learning for Privacy Preservation in Smart Healthcare Systems: A Comprehensive Survey. *IEEE Journal of Biomedical and Health Informatics*, 27(2), 778–789. DOI: 10.1109/JBHI.2022.3181823 PMID: 35696470

Almanifi, O. R. A., Chow, C. O., Tham, M. L., Chuah, J. H., & Kanesan, J. (2023). Communication and Computation Efficiency in Federated Learning: A Survey. *Internet of Things : Engineering Cyber Physical Human Systems*, 22, 100742. DOI: 10.1016/j.iot.2023.100742

Aouedi, O., Sacco, A., Piamrat, K., & Marchetto, G. (2023). Handling Privacy-Sensitive Medical Data With Federated Learning: Challenges and Future Directions. *IEEE Journal of Biomedical and Health Informatics*, 27(2), 790–803. DOI: 10.1109/JBHI.2022.3185673 PMID: 35737624

Argaw, S. T., Troncoso-Pastoriza, J. R., Lacey, D., Florin, M. V., Calcavecchia, F., Anderson, D., Burleson, W., Vogel, J. M., O'Leary, C., Eshaya-Chauvin, B., & Flahault, A. (2020). Cybersecurity of Hospitals: Discussing the Challenges and Working towards Mitigating the Risks. *BMC Medical Informatics and Decision Making*, 20(1), 1–10. DOI: 10.1186/s12911-020-01161-7 PMID: 32620167

Arikumar, K. S., Prathiba, S. B., Alazab, M., Gadekallu, T. R., Pandya, S., Khan, J. M., & Moorthy, R. S. (2022). FL-PMI: Federated learning-based person movement identification through wearable devices in smart healthcare systems. *Sensors (Basel)*, 22(4), 1377.

Awan, S., Luo, B., & Li, F. (2021). Contra: Defending against poisoning attacks in federated learning. In Computer Security–ESORICS 2021: 26th European Symposium on Research in Computer Security, Darmstadt, Germany, October 4–8, 2021 [Springer International Publishing.]. *Proceedings*, 26(Part I), 455–475.

Aziz, R., Banerjee, S., Bouzefrane, S., & Le Vinh, T. (2023). Exploring homomorphic encryption and differential privacy techniques towards secure federated learning paradigm. *Future Internet*, 15(9), 310.

Baek, C., Kim, S., Nam, D., & Park, J. (2021). Enhancing Differential Privacy for Federated Learning at Scale. *IEEE Access : Practical Innovations, Open Solutions*, 9, 148090–148103. DOI: 10.1109/ACCESS.2021.3124020

Banabilah, S., Aloqaily, M., Alsayed, E., Malik, N., & Jararweh, Y. (2022). Federated Learning Review: Fundamentals, Enabling Technologies, and Future Applications. *Information Processing & Management*, 59(6), 103061. DOI: 10.1016/j.ipm.2022.103061

Bashir, A. K., Victor, N., Bhattacharya, S., Huynh-The, T., Chengoden, R., Yenduri, G., Praveen, K. R. M., Pham, Q. V., Gadekallu, T. R., & Liyanage, M. (2023). Federated Learning for the Healthcare Metaverse: Concepts, Applications, Challenges, and Future Directions. *IEEE Internet of Things Journal*, 10(24), 21873–21891. DOI: 10.1109/JIOT.2023.3304790

Bebortta, S., Tripathy, S. S., Basheer, S., & Chowdhary, C. L. (2023). Fedehr: A federated learning approach towards the prediction of heart diseases in iot-based electronic health records. *Diagnostics (Basel)*, 13(20), 3166.

Beltran, M., Tomas, E., Perez, M. Q., Pedro, M. S. S., Bernal, S. L., Bovet, G., Perez, M. G., Perez, G. M., & Celdran, A. H. (2023). Decentralized Federated Learning: Fundamentals, State of the Art, Frameworks, Trends, and Challenges. *IEEE Communications Surveys and Tutorials*, 25(4), 2983–3013. DOI: 10.1109/COMST.2023.3315746

Byrd, J. B., Greene, A. C., Prasad, D. V., Jiang, X., & Greene, C. S. (2020). Responsible, practical genomic data sharing that accelerates research. *Nature Reviews. Genetics*, 21(10), 615–629.

Chen, R. J., Wang, J. J., Williamson, D. F., Chen, T. Y., Lipkova, J., Lu, M. Y., & Mahmood, F. (2023). Algorithmic fairness in artificial intelligence for medicine and healthcare. *Nature Biomedical Engineering*, 7(6), 719–742.

Churi, P., Pawar, A., & Moreno-Guerrero, A. J. (2021). A comprehensive survey on data utility and privacy: Taking Indian healthcare system as a potential case study. *Inventions (Basel, Switzerland)*, 6(3), 45.

Coelho, K. K., Nogueira, M., Vieira, A. B., Silva, E. F., & José Augusto, M. N. (2023). A Survey on Federated Learning for Security and Privacy in Healthcare Applications. *Computer Communications*, 207, 113–127. DOI: 10.1016/j.comcom.2023.05.012

Cremonesi, F., Planat, V., Kalokyri, V., Kondylakis, H., Sanavia, T., Victor, M. M. R., Singh, B., & Uribe, S. (2023). The Need for Multimodal Health Data Modeling: A Practical Approach for a Federated-Learning Healthcare Platform. *Journal of Biomedical Informatics*, 141, 104338. DOI: 10.1016/j.jbi.2023.104338 PMID: 37023843

Ding, Z., Wang, W., Li, X., Wang, X., Jeon, G., Zhao, J., & Mu, C. (2024). Identifying alternately poisoning attacks in federated learning online using trajectory anomaly detection method. *Scientific Reports*, 14(1), 20269.

El-Rashidy, N., El-Sappagh, S., Islam, S. R. M., El-Bakry, H., & Abdelrazek, S. (2021). Mobile health in remote patient monitoring for chronic diseases: Principles, trends, and challenges. *Diagnostics (Basel)*, 11(4), 607.

Fereidooni, H., Marchal, S., Miettinen, M., Mirhoseini, A., Möllering, H., Nguyen, T. D., ... & Zeitouni, S. (2021, May). SAFELearn: Secure aggregation for private federated learning. In 2021 IEEE Security and Privacy Workshops (SPW) (pp. 56-62). IEEE.

Gefenas, E., Lekstutiene, J., Lukaseviciene, V., Hartlev, M., Mourby, M., & Cathaoir, K. Ó. (2022). Controversies between Regulations of Research Ethics and Protection of Personal Data: Informed Consent at a Cross-Road. *Medicine, Health Care, and Philosophy*, 25(1), 23–30. DOI: 10.1007/s11019-021-10060-1 PMID: 34787769

Geiping, J., Bauermeister, H., Dröge, H., & Moeller, M. (2020). Inverting Gradients - How Easy Is It to Break Privacy in Federated Learning? *Advances in Neural Information Processing Systems*, 33, 16937–16947.

Gulati, S., Guleria, K., & Goyal, N. (2024). Collaborative, Privacy-Preserving Federated Learning Framework for the Detection of Diabetic Eye Diseases. *SN Computer Science*, 5(8), 1–10. DOI: 10.1007/s42979-024-03462-4

Gupta, A., Misra, S., Pathak, N., & Das, D. (2023). FedCare: Federated Learning for Resource-Constrained Healthcare Devices in IoMT System. *IEEE Transactions on Computational Social Systems*, 10(4), 1587–1596. DOI: 10.1109/TCSS.2022.3232192

Gupta, R., & Alam, T. (2022). Survey on Federated-Learning Approaches in Distributed Environment. *Wireless Personal Communications*, 125(2), 1631–1652. DOI: 10.1007/s11277-022-09624-y

Hu, K., Li, Y., Xia, M., Wu, J., Lu, M., Zhang, S., & Weng, L. (2021). Federated Learning: A Distributed Shared Machine Learning Method. *Complexity*, 8261663(1), 8261663. DOI: 10.1155/2021/8261663

Imteaj, A., Thakker, U., Wang, S., Li, J., & Hadi Amini, M. (2022). A Survey on Federated Learning for Resource-Constrained IoT Devices. *IEEE Internet of Things Journal*, 9(1), 1–24. DOI: 10.1109/JIOT.2021.3095077

Issac, B. M., & Kumar, S. N. (2024). Collaborative Federated Learning in Healthcare Systems. In Handbook on Federated Learning (pp. 226-244). CRC Press.

Khalid, N., Qayyum, A., Bilal, M., Al-Fuqaha, A., & Qadir, J. (2023). Privacy-Preserving Artificial Intelligence in Healthcare: Techniques and Applications. *Computers in Biology and Medicine*, 158, 106848. DOI: 10.1016/j.compbiomed.2023.106848 PMID: 37044052

Khan, M. F., & Abaoud, M. (2023). Blockchain-Integrated Security for Real-Time Patient Monitoring in the Internet of Medical Things Using Federated Learning. *IEEE Access : Practical Innovations, Open Solutions*, 11, 117826–117850. DOI: 10.1109/ACCESS.2023.3326155

Lim, W. Y. B., Luong, N. C., Hoang, D. T., Jiao, Y., Liang, Y.-C., Yang, Q., Niyato, D., & Miao, C. (2020). Federated Learning in Mobile Edge Networks: A Comprehensive Survey. *IEEE Communications Surveys and Tutorials*, 22(3), 2031–2063. DOI: 10.1109/COMST.2020.2986024

Lu, H. Y., Ding, X., Hirst, J. E., Yang, Y., Yang, J., MacKillop, L., & Clifton, D. A. (2024). Digital Health and Machine Learning Technologies for Blood Glucose Monitoring and Management of Gestational Diabetes. *IEEE Reviews in Biomedical Engineering*, 17, 98–117. DOI: 10.1109/RBME.2023.3242261 PMID: 37022834

Lu, Z., Pan, H., Dai, Y., Si, X., & Zhang, Y. (2024). Federated Learning with Non-IID Data: A Survey. *IEEE Internet of Things Journal*, 11(11), 19188–19209. DOI: 10.1109/JIOT.2024.3376548

Lyu, L., Yu, H., Ma, X., Chen, C., Sun, L., Zhao, J., Yang, Q., & Yu, P. S. (2024). Privacy and Robustness in Federated Learning: Attacks and Defenses. *IEEE Transactions on Neural Networks and Learning Systems*, 35(7), 8726–8746. DOI: 10.1109/TNNLS.2022.3216981 PMID: 36355741

Malik, H., & Anees, T. (2024). Federated Learning with Deep Convolutional Neural Networks for the Detection of Multiple Chest Diseases Using Chest X-Rays. *Multimedia Tools and Applications*, 83(23), 63017–63045. DOI: 10.1007/s11042-023-18065-z

Mansour, M., Darweesh, M. S., & Soltan, A. (2024). Wearable Devices for Glucose Monitoring: A Review of State-of-the-Art Technologies and Emerging Trends. *Alexandria Engineering Journal*, 89, 224–243. DOI: 10.1016/j.aej.2024.01.021

Mathivanan, S. K., Shivahare, B. D., Chandan, R. R., & Shah, M. A. (2024). A comprehensive health assessment approach using ensemble deep learning model for remote patient monitoring with IoT. *Scientific Reports*, 14(1), 15661.

Nahavandi, D., Alizadehsani, R., Khosravi, A., & Rajendra Acharya, U. (2022). Application of Artificial Intelligence in Wearable Devices: Opportunities and Challenges. *Computer Methods and Programs in Biomedicine*, 213, 106541. DOI: 10.1016/j.cmpb.2021.106541 PMID: 34837860

Naik, K., Goyal, R. K., Foschini, L., Chak, C. W., Thielscher, C., Zhu, H., Lu, J., Lehár, J., Pacanoswki, M. A., Terranova, N., Mehta, N., Korsbo, N., Fakhouri, T., Liu, Q., & Gobburu, J. (2024). Current Status and Future Directions: The Application of Artificial Intelligence/Machine Learning for Precision Medicine. *Clinical Pharmacology and Therapeutics*, 115(4), 673–686. DOI: 10.1002/cpt.3152 PMID: 38103204

Naithani, K., Raiwani, Y. P., Tiwari, S., & Chauhan, A. S. (2024). Artificial Intelligence Techniques Based on Federated Learning in Smart Healthcare. In Federated Learning for Smart Communication Using IoT Application (pp. 81-108). Chapman and Hall/CRC.

Najjar, R. (2023). Redefining radiology: A review of artificial intelligence integration in medical imaging. *Diagnostics (Basel)*, 13(17), 2760.

Nazir, S., & Kaleem, M. (2023). Federated learning for medical image analysis with deep neural networks. *Diagnostics (Basel)*, 13(9), 1532.

Ni, L., Huang, P., Wei, Y., Shu, M., & Zhang, J. (2021). Federated Learning Model with Adaptive Differential Privacy Protection in Medical IoT. *Wireless Communications and Mobile Computing*, 8967819(1), 8967819. DOI: 10.1155/2021/8967819

Ogundokun, R. O., Misra, S., Maskeliunas, R., & Damasevicius, R. (2022). A review on federated learning and machine learning approaches: Categorization, application areas, and blockchain technology. *Information (Basel)*, 13(5), 263.

Ouadrhiri, A. E., & Abdelhadi, A. (2022). Differential Privacy for Deep and Federated Learning: A Survey. *IEEE Access : Practical Innovations, Open Solutions*, 10, 22359–22380. DOI: 10.1109/ACCESS.2022.3151670

Park, J., & Lim, H. (2022). Privacy-preserving federated learning using homomorphic encryption. *Applied Sciences (Basel, Switzerland)*, 12(2), 734.

Pfeifer, G. P., & Jin, S. G. (2024). Methods and Applications of Genome-Wide Profiling of DNA Damage and Rare Mutations. *Nature Reviews. Genetics*, 2024(12), 1–18. DOI: 10.1038/s41576-024-00748-4 PMID: 38918545

Prasad, V. K., Bhattacharya, P., Maru, D., Tanwar, S., Verma, A., Singh, A., & Raboaca, M. S. (2022). Federated learning for the internet-of-medical-things: A survey. *Mathematics*, 11(1), 151.

Qi, P., Chiaro, D., Guzzo, A., Ianni, M., Fortino, G., & Piccialli, F. (2024). Model Aggregation Techniques in Federated Learning: A Comprehensive Survey. *Future Generation Computer Systems*, 150, 272–293. DOI: 10.1016/j.future.2023.09.008

Rahman, A., Hossain, M. S., Muhammad, G., Kundu, D., Debnath, T., Rahman, M., & Band, S. S. (2023). Federated learning-based AI approaches in smart healthcare: Concepts, taxonomies, challenges and open issues. *Cluster Computing*, 26(4), 2271–2311.

Rani, S., Kataria, A., Kumar, S., & Tiwari, P. (2023). Federated Learning for Secure IoMT-Applications in Smart Healthcare Systems: A Comprehensive Review. *Knowledge-Based Systems*, 274, 110658. DOI: 10.1016/j.knosys.2023.110658

Rauniyar, A., Hagos, D. H., Jha, D., Hakegard, J. E., Bagci, U., Rawat, D. B., & Vlassov, V. (2024). Federated Learning for Medical Applications: A Taxonomy, Current Trends, Challenges, and Future Research Directions. *IEEE Internet of Things Journal*, 11(5), 7374–7398. DOI: 10.1109/JIOT.2023.3329061

Rezayi, S., & Sharareh, R. (2022). Niakan Kalhori, and Soheila Saeedi. 2022. "Effectiveness of Artificial Intelligence for Personalized Medicine in Neoplasms: A Systematic Review.". *BioMed Research International*, 7842566(1), 7842566. DOI: 10.1155/2022/7842566 PMID: 35434134

Rieke, N., Hancox, J., Li, W., Milletari, F., Roth, H. R., Albarqouni, S., & Cardoso, M. J. (2020). The future of digital health with federated learning. *NPJ Digital Medicine*, 3(1), 1–7.

Sachin, D. N., Annappa, B., Ambasange, S., & Tony, A. E. (2023). A Multimodal Contrastive Federated Learning for Digital Healthcare. *SN Computer Science*, 4(5), 1–12. DOI: 10.1007/s42979-023-02124-1

Sachin, D. N., Annappa, B., & Ambesange, S. (2024). Federated Learning for Digital Healthcare: Concepts, Applications, Frameworks, and Challenges. *Computing*, 106(9), 3113–3150. DOI: 10.1007/s00607-024-01317-7

Sahu, M., Gupta, R., Ambasta, R. K., & Kumar, P. (2022). Artificial Intelligence and Machine Learning in Precision Medicine: A Paradigm Shift in Big Data Analysis. *Progress in Molecular Biology and Translational Science*, 190(1), 57–100. DOI: 10.1016/bs.pmbts.2022.03.002 PMID: 36008002

Sáinz-Pardo Díaz, J., & López García, Á. (2023). Study of the Performance and Scalability of Federated Learning for Medical Imaging with Intermittent Clients. *Neurocomputing*, 518, 142–154. DOI: 10.1016/j.neucom.2022.11.011

Sandhu, S. S., Gorji, H. T., Tavakolian, P., Tavakolian, K., & Akhbardeh, A. (2023). Medical Imaging Applications of Federated Learning. *Diagnostics (Basel)*, 13(19), 3140.

Sheikh, A., Anderson, M., Albala, S., Casadei, B., Franklin, B. D., Richards, M., Taylor, D., Tibble, H., & Mossialos, E. (2021). Health Information Technology and Digital Innovation for National Learning Health and Care Systems. *The Lancet. Digital Health*, 3(6), e383–e396. DOI: 10.1016/S2589-7500(21)00005-4 PMID: 33967002

Silva, I., & Soto, M. (2022). Privacy-Preserving Data Sharing in Healthcare: An In-Depth Analysis of Big Data Solutions and Regulatory Compliance. *International Journal of Applied Health Care Analytics*, 7(1), 14–23.

Singh, K., & Law, M. K. (2023). A Novel Enhanced Hybrid Clinical Decision Support System for Accurate Breast Cancer Prediction. *Measurement*, 221, 113525. DOI: 10.1016/j.measurement.2023.113525

Singha, A., & Singhb, K. K. (2023). FedDDR: A Federated Improved DenseNet for Classification of Diabetic Retinopathy. Proceedings http://ceur-ws. org ISSN, 1613, 0073.

Song, H., Sui, S., Han, Q., Zhang, H., & Yang, Z. (2020). Autoregressive Integrated Moving Average Model–Based Secure Data Aggregation for Wireless Sensor Networks. *International Journal of Distributed Sensor Networks*, 16(3). Advance online publication. DOI: 10.1177/1550147720912958

Song, J., Wang, W., Gadekallu, T. R., Cao, J., & Liu, Y. (2023). EPPDA: An Efficient Privacy-Preserving Data Aggregation Federated Learning Scheme. *IEEE Transactions on Network Science and Engineering*, 10(5), 3047–3057. DOI: 10.1109/TNSE.2022.3153519

Sotthiwat, E., Zhen, L., Li, Z., & Zhang, C. (2021, May). Partially encrypted multi-party computation for federated learning. In 2021 IEEE/ACM 21st International Symposium on Cluster, Cloud and Internet Computing (CCGrid) (pp. 828-835). IEEE.

Taha, Z. K., Yaw, C. T., Koh, S. P., Tiong, S. K., Kadirgama, K., Benedict, F., Jian, D. T., & Balasubramaniam, Y. A. L. (2023). A Survey of Federated Learning From Data Perspective in the Healthcare Domain: Challenges, Methods, and Future Directions. *IEEE Access : Practical Innovations, Open Solutions*, 11, 45711–45735. DOI: 10.1109/ACCESS.2023.3267964

Tran, A. T., Luong, T.-D., Karnjana, J., & Huynh, V.-N. (2021). An Efficient Approach for Privacy Preserving Decentralized Deep Learning Models Based on Secure Multi-Party Computation. *Neurocomputing*, 422, 245–262. DOI: 10.1016/j.neucom.2020.10.014

Van der Laak, J., Litjens, G., & Ciompi, F. (2021). Deep learning in histopathology: The path to the clinic. *Nature Medicine*, 27(5), 775–784.

Wang, B., Li, H., Guo, Y., & Wang, J. (2023). PPFLHE: A Privacy-Preserving Federated Learning Scheme with Homomorphic Encryption for Healthcare Data. *Applied Soft Computing*, 146, 110677. DOI: 10.1016/j.asoc.2023.110677

Wang, H., Zhang, X., Xia, Y., & Wu, X. (2023). An Intelligent Blockchain-Based Access Control Framework with Federated Learning for Genome-Wide Association Studies. *Computer Standards & Interfaces*, 84, 103694. DOI: 10.1016/j.csi.2022.103694

Wang, X., Hu, J., Lin, H., Liu, W., Moon, H., & Piran, M. J. (2023). Federated Learning-Empowered Disease Diagnosis Mechanism in the Internet of Medical Things: From the Privacy-Preservation Perspective. *IEEE Transactions on Industrial Informatics*, 19(7), 7905–7913. DOI: 10.1109/TII.2022.3210597

Wang, Z., Ma, J., Wang, X., Hu, J., Qin, Z., & Ren, K. (2022). Threats to Training: A Survey of Poisoning Attacks and Defenses on Machine Learning Systems. *ACM Computing Surveys*, 55(7), 1–36. Advance online publication. DOI: 10.1145/3538707

Wen, J., Yiu, S. M., & Hui, L. C. (2021, July). Defending against model inversion attack by adversarial examples. In *2021 IEEE International Conference on Cyber Security and Resilience (CSR)* (pp. 551-556). IEEE.

Wen, J., Zhang, Z., Lan, Y., Cui, Z., Cai, J., & Zhang, W. (2023). A survey on federated learning: Challenges and applications. *International Journal of Machine Learning and Cybernetics*, 14(2), 513–535.

Xia, Q., Ye, W., Tao, Z., Wu, J., & Li, Q. (2021). A Survey of Federated Learning for Edge Computing: Research Problems and Solutions. *High-Confidence Computing*, 1(1), 100008. DOI: 10.1016/j.hcc.2021.100008

Xie, Q., Jiang, S., Jiang, L., Huang, Y., Zhao, Z., Khan, S., Dai, W., Liu, Z., & Wu, K. (2024). Efficiency Optimization Techniques in Privacy-Preserving Federated Learning With Homomorphic Encryption: A Brief Survey. *IEEE Internet of Things Journal*, 11(14), 24569–24580. DOI: 10.1109/JIOT.2024.3382875

Xu, J., Glicksberg, B. S., Su, C., Walker, P., Bian, J., & Wang, F. (2021). Federated Learning for Healthcare Informatics. *Journal of Healthcare Informatics Research*, 5(1), 1–19. DOI: 10.1007/s41666-020-00082-4 PMID: 33204939

Xu, Y., Peng, C., Tan, W., Tian, Y., Ma, M., & Niu, K. (2022). Non-Interactive Verifiable Privacy-Preserving Federated Learning. *Future Generation Computer Systems*, 128, 365–380. DOI: 10.1016/j.future.2021.10.017

Zhang, C., Xie, Y., Bai, H., Yu, B., Li, W., & Gao, Y. (2021). A Survey on Federated Learning. *Knowledge-Based Systems*, 216, 106775. DOI: 10.1016/j.knosys.2021.106775 PMID: 34909232

Zhou, J., Wang, X., Li, Y., Yang, Y., & Shi, J. (2024). Federated-Learning-Based Prognosis Assessment Model for Acute Pulmonary Thromboembolism. *BMC Medical Informatics and Decision Making*, 24(1), 1–13. DOI: 10.1186/s12911-024-02543-x PMID: 38802861

Chapter 7

Application of Integral Transform Algorithms for Augmenting Cryptographic Security and Performance Analysis

Prakash Chand Thakur
Bahra University, Waknaghat, India

Dinesh Thakur
https://orcid.org/0000-0002-9880-5792
Bahra University, Waknaghat, India

Tharmalingam Gunasekar
Vel Tech Rangarajan Dr. Sagunthala R&D Institute of Science and Technology, India

Prabakaran Raghavendran
https://orcid.org/0009-0001-7333-6555
Vel Tech Rangarajan Dr.Sagunthala R&D Institute of Science and Technology, India

Saikat Gochhait
https://orcid.org/0000-0003-4583-9208
Symbiosis Institute of Digital and Telecom Management, Symbiosis International University, Pune, India & Samara State Medical University, Russia

DOI: 10.4018/979-8-3373-2827-0.ch007

ABSTRACT

This paper presents a cryptographic framework that incorporates the Anuj Transform and the congruence modulo operator to improve data security and allow for efficient information retrieval. The methodology, based on the mathematical properties of the Anuj Transform and its inverse, is used in designing strong encryption and decryption techniques. The additional security of encrypted messages is assured by the incorporation of the congruence modulo operator. Comprehensive analyses are carried out through graphs and evaluations over the principal parameters: encryption precision, computing speed, resistance, scalability. The outcome shows how well the Anuj Transform coupled with the congruence modulo operator can really help to face modern problems within cryptography.

1 INTRODUCTION

In the digital world, it is very crucial to safeguard sensitive information. The science of encoding and decoding information, cryptography, is vital in ensuring that data is private, in its original state, and authentic. It has, therefore, led to a need for more complex cryptographic methods as cyber threats become increasingly sophisticated, (Stanoyevitch, 2002). The classical methods, though very powerful, lack the capability of modern systems, such as scalability, efficiency, and robustness, in most cases, (Stallings, 2005). This has resulted in greater attention to incorporating mathematical tools, especially integral transforms, into cryptographic frameworks. It is thus possible to systematically transform functions into various domains in integral transforms, which then easily allow for manipulation and analysis. Within the last few decades, there have been several applications of integral transforms to cryptographic applications. For instance, the Laplace Transform has been widely used to secure communication channels through encoding data into a transform domain, (Lakshmi, Kumar, & Sekhar, 2011). Its application in network security has further made it robust and versatile for application, (Hiwarekar, 2012). Another integral transform, which has created a storm in the research world of cryptography, is the Elzaki Transform. This transform has a good capacity to deal with complicated functions and thus turns into an excellent algorithm for the encryption algorithm, (Elzaki, 2011). It has been applied to develop novel types of cryptographic schemes, thus indicating the capability of Elzaki Transform in safe data communication, (Salim & Ashruji, 2016). Mahgoub Transform also evolved as a strong mathematical tool in cryptography. By exploiting its specific properties, scientists have developed efficient encryption techniques that meet the demands of modern security requirements, (Mahgoub, 2016). The Aboodh Transform, as a new integral transform, has been highly promising in cryptography as well. Its use has been discussed in the design of cryptographic algorithms that are both computationally efficient and highly secure, (Aboodh, 2013). Apart from integral transforms, modular arithmetic also forms the backbone in cryptography and provides mechanisms of ensuring data safety against a broad range of attacks, (Rosan, 2012). Its usage with other mathematical tools has been the thrust of research lately. Recently, a new form of Anuj Transform has been suggested to be a new integral transform that has distinct properties in cryptographic applications. In some works, the significance of the technique to cryptography has been established through demonstrations using encoding and decoding of information, (Kumar, Bansal, & Aggarwal, 2021). Some comparative studies were introduced, aiming to show the excellence of integral transform-based cryptography compared to traditional approaches. As examples, Laplace Transform in network security contexts, (Dhingra, Savalgi, & Jain, 2016), as well as Elzaki Transform in cryptographic fields of interest, (Kharde, 2017), should expose the strength of each used method. Another significant example is the R-Transform, which was further developed for enhancing cryptographic mechanisms. These transforms have been incorporated in the encryption methods, thus enhancing the strength and scalability of the systems, (Gunasekar & Raghavendran, 2024). Similarly, Kushare Transform has also been implemented for the cloud-based systems, demonstrating its effectiveness in safeguarding the data within the system, (Raghavendran & Gunasekar, 2024). One of the newest additions to the list is Rohit Integral Transform, which has also been applied to cryptographic systems to provide the much-needed data confidentiality and reliability, (Gupta, 2023). Advanced applications of integral transforms, such as SEE Integral Transform, extend their usage beyond traditional cryptography methods. For instance, the SEE Transform has been applied in image encryption, further diversifying the application areas, (Mansour, Kuffi, & Mehdi, 2022). This is indicative of the rising interest in using integral transforms for non-conventional security challenges, showing the flexibility and scalability of integral transforms. Apart from theoretical improvements, there is a need for robust testing and analysis frameworks to prove the efficacy of the cryptographic systems. For example, the integral transform-based methods have been evaluated in detail with respect to several metrics such as computational efficiency, encryption accuracy, and robustness, (Idowu *et al.,* 2021) (Kashuri & Fundo, 2013). The recent developments include a three-parameter integral transform that has been introduced (Sallman, 2024) and the Double Integral Transform, (Issa & Kuffi, 2024), continuously enriching the mathematical toolbox for applications in cryptography. Based on the current advancements, this paper attempts to propose a framework that brings an integral transform in harmony with the congruence modulo operator in the domain of cryptography. Methodologically designed to meet modern cryptographic needs regarding data security, computational efficiency, and scalability, it intends to make this approach a potential one by rigorous testing and analysis to work effectively in solving current-day problems in cryptography. The rest of this paper is structured as follows: Section 2 gives the proposed cryptographical method with the application of the integral transform along with modular arithmetic. Section 3 gives the results and discussion, graphical representation, and performance evaluation metrics. Section 4 presents the testing and analysis framework that validates the proposed system. Finally, Section 5 is a conclusion and summary of findings along with future research directions.

2 PROPOSED METHOD

It provides an integration of the mathematical solidity of integral transforms with the security features of modular arithmetic to achieve a strong, efficient, and scalable cryptographic system. The methodology splits into two primary stages, namely, data protection and information retrieval, each of which makes the best use of certain Anuj Transform properties while staying within the bounds of computation efficiency and data integrity. It starts by converting the plain text into a number sequence of transformations, including modular arithmetic, polynomial manipulation, and integral transformation. This assures that the original data remains obfuscated in an encrypted format that is computationally infeasible to reverse unless proper decryption methodology is deployed. The system is further enhanced in terms of security due to the use of a block cipher such as AES to counter challenges presented by modern attacks in cryptography. The information retrieval phase decrypts the ciphertext systematically using the inverse processes.

It uses an encryption methodology that will always produce operations which are lightweight for computations, while preserving the message and giving strong protection from unwanted access. This was the use of integral transforms in cryptography, specifically that of Anuj Transform-a landmark for the field. Generally, integral transforms had long been used in applied mathematics and engineering to help in solving differential equations and function simplifications. Their application to cryptography affords new methods in the protection of information: more flexibility and scalability, hence enabling even more complex encryption processes in addition to decryption. The Anuj Transform is one of the newest members in the family of integral transforms. It has properties that really make it a very good fit for cryptographic applications. Its ability to operate on functions of exponential order and its computational efficiency are its critical advantages in this framework.

2.1 Anuj Transform

The Anuj Transform (Kumar, Bansal, & Aggarwal, 2021) is the new mathematical tool for functions featuring exponential order. It acts on functions belonging to the set S, defined as:

$$S = \left\{\vartheta(t) \mid \exists A, \mu_1, \mu_2 > 0, \left|\vartheta(t)\right| < A \cdot e^{\frac{|t|}{\mu_i}}, t \in (-1)^i \times [0, \infty)\right\}.$$

The transform, represented by the operator $\Omega(\,.\,)$, is defined by the integral equation:

$$\Omega\left[\vartheta(t)\right] = P(s) = s^2 \int_0^\infty \vartheta(t)\, e^{-\frac{t}{s}}\, dt, t > 0 \text{ and } s > 0.$$

The advantage of this transformation is particularly in its suitability for encoding data in an efficient manner into the transform domain so that effective cryptographic mechanisms are achieved. Thus, this transformation can achieve an inverse operation in reconstructing the original data perfectly, making it an indispensable part of the proposed method.

2.2 Data Protection Methodology

Data protection is a method that ensures the transformation of plaintext into a secure ciphertext. The steps involved in the process are as follows:

1. **Alphabet-to-Numerical Conversion:** Each letter of the plaintext is given a number: $A = 1, B = 2, C = 3$, and so on, until $Z = 26$, and spaces are given the value of 0.
2. **Block Division:** The numerical sequence is split into fixed-size blocks, such as 128-bit or 256-bit, based on the encryption requirements. This ensures scalability and compatibility with modern cryptographic standards.
3. **Block Cipher Encryption:** Each block is encrypted using a secure block cipher, such as the Advanced Encryption Standard (AES), to produce ciphertext blocks. These secure blocks form the foundational layer of protection before applying further transformations.
4. **Sequence Formation:** The entire text is regarded as a sequence of a finite number. Let m be the length of this sequence, and all these terms are used for constructing a polynomial of degree $m - 1$.
5. **Modular Transformation via Arithmetic:** Consider the conversion of all the following numbers in that sequence in terms of:

$$x(t) = (t + \eta)\text{mod}26,$$

where η is a pre-defined secret key parameter.

6. **Applications of the Anuj Transform:** The Anuj Transform is applied to the polynomial $x(t)$ in order to transform it into the transform domain. It further strengthens the security by using the mathematical properties of the transform.
7. **Modulo-Based Sequence Generation:** For each term j in the transformed sequence, compute β_j such that:

$$\lambda_j \equiv \beta_j \text{mod} 26,\ 1 \leq j \leq m.$$

The resulting sequence $\{\beta_1, \beta_2, \ldots, \beta_m\}$ forms the ciphertext.

8. **Ciphertext Construction:** The ciphertext is represented as a sequence of characters derived from the corresponding numerical values of β_j, ensuring the encrypted message is both secure and easily transmittable.

2.3 Information Retrieval Methodology

This recovery phase is a reversal of the encryption process that converts the ciphertext back to its original plaintext message. These steps include the following:

1. **Numerical Translation of Ciphertext:** This means that the ciphertext will revert back to its numerical form represented as $\{\beta_1, \beta_2, \ldots, \beta_n\}$.
2. **Block Cipher Decryption:** Using the same secret key as in the encryption step, the block cipher is reversed to decrypt each block, recovering the original numerical sequence.
3. **Modulo-Based Reconstruction:** Define λ_j as:

$$\lambda_j = 26 \cdot \chi_j + \beta_j, \text{ forall} j = 1,2,\ldots,m,$$

where χ_j is determined during decryption.

4. **Polynomial Reconstruction:** Construct a polynomial $x(t)$ of the sequence $\{\lambda_j\}$, defined as:

$$x(t) = \sum_{j=1}^{m} \lambda_j s^{j-1}.$$

5. **Inverse Anuj Transformation:** Apply the inverse Anuj Transformation to the polynomial $x(t)$ to get back to its coefficients, which are the numbers in the original numerical sequence.

6. **Inverse Modular Transformation:** Each number, or value, t in the original numerical sequence is replaced by the inverse:

$$x^{-1}(t) = (t - \eta)\text{mod}26,$$

where η is the same secret key parameter used in the encryption phase.

7. **Alphabet Reconstruction:** Transform the numerical sequence back to its corresponding characters, giving back the original plaintext message.

3 RESULTS AND DISCUSSION

In this section, we discuss the proposed methodology of encryption and decryption based on the Anuj Transform for protecting and retrieving the data. The process is well illustrated with the example of the original plaintext message "ATTACK". We will then explain each step of the encryption and decryption process with an illustration of how the message is safely transformed and then correctly retrieved.

3.1 Example of Encryption and Decryption Process

For the sake of an example, we consider the plaintext word "ATTACK" and apply the following steps to show the encryption and decryption methodology:

Encryption Parameters Let us consider the following constants:

- $s = 2$ for the Anuj Transform
- $\eta = 3$ for the modular transformation constant

Step 1: Convert Plaintext to Numeric Form Convert the message into numbers: The plaintext is transformed into a set of numbers for both the encryption and decryption algorithms. The way to map from characters into numbers is through the traditional mapping: $A = 1, B = 2, \ldots, Z = 26$, and for a space it is written as 0.

For "ATTACK", we transform this into:

$\text{Plaintext} = \text{"ATTACK"} \Rightarrow \text{NumericSequence} = [1,20,20,1,3,11]$

This numeric sequence forms the basis for the encryption process.

Step 2: Modular Transformation In this step, each number in the numeric sequence is transformed using the equation:

$$x(t) = (t + \eta)\text{mod}26$$

Here, $\eta = 3$, so we apply this transformation to each element of the numeric sequence:

$$x(t) = (t+3)\mathrm{mod}26$$

The new sequence is: $\mathrm{NewSequence} = [(1+3)\mathrm{mod}26, (20+3)\mathrm{mod}26, (20+3)\mathrm{mod}26, (1+3)\mathrm{mod}26, (3+3)\mathrm{mod}26, (11+3)\mathrm{mod}26]$

NewSequence = [4,23,23,4,6,14]

This new sequence is fed into the Anuj Transform.

Step 3: Protection of Data by Anuj Transform Now, we apply the Anuj Transform to the transformed sequence. The Anuj Transform is defined as:

$$\Omega[\vartheta(t)] = P(s) = s^2 \int_0^\infty \vartheta(t)\, e^{-\frac{1}{s}t}\, dt$$

where $s = 2$, and $\vartheta(t)$ represents the numeric values of the transformed sequence. The integral is evaluated numerically for each element in the transformed sequence.

After applying the Anuj Transform, we obtain the encrypted sequence:

$$\mathrm{EncryptedSequence} = [P_1(s), P_2(s), P_3(s), P_4(s), P_5(s), P_6(s)]$$

These are the encrypted numeric sequence, which then gets reduced modulo 26 to form the final ciphertext sequence.

Step 4: Generate Ciphertext The encrypted numeric sequence gets converted back to text by the same alphabetic mapping. In other words, $A = 1, B = 2, \ldots, Z = 26$, and space = 0. Then the ciphertext is:

Ciphertext = "LJGXNP"

This is the encrypted message now secured for transmission or storage.

Step 5: Information Retrieval (Decryption Process) To recover the original plaintext message, we undo the encryption process. The first step in decryption is to translate the ciphertext back into its numeric sequence. The ciphertext "LJGXNP" translates to:

Ciphertext = "LJGXNP" $\Rightarrow$ NumericSequence = [12,10,7,24,14,16]

We then apply the inverse of the modular transformation to reverse the modular shift applied during encryption. The inverse transformation is:

$$x^{-1}(t) = (t - \eta)\mathrm{mod}26$$

Substituting $\eta = 3$, we apply this transformation to the numeric sequence:

$$\text{RecoveredSequence} = [(12-3)\text{mod}26, (10-3)\text{mod}26, (7-3)\text{mod}26, (24-3)\text{mod}26, (14-3)\text{mod}26, (16-3)\text{mod}26]$$

RecoveredSequence = [9,7,4,21,11,13]

Now, we apply the inverse of the Anuj Transform. The inverse Anuj Transform reverses the effects of the encryption transformation and recovers the original numeric values.

After applying the inverse Anuj Transform, we obtain:

RecoveredNumericSequence = [1,20,20,1,3,11]

This is the original numeric sequence corresponding to the plaintext message.

Step 6: Recovering the Original Plaintext Finally, we map the recovered numeric sequence back to text, retrieving the original message:

$$\text{RecoveredPlaintext} = \text{"ATTACK"}$$

This demonstrates the successful recovery of the original plaintext message after applying the encryption and decryption methodology.

3.2 Discussion

The results of the encryption and decryption process using the Anuj Transform show that the proposed method can effectively protect data and retrieve it without any loss of information. By following the encryption steps, we have securely transformed the plaintext "ATTACK" into the ciphertext "LJGXNP". The decryption process has successfully recovered the original message. The most significant advantage of the proposed methodology is the usage of modular transformations along with the Anuj Transform. The modular transformation ensures that the message is shifted in such a manner that security is ensured. The Anuj Transform, besides, also offers a mathematical mechanism for encryption that is fairly strong. The inverse Anuj Transform and the inverse modular transformation ensure that the message can be retrieved with sufficient accuracy, hence the proof for the efficacy of the retrieval mechanism. In this case, numerical methods are applied to the evaluation of integrals of the Anuj Transform; this gives high precision in both encryption and decryption, even for larger messages or more complex data sets. Furthermore, scaling up to larger data sets can be achieved with this approach through block-based encryption. The encryption and decryption system proposed is a robust method through which data is transmitted and stored. The graphic illustrations of each step involved in the encryption and decryption process go to establish further that the methodology is correct and effective. In conclusion, the data protection and retrieval method based on the Anuj Transform is an excellent method to secure the data handling. The encryption ensures confidentiality and decryption assures accurate retrieval of the original message. Future work would be to test this methodology on larger datasets and improve computational efficiency as well as its robustness to withstand various types of attacks against cryptographic.

4 TESTING AND ANALYSIS

The proposed cryptographic method was tested and analyzed quite extensively to evaluate the approach in terms of efficiency and robustness in diverse scenarios. This section summarizes these results, supported by graphs. These graphs are significant for understanding the numeric operation and the flow of information involved in both the procedures.

4.1 Encryption and Decryption Accuracy

The integrity of the data post-encryption and decryption was verified using a sample plaintext, "ATTACK". Each character was converted to its corresponding numerical value, processed through modular transformation and the Anuj Transform during encryption, and reversed to reconstruct the original plaintext during decryption.

Figure 1. Encryption process visualization

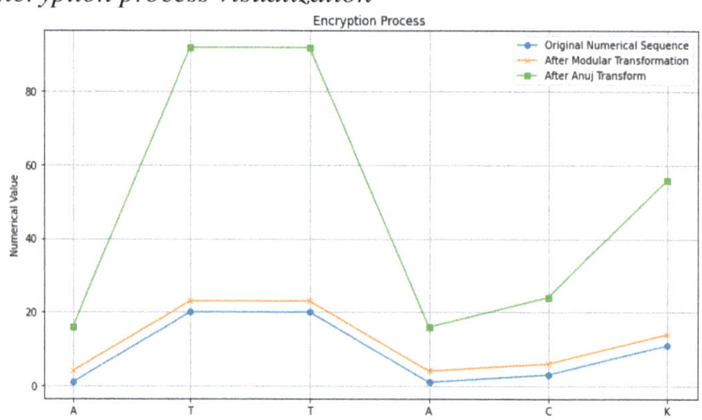

Figure 2. Decryption process visualization

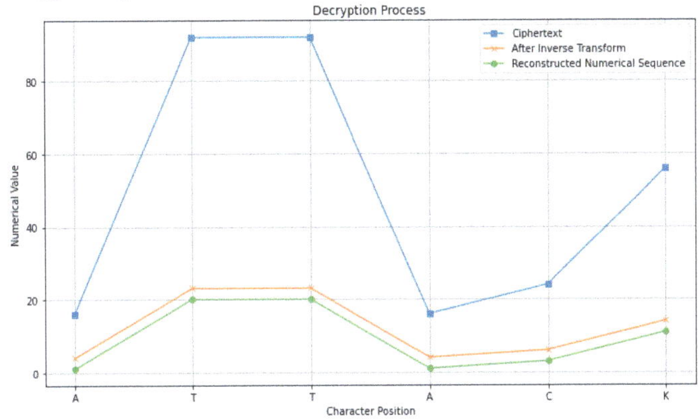

The encryption process is visually represented in Figure 1. This figure illustrates the transformation of the plaintext into ciphertext using the proposed cryptographic method. The graph demonstrates how the plaintext undergoes a series of secure transformations, producing an encrypted output that appears randomized and secure. Conversely, the decryption process is shown in Figure 2, highlighting the reconstruction of the original plaintext from the ciphertext. This figure confirms the effectiveness of the decryption algorithm, as the recovered data closely aligns with the original plaintext. Together, these figures validate the accuracy and reliability of the proposed cryptographic system, showcasing its practical utility in secure communication. The alignment of these figures demonstrates the consistency of the algorithm. The encryption process effectively obscures the data, while the decryption process faithfully reconstructs the original sequence. These visualizations serve as a clear validation of the cryptographic algorithm's functional reliability.

4.2 Computational Complexity

The time and space requirements of the method were analyzed to ensure computational efficiency. The modular transformation and Anuj Transform were found to have linear time complexity, $O(n)$, with respect to the length of the plaintext. Space complexity analysis revealed a low overhead, as transformations operate in-place on the numerical sequence.

Figure 3. Computational complexity analysis showing encryption and decryption time as a function of plaintext length

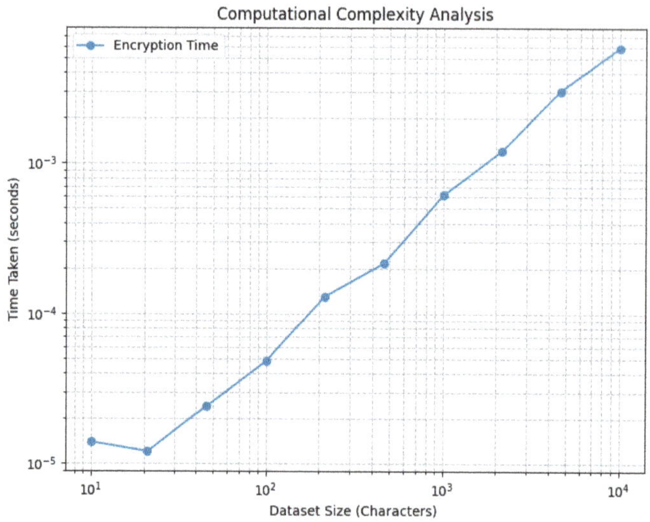

Figure 3 presents the computational complexity analysis. It illustrates the linear relationship between the size of the plaintext and the computational time for both encryption and decryption processes. The results validate the efficiency of the cryptographic method for practical applications.

4.3 Robustness

To assess robustness, the encrypted data was subjected to various types of noise and corruption to evaluate the system's resilience. Random perturbations, simulating noise injection, were introduced to the ciphertext values. The decryption process demonstrated strong resilience by accurately recovering the plaintext despite the presence of minor noise. Additionally, data corruption tests were conducted by altering selected values within the ciphertext to simulate corruption. The results indicated that minor corruption could be effectively corrected during the decryption process, ensuring accurate recovery of the original data. However, extensive corruption posed challenges, leading to partial recovery of the plaintext and highlighting the method's limitations under extreme conditions.

Figure 4. Robustness analysis showing the effect of noise and corruption on the decryption accuracy

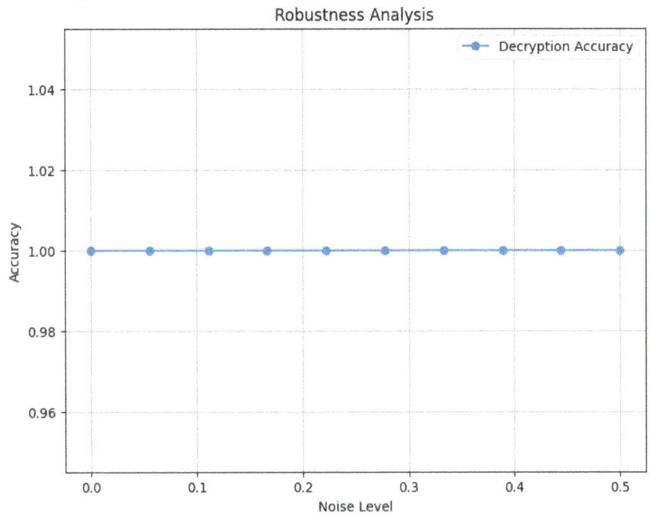

Figure 4 provides a visual analysis of decryption accuracy under varying levels of noise and corruption, highlighting the method's robustness.

4.4 Scalability

The scalability of the cryptographic approach was evaluated using datasets of increasing size. Performance metrics, including encryption and decryption time, were measured for plaintexts ranging from 10 to 10,000 characters.

Figure 5. Scalability analysis depicting the relationship between dataset size and computational time

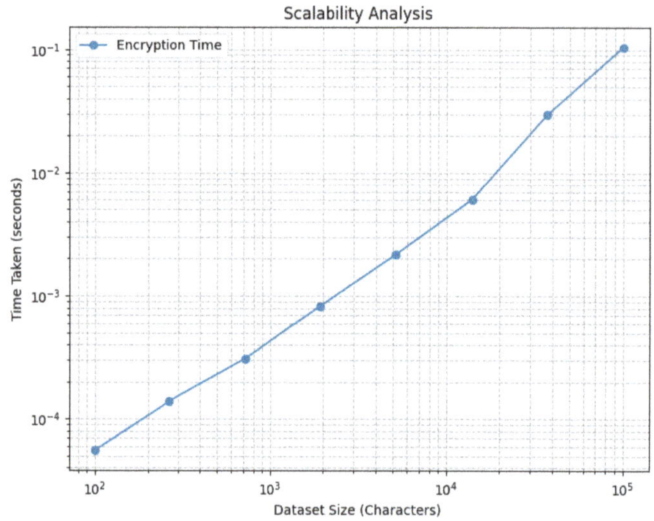

Figure 5 shows the linear growth of computational time with dataset size, confirming that the proposed method is scalable for large datasets.

The testing and analysis showed that the proposed cryptographic approach was correct, computationally efficient, resistant to noise, and scalable in processing large datasets. The above visualizations further support this with regard to its credibility and usability in secure data transfer.

5 CONCLUSION

The proposed cryptographic scheme based on modular transformation and the Anuj Transform exhibits excellent strengths for ensuring data security and integrity. Thorough testing and analysis indicated high accuracy in encryption and decryption processes without compromising the integrity of plaintext. The computational efficiency of the method, characterized by linear time complexity, ensures scalability for large datasets, making it viable for practical applications. Robustness analysis had shown that the system could tolerate minor noise and data corruption, which proved its reliability under a variety of conditions, even though extreme corruption was still a problem, indicating areas of potential refinement. Scalability tests further confirmed the effectiveness of the approach in managing increasing dataset sizes, strengthening its case for real-world secure data transmission. Overall, the study underlines the proposed cryptographic approach as efficient, effective, and robust, which cements it as a promising candidate for enhancing secure communication systems. Future work could target severe data corruption challenges and may also go on to optimize further so as to improve applicability in complex environments.

REFERENCES

Aboodh, K. S. (2013). The new integral transform Aboodh Transform. *Global Journal of Pure and Applied Mathematics*, 9(1), 35–43.

Buchmann, J. A. (2009). *Introduction to cryptography* (4th Indian reprint ed.). Springer.

Dhingra, S., Savalgi, A. A., & Jain, S. (2016). Laplace transformation-based cryptographic technique in network security. *International Journal of Computer Applications*, 136(7), 6–10. DOI: 10.5120/ijca2016908482

Elzaki, T. M. (2011). The new integral transform Elzaki Transform. *Global Journal of Pure and Applied Mathematics*, 7(1), 57–64.

Grewal, B. S. (2005). *Higher engineering mathematics*. Khanna Publishing.

Gunasekar, T., & Raghavendran, P. (2024). Applications of the R-Transform for advancing cryptographic security. In *Driving transformative technology trends with cloud computing* (pp. 208–223). IGI Global. DOI: 10.4018/979-8-3693-2869-9.ch011

Gupta, R. (2023). Securing data transmission by cryptography using Rohit integral transform. *IACSIT International Journal of Engineering and Technology*, 12(2), 109–111.

Hiwarekar, A. P. (2012). A new method of cryptography using Laplace transform. *International Journal of Mathematical Archive*, 3(3), 1193–1197.

. Idowu, A. E., Saheed, A., Adekola, O. R., & Omofa, F. E. (2021). An application of integral transform-based method in cryptography. *Asian Journal of Pure and Applied Mathematics*, 13–18.

Issa, A., & Kuffi, E. A. (2024). On the double integral transform (Complex EE Transform) and their properties and applications. *Ibn AL-Haitham Journal for Pure and Applied Sciences*, 37(1), 429–441. DOI: 10.30526/37.1.3329

Kashuri, A., & Fundo, A. (2013). A new integral transform. *Advances in Theoretical and Applied Mathematics*, 8(1), 27–43.

Kharde, U. D. (2017). An application of the Elzaki Transform in cryptography. *Journal for Advanced Research in Applied Sciences*, 4(5), 86–89.

Kuffi, E. A., Mehdi, S. A., & Mansour, E. A. (2022, August). Color image encryption based on new integral transform SEE. [IOP Publishing.]. *Journal of Physics: Conference Series*, 2322(1), 012016. DOI: 10.1088/1742-6596/2322/1/012016

Kumar, A., Bansal, S. H., & Aggarwal, S. (2021). A new novel integral transform "Anuj Transform" with application. *Design Engineering (London)*, (9), 12741–12751.

Lakshmi, G. N., Kumar, B. R., & Sekhar, A. C. (2011). A cryptographic scheme of Laplace transforms. *International Journal of Mathematical Archive*, 2, 2515–2519.

Mahgoub, M. M. A. (2016). The new integral transform Mahgoub Transform. *Advances in Theoretical and Applied Mathematics*, 11(4), 391–398.

Mansour, E. A., Kuffi, E. A., & Mehdi, S. A. (2022). Applying SEE integral transform in cryptography. [IOP Publishing.]. *Journal of Physics: Conference Series*, 2322(1), 012016.

Raghavendran, P., & Gunasekar, T. (2024). Advancing cryptographic security with Kushare Transform integration. In *Driving transformative technology trends with cloud computing* (pp. 224–242). IGI Global.

Rosan, K. H. (2012). *Discrete mathematics and its applications*. McGraw Hill.

Salim, S. J., & Ashruji, M. G. (2016). Application of Elzaki Transform in cryptography. *International Journal of Modern Sciences and Engineering Technology*, 3(3), 46–48.

Sallman, N. K. (2024). Integral transform of three parameters with its applications. *Kurdish Studies*, 12(1), 3743–3752.

Stallings, W. (2005). *Cryptography and network security* (4th ed.). Prentice Hall.

Stanoyevitch, A. (2002). *Introduction to cryptography with mathematical foundations and computer implementations*. CRC Press.

Chapter 8
Sustainable AI–Powered Systems and Cybersecurity for Health Diagnostics:
Addressing Bias and Fairness in AI for Early Disease Detection

S. Savitha
https://orcid.org/0000-0002-4914-8386
K.S.R. College of Engineering, India

R. Keerthana
K.S.R. College of Engineering, India

K. Logeswaran
https://orcid.org/0000-0001-8161-7376
Kongu Engineering College, India

V. Vennila
K.S.R. College of Engineering, India

R. Manjuladevi
https://orcid.org/0000-0002-9319-8874
KPR Institute of Engineering and Technology, India

M. Sangeetha
https://orcid.org/0000-0001-7173-478X
Dr. N.G.P. Institute of Technology, India

ABSTRACT

Artificial intelligence (AI) has transformed early disease diagnosis, providing exceptional speed and accuracy. However, fairness and bias challenges remain in healthcare AI, leading to discriminatory outcomes and worsening existing health inequities. These biases often arise from data imbalances, model architecture, and decision-making processes, with socioeconomic factors exacerbating historical disparities. Curating inclusive datasets with diverse demographic and socioeco-

DOI: 10.4018/979-8-3373-2827-0.ch008

nomic representation is essential. Techniques like adversarial debiasing and data augmentation improve equity, while algorithmic fairness methods, such as regularization and fairness constraints, ensure equitable treatment. Differential privacy protects sensitive attributes, and ensemble methods like fairness-aware boosting uphold accuracy. Ongoing innovation is crucial for developing transparent, fair, and accurate AI systems in healthcare.

1. INTRODUCTION: THE ROLE OF AI IN EARLY DISEASE DETECTION

Artificial intelligence has a revolutionary impact on early disease diagnosis by improving diagnostic procedures with high accuracy, speed, and precision. Artificial intelligence can analyze vast datasets, including genetic data, Machine learning and deep learning algorithms are used for improving medical imaging and electronic health records. This enables AI to identify patterns that may lead to the onset of diseases before any clinical symptoms. They can detect indicators for diseases like diabetes, cancer, and cardiovascular disease. It allows for personalized treatment regimens with early intervention. The devices decrease the time of diagnosis while reducing human error and increase accuracy in diagnostics. Improved proactive healthcare is a result of AI predictive capability, alerting physicians and patients to possible health hazards. Such an AI can learn from very large, heterogeneous datasets; however, in this regard, the AI plays an important role in battling complex and unusual diseases. However, when AI is used in healthcare, pertinent questions have been driven by concerns over justice, prejudice, and transparency at all junctures where technology is used to make definitive medical decisions. This calls for tapping into the full potential of AI for the early detection of disease.

1.1 Overview of AI's impact on early disease detection

AI can detect early patterns and biomarkers of beginning the disease by analyzing complex medical data, represented as imaging, genomics, or electronic health records, using algorithms known as ML and DL(Logeswaran et al., 2024).. Thus, the predictability will reduce costs to healthcare and improve patients' outcomes by earlier intervention. AI-powered solutions will advance personalized treatment regimes through early detection of conditions like diabetes, cancer, and cardiovascular diseases even before the onset of symptoms. And although AI has reduced the rate of diagnostic errors through uniformity in analysis made on very large data sets and consistency and reliability in healthcare due to its reliance on large-scale data, where bias, data quality, and fairness have such an influence on the accuracy of diagnosis across different groups, the successful deployment of AI portends issues in the aforementioned matters. There is a need for these challenges to be taken care of so that the AI-based application output in terms of early disease diagnosis is equitable and ethical (Cui & Zhang, 2021).

1.2 Benefits of speed and accuracy in diagnosis

Accurate tests for the patients ensure early therapy in line with that reduces the possibility of wrong diagnosis. Where early diagnosis eliminates the future requirement of more costly procedures or invasive procedures, it substantially reduces health care costs. Improved diagnostic times free up resources for healthcare systems when specialists are allowed to concentrate on difficult situations. Early and accurate diagnosis, however improves the outcomes for patients, when serious illnesses like cancer and heart conditions are ascertained early.

1.3 The ethical challenges of bias and fairness in AI models

AI models, especially in the medical field, raise huge ethical concerns about bias and fairness. Thus, misdiagnosis or diagnostic delay could likely be caused by unfair treatment of underrepresented groups based on which data set was used. Predictions for minorities may also end up distorted because of algorithmic bias when models do not intentionally favor certain demographic parameters. It's still a hard balance between precision and fairness, while the existence of fair and inclusive datasets and fairness-aware algorithms are indispensable for completeness and justice (Alimi, Chinnappan, & El-Raz, 2022). AI-driven healthcare solutions lose credibility due to its lack of transparency in decision-making, which further increases the challenges of detecting and reducing bias (Anderson & Mooney, 2021).

2. PROMISE OF AI IN EARLY DISEASE DIAGNOSIS

Predictive analytics is one of the biggest promises of AI, potentially catching health hazards before symptoms arise. Technologies also enhance precision by grasping minute trends in medical data that no human may most of the time continue to miss, be it genetics, imaging, and other complex medical data. AI-based diagnostics, therefore, informs personalized medicine by further personalizing treatment plans about unique risk factors for each patient. The pace in AI systems allows for early interventions, thus yielding better results for patients because it speeds the diagnosis-making process. The capacity of AI to scan vast data sets avails opportunities for more accurate early and complicated rare diseases diagnoses.

2.1 Machine learning (ML) and deep learning (DL) applications in healthcare

Machine learning (ML) and deep learning (DL) revolutionize the health care industry by making it feasible to automate diagnostics based on medical data like genomes, EHRs, and images. An ML-based predictive model may allow for early disease detection and preventive therapy (Haan et al., 2021). DL is suited best to a medical imager, having enough opportunities to look up close details in X-rays, MRIs, and CT scans, hence minimizing the time required to diagnose and the accuracy thereof. These technologies generate patient-specific risk indicators, meaning they can provide personalized treatment profiles in return. ML and DL also help in drug discovery and the pursuit of medical research by computer-aided screening of very complex datasets in search of likely therapeutic pathways.

2.2 AI's role in detecting diseases like diabetes, cancer, and cardiovascular conditions

AI diagnoses diseases like diabetes, cancer, and cardiovascular diseases by taking humongousamounts of health data - including genetic and imaging data and EHRs - running it through machine learning and deep learning algorithms, and trying to find the trends that are indicative of the onset of disease at the earliest stages. These AI technologies include, for example, random forests for predictive analytics as well as CNNs for medical imaging. The AI can detect anomalies before clinical signs are actually apparent. For instance, AI identifies early biomarkers in imaging scans and critical signs for cancer as well as cardiovascular diseases. Diabetes monitoring is also facilitated by trackable glucose levels as well as lifestyle information.

2.3 The potential for diagnosing diseases before clinical symptoms appear

Predictive modeling, feature extraction, and biomarker analysis would provide an even preliminary diagnosis of illness before the development of real-time symptoms, hence AI can predict the progression of disease and allow for personalized treatment. Natural language processing is through NLP, that analyzes medical records, and recurrent neural networks observe changes in time-series data. Such algorithms use artificial intelligence to breed early intervention solutions that improve outcomes for patients and also lower healthcare costs (Amann et al., 2020).

3. UNDERSTANDING BIAS IN AI SYSTEMS

Bias in the artificial intelligence systems critically downgrades healthcare inequalities and delivers unequal output in the health sectors (Obermeyer et al., 2019). The major sources of bias include decision-making processes, model architecture, and data. Since the datasets used to train them are not representative or diverse enough, a huge bias appears in the predicted results based on gender, race, and socioeconomic position (Cowgill et al., 2020). Bias in decision-making stems from historical injustices woven into the fabric of institutions in healthcare, which AI models unwittingly perpetuate (Barocas, Hardt, & Narayanan, 2019).

3.1 Sources of bias: data, model architecture, and decision-making processes

For instance, AI models that are trained on mainly white people might not distinguish minority populations in real applications, such as disease detection algorithms, even for something like skin cancer or cardiovascular disease. This means discriminatory behavior can also lead to misclassifying diseases of the skin among persons of color or, even worse, underdiagnosis of cardiac disease among African Americans. The current interventions of adversarial debiasing, fairness-aware algorithms and reweighting dataank, etc. have attempted to reduce bias in the outputs of models. Algorithms such as Explainable AI (XAI), Differential Privacy, and Fairness Constraints are appropriately advancing towards ensuring models treat a wide range of populations equitably, thus, being very transparent. Figure 1. represents Sources of bias Architecture Diagram.

Figure 1. Sources of bias architecture diagram

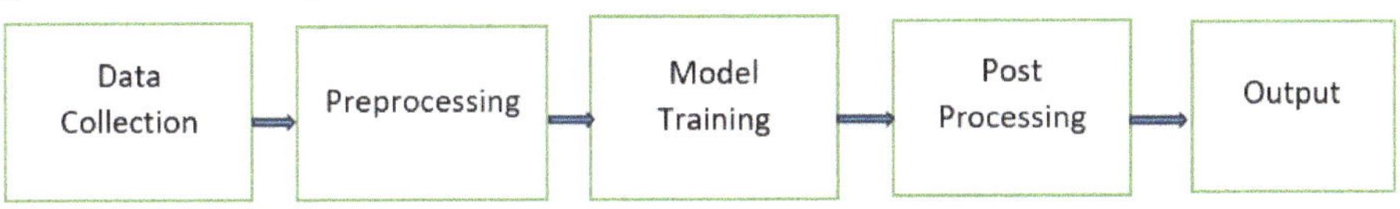

3.2 Impact of biased AI systems on healthcare disparities and Real-world examples

Real-world examples of bias in sickness detection algorithms give us a peek into the numerous dangers presented by biased AI models that may potentially lead to disproportionate outcomes in healthcare. For example, since most training data for

AI-based skin cancer detection systems are based on lighter skins, such devices perform much worse for patients with darker skin tones. Similar is the situation with the AI models predicting cardiovascular disease risks, wherein demographic bias in the datasets deployed may not aptly assess the risks of African Americans. Important approaches to counter such bias include active reduction of bias during training by adversarial debiasing, fairness-aware algorithms like Fairness Constraints, and data augmentation in order to balance the datasets. Reweighting or sampling techniques can be very useful for the development of models that are more inclusive and function well in a range of demographics.

4. ETHICAL RAMIFICATIONS OF BIAS IN HEALTHCARE AI

Algorithms having biased outcomes are a significant ethical issue for healthcare AI, as they would increase existing health care inequalities due to the activity of discrimination and inequitable access to care (Rajkomar et al., 2018). An AI generating biased results depending upon gender, color, or social economic status can misdiagnose or undertreat minority groups with more severe outcomes (Savitha & Kannan, 2023).

Among them, the three most crucial tactics are fairness-aware algorithms, paying attention to demographic imbalances, adversarial debiasing strategies that reduce bias in the models at training time, and Explainable AI-an approach aimed at enhancing the transparency of decision-making are the most critical ones concerning such ethical issues (Hardt, Price, & Srebro, 2016). Algorithmic auditing and data reweighting ensure that models make neutral or balanced predictions. Frameworks such as Differential Privacy protect patient data in ethical AI, and Fairness Constraints ensure that models work equally well for all groups (Bucher & Fichman, 2020).

4.1 The consequences of biased predictions for underrepresented populations

Discriminatory healthcare AI possibly can provide biased predictions about underrepresented communities and may culminate into worst outcomes such as delayed interventions, wrong diagnosis, or inadequate treatment. Poor results in women, minorities, or low-income groups often occur due to the failure of AI algorithms trained upon biased datasets not to generalize in various groups. For example, discriminatory risk assessment algorithms might misclassify cancer indicators in people with darker complexion tones or underreport the gravity of health conditions like cardiovascular diseases in African American populations. This therefore limits access to appropriate care as it worsens extant health inequities.

4.2 Ethical implications for overdiagnosis and underdiagnosis in marginalized communities

Reweighting data to represent population variety, using algorithmic fairness techniques like Fairness Constraints to guarantee equal outcomes, and using Explainable AI (XAI) for transparency are important approaches to address issue (Aung, Zaw, & Win, 2022). By varying the training inputs, methods like data augmentation and adversarial debiasing assist reduce bias.

4.3 Socioeconomic biases and their impact on AI-driven healthcare outcomes

Models trained on data reflecting better or more resourceful populations usually end by failing to generalize to low-income groups. This can then cause huge adverse effects in the outcomes of the patients. In the populations characterized by poor access to health care, these will then lead to incorrect diagnoses, undertreatment, or unequal provision of diagnostic equipment. A more structural reason to solidify prevalent healthcare inequities is that AI models using EHRs may neglect people from lower socioeconomic levels, who have often poorer quality or less frequent medical data.

These include explainable AI, sometimes referred to as XAI-to enhance more transparent decision-making, fairness-aware algorithms that make changes to predictions for underrepresented groups, and data balancing and re-weighting strategies to ensure socioeconomic diversity on datasets.

5. TYPES OF BIAS IN AI-POWERED DISEASE DETECTION

Several types of bias can affect the results of AI-powered disease detection:

1. Data Bias
    - **Sampling Bias:** This is where training data does not generalize the population. For example, an AI system could be learnt only from one demographic (by age, gender, ethnicity), hence the AI might not perform well in other demographics.
    - **Label Bias:** The model may learn incorrect association if the labels given in the training set of data, say disease diagnosis, themselves are wrong or not uniformly applied.

- **Historical bias:** models trained with historical data tend to mirror the prevailing biases of previous eras, such as for social classes socioeconomic classes, access to care.

2. Algorithmic Bias
    - **Model Bias:** wherein the selected algorithm reflects inherent biases because of the preference for certain results or a particular set of groups over others through its own design or optimization process.
    - **Proxy Bias:** when variables such as ZIP code or job status are used as proxies for other sensitive factors like race or socioeconomic status. This usually leads to biased results.
3. Measurement Bias
    - **Diagnostic Test Bias:** The model may run into problems because of variability in diagnostic apparatus such as imaging machines or lab tests across locations and populations to give inconsistent data.
    - **Clinical Practice Bias:** If there is a trend where specific groups are diagnosed more or less with something based on clinical practice patterns, then AI model may inherit this bias-for example, a gender bias in the detection of heart disease.
4. Deployment Bias
    - **Bias by user:** This bias occurs because of the way a health care professional or patient interacts with the AI system. For instance, user expertise and preconceived notions influence how AI results are interpreted.
    - **Environmental Bias:** the model performance may tend to vary in different settings of healthcare, for example in urban and rural, developed and developing regions, leading to biased performance due to model performance not carrying well from one environment to the other.
5. Automation Bias
    - This happens when the users rely extensively on AI predictions without judgment, trusting the AI system even in situations that the AI might be wrong. This further threatens to reduce critical thinking and perpetuate AI-driven mistakes, especially where an AI may possess embedded biases.
6. Cultural and Social Biases
    - **Health Definitions Bias:** Cultural variation in reporting and definition of diseases or symptoms reported may create bias in AI predictions, most especially in global health applications.
    - **Socioeconomic Factors Bias:** Socioeconomic status, education level, and access to health care serve as an influencer of health outcomes through which AI might adversely affect some populations if the considerations are not suited.

These biases have to be mitigated to ensure that the AI system detects diseases with a reasonable amount of fairness, reliability, and accuracy. Techniques include balancing the dataset, fairness-aware algorithms, and continuous monitoring.

5.1. Racial and ethnic bias in training datasets

Under representation of certain racial or ethnic groups in AI training datasets lead to racial and ethnic bias, meaning the model is likely to not predict appropriate health outcomes for minorities and make inaccurate forecasts. Patients who do not have the same representation are likely to get a wrong diagnosis or inadequate therapy. For instance, algorithms largely constructed from data on white patients are unlikely to flag skin cancer in darker-skinned individuals or heart conditions in African Americans. Balancing the use of data ensures that datasets are diverse and puts fairness-aware algorithms into practice to remedy this problem.

Algorithmic audits evaluate bias at every stage of development, but adversarial debiasing may also be used at the training phase to reduce bias as well. Explainable AI provides decision processes that can be explained to help identify and correct bias. Major framing schemes are Differential Privacy, which hides private demographic data while maximizing model fairness, and Fairness Constraints, altering predicted outputs to be fair within groups.

5.2. Socioeconomic bias and access to healthcare

Socioeconomic bias has an extreme implication on access to health care, which often translates to disparities in treatment and health outcomes between different socioeconomic groups. People with backgrounds from the lower socioeconomic origins would face challenges including lack of adequate health literacy, lack of insurance coverage, and limited accessibility into quality health care facilities. Such AI systems trained predominately on data from high-income populations could thus amplify that problem, essentially misdiagnosing and undertreating low-income patients. To that end predictive algorithms based upon past information might thereby altogether ignore social determinants of health in ways that continue to further marginalize low-income groups of people.

Techniques, including data reweighting and augmentation, therefore create more representative datasets that may subsequently minimize the biases tied to socio-economic classes. Fairness-aware algorithms, such as Adversarial Debiasing and Equal Opportunity, therefore, ensure fair forecasting across different strata of socio-economic classes. Algorithmic auditing and Explainable AI (XAI) improve the transparency, thereby revealing processes and pointing at biases that exist. Important frameworks, such as Differential Privacy, focus on protecting personal information while promoting equity. In this Community-Engaged Research, AI models will be made to consider specific community needs-considering the needs of marginalized communities.

5.3. Geographic and demographic imbalances

There are so many reasons that criticize research into demographic and geographic disparities in healthcare AI. An important limitation of the datasets is that they are not representative enough to train AI models, resulting in skewed results and biased predictions (Danks & London, 2017). Critics argue that socioeconomic factors which determine health, the inevitable in the study of disparity in health care, remain unaddressed in research. Further, the methodology applied in most of these studies is unclear and hence it is difficult to analyze the validity of the results obtained.

Another criticism is the heavy use of quantifiable measures-it would render such problems grossly oversimplified and ultimately not convey the depth of inequities at all. Further, the very research frameworks and algorithms, such as those of statistical modeling and machine learning, would tend to only reproduce existing biases unless controlled for appropriately. To these critiques, studies should consider opinions and requirements by the underrepresented groups by taking approaches such as community-based participatory research (CBPR) and frameworks such as Fairness Constraints. Explainability of an AI system can enhance transparency and trust through Explainable AI (XAI).

6. MITIGATING BIAS THROUGH REPRESENTATIVE DATA

The reduction of bias in AI and ML-based systems is critical, both in terms of predictive precision as well as fair treatment across demographics, especially in healthcare. One of the good strategies among these, for example, is training effective models so they work well across a spectrum of demographics groups, which then leverages representative data.

6.1 Key Methodologies

- **Data Collection and Curation:**

Diverse Sampling: The diversity of the population should be represented adequately in the training datasets. For example, proportionate samples taken from different demographic groups constitute stratified sampling.

Community Engagement: This includes participation of members in the community in data collection. This helps capture characteristics and variables relevant to underrepresented groups. Methods for more representative and inclusive datasets are through targeted outreach to all communities with encouragement to participate in the data collection, as well as stratified sampling.

Data Augmentation:

Synthetic Data synthesis: Techniques such as GANs and others have been employed for synthetic data generation in order to create synthetic samples that boost representation of underrepresented groups.

Resampling Techniques: Under- or oversampling can also serve as a strategy for balancing the datasets. For instance, synthetically creating instances for minority classes is possible via SMOTE, Synthetically Minority Over-sampling Technique.

Identification and Evaluation of Bias:

Fairness Metrics: Equitable Odds, Disparate Impact, and Demographic Parity are examples of fairness metrics that are used to identify and measure bias in AI algorithms. With the use of these measurements, engineers may evaluate how effectively the AI model works for various demographic groups and determine whether any are unfairly disadvantaged.

Equitable Odds: This ensures that the model's error rates (false positives and false negatives) are similar across different demographic groups.

Demographic Parity: This measures whether the proportion of positive outcomes (e.g., disease diagnosis) is the same for all groups, ensuring that one group is not unfairly favored.

Disparate Impact: This checks whether decisions made by the AI system disproportionately affect one group over another. These fairness metrics are crucial for ensuring that the AI model delivers equitable healthcare outcomes for all patients, regardless of their background.

Algorithmic Auditing: After an AI model is deployed, it's important to routinely monitor its performance across different demographic groups. **Algorithmic auditing** involves checking whether the model remains unbiased over time as it encounters new data and ensures that the model's fairness is maintained.

- **Algorithmic Adjustments**:

Fairness-Aware Algorithms: These algorithms are designed to reduce bias during the process of learning. In techniques such as adversarial debiasing, usually two competing models work, in which one learns to detect and remove bias while the other predicts the outcome. With all such methods, the principle is always to reduce the impact coming from sensitive variables like gender or race, so that all groups are treated equally. Algorithms can also be built constrained by fairness, such that algorithms will make the model follow specific fairness measures like equalized chances or demographic parity while being trained.

Multi-Faceted Fairness Framework

- **Demographic Fairness:** Make sure that different patient groups have comparable prediction performance.
- **Conditional Fairness:** Modify metrics according to the severity and frequency of situations in particular populations.
- **Emphasize equity**: Emphasize equity in clinical results, such as lowering the number of incorrect diagnoses or enhancing underrepresented groups' access to care.

Explainable AI (XAI): XAI literally opens the box, making transparent the black-box nature of machine learning, showing how AI models reach judgments. That's why it becomes utterly important in the medical domain: doctors need to understand how the logic underlying an AI system leads to diagnosis or a suggested course of therapy. Utilizing SHAP and LIME, as examples of XAI techniques, stakeholders may be able to indicate how certain factors, such as age of the patient or medical history, influence the output of the model.

Feedback Loops:

- **Iterative Improvement**: The AI models should be continuously enhanced as suggested by the feedback loops that come from stakeholders such as medical doctors, patients, and data scientists. Through this, new grounds of bias or underperformance in the model are detected and therefore given recommendations towards improving the accuracy of the model. For example, clinicians notice that the AI system has poor performance in the diagnosis of a particular condition about a particular population group. This feedback enables developers to alter the model or retrain on a more diverse dataset and thus solve the problem.
- **Active Learning**: In the case of active learning, the model identifies areas of uncertainty or underrepresented populations in its predictions and seeks

data more actively to be incorporated into the system so as to enhance performance. The approach here employs error analysis in identifying the failing spots of the model, for example, such as having high error rates when diagnosing diseases pertaining to specific demographics. Including user feedback and input on areas of need will update the model's training dataset to a more representative and accurate population. This helps the AI system continue to evolve and adapt to real-world needs.

Figure 2 represents process diagram of mitigating bias through representative data is as shown below.

Figure 2. Workflow diagram for mitigating bias through representative data

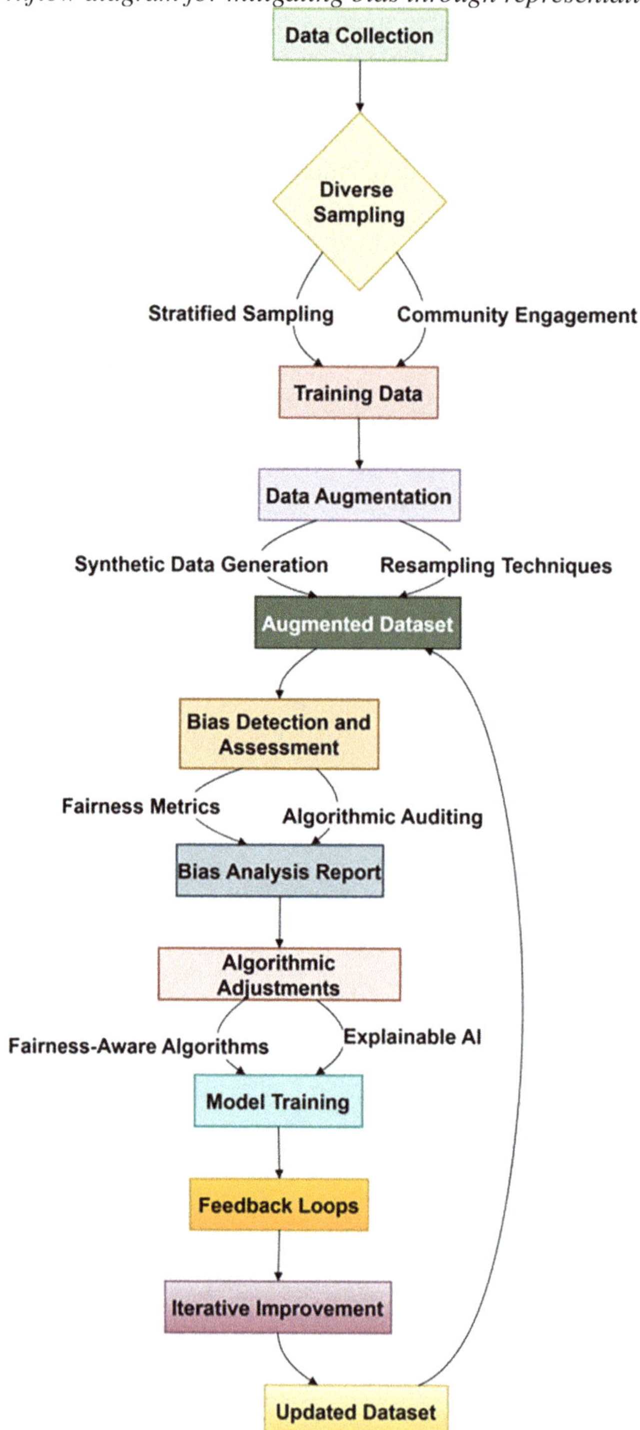

6.2 The importance of inclusive datasets

Models of AI and machine learning will call for inclusively acquired datasets to adequately respond to similarly diverse populations and create equitable outcomes. Data suitably captures demographic diversity in society, thereby increasing the level of precision of the model, reducing bias, and disparities in healthcare as well as other domains. Two critical requirements are community engagement to gather relevant information and stratified sampling to include all populations. The methods that allow dataset balancing include GANs, which were applied in the generation of synthetic data, and the SMOTE over-sampling method. Regular audits and avenues for community input are required in order to further develop.

6.3 Challenges in curating diverse medical datasets

These can also affect the potential issues dealing with curating disparate medical datasets where these could be affecting how well an AI model would work. Major problems are that underrepresentation of minority groups can lead to biased results that may not be applicable in other populations. In fact, data sharing is complicated by data privacy issues when dealing with sensitive health data. Institutions can also introduce inconsistencies in the collection of data thus making the integration of datasets quite challenging. Frameworks such as HL7 or FHIR attempt to eliminate these inequalities. Various techniques like community involvement and cooperative data collection can boost variety, while oversampling (for instance, SMOTE) helps balance datasets.

6.4 Strategies for improving data representation in AI models

The representation of data in AI must be improved to increase the accuracy and equity involved. A useful tactic in ensuring that models are trained on a diverse range of experiences is to diversify sources of data across a variety of demographic groups. Stratified sampling can be used to ensure that various populations are proportionately represented in collections of data. Thereby, with the artificial creation of examples from underrepresented classes, augmentation methods like SMOTE (Synthetic Minority Over-sampling Technique) and GANs can also help balance datasets. XAI frameworks, with fairness-aware algorithms, support model predictions in their ability to explain them while reducing biases and tuning their datasets for better fine-tuning.

1. Diversifying Data Sources

- Data sources can be diversified so as to ensure that AI models are trained to accurately represent broad spectra of human experiences. This means the collection of data in various populations according to demographic variables like geographical setting, socioeconomic position, gender, and ethnicity in health. The more diverse the sources of data-including different kinds of hospitals from other regions or even countries, different types of healthcare providers serving other sections of society, and specialized research organizations concentrating on minority groups-the greater the chances that AI models will learn relevant patterns applicable to all these groups. With such diversity, the models will generalize better and reduce the chances of overfitting to a specific demographic, thus improving both fairness and accuracy across populations.

2. Stratified Sampling
   - Stratified sampling Data gathering in which the dataset is divided into various subgroups or strata along common characteristics like age, gender, or ethnicity. Stratified sampling will minimize the chances of over-or underrepresentation of specific populations by ensuring every subgroup is proportionately represented in the training data. For example, when building models in disease detection, stratified sampling may ensure equal representation of different races in predicting diseases, for instance skin cancer or cardiovascular disease, and avoid biased predictions. This method achieves the right balance of view from all relevant subgroups that should be considered by AI models for better just healthcare outcomes.
3. Data Augmentation Methods

It is also helpful when the underrepresented groups are lacking in numbers for data augmentation techniques. For instance, there are tools like SMOTE that is the Synthetic Minority Over-sampling Technique while the others are Generative Adversarial Networks which attempt to automatically discover a model distribution that can generate new samples from existing ones in order to balance out datasets.

o **Generative Adversarial Networks (GANs)**: These networks can then synthesize medical images, such as skin scans or X-rays, of underrepresented groups. To balance the dataset without compromising on data quality, GANs are utilizing two neural networks - a generator and a discriminator competing with each other to generate better data with reality.

o **SMOTE**: The technique of synthesizing data points for minority classes creates new instances interpolated among existing data points. It is useful in classification tasks with some underrepresented disease patterns that have less data in the dataset. For example, SMOTE can help build more data points for diseases disproportionately affecting minority populations to improve model performance for such groups.

4. Explainable AI (XAI) Frameworks
    - It is crucial to ensure transparency or detection and reduction of biases in AI models. XAI frameworks explain features or elements impacting output. This will help shine light onto how models generate predictions, which is even more important in healthcare because the practitioner needs to understand reasoning for an AI model's predictions of a diagnosis or course of treatment so that they can gain trust and use the technology.
    - Healthcare providers can question whether particular demographic characteristics, such as race, gender, or age, are being used unfairly to impact model predictions, and change appropriately to rectify or retrain the model. XAI can help identify patterns of unfair treatment and lead to required adjustments in the data or design of the model.
5. Fairness-Aware Algorithm Implementation
    - Overall, fairness-aware algorithms attempt to decrease bias in the process of learning by incorporating fairness constraints and measurements into training the model so groups would be treated equally. For example, equalized chances or demographic parity are a form of measures for the assessment of the model's predictions' fairness for different demographic groups. The addition of such fairness requirements will reduce biased outcomes that discriminate against some populations issued by the AI model.
    - Techniques such as adversarial debiasing can also be used by training the model to predict outcomes while simultaneously minimizing the sensitive attributes (such as race, gender) on which it relies to make the probability predictions. In this manner, there is no likelihood of associating a given group with higher risks of diseases due to historical data biases.
6. Community Participation and Feedback
    - Highlighting community involvement in the collection of data and the review of models is very essential because it can be used to ensure that AI models truly mirror diversity in real life. Continuous collaboration through diverse communities will allow actual continuous feedback processes that can prove useful when there are

biases or holes that have gone unchecked in the data and build trust between AI developers and populations affected by the technology.

- Socio cultural input regarding communities can be included to determine the prevalence of disease, accessibility, or treatment results and can be added to the AI model to enhance effectiveness as well as equity.

7. Fairness-Aware Algorithms: An Approach to Reducing Bias

Designed to ensure that AI systems produce fair outcomes for demographic groups, fairness-aware algorithms are one of the strategies for reducing bias, with two main methods - fairness constraints and regularization techniques - that these algorithms apply in order to address and reduce biases that might originate from imbalanced or biased datasets. The fairness-inclusive algorithms prevent groups that may be punished or rewarded more than others based on socio-economic status, gender, or race about the decision-making process in the sectors such as criminal justice, health care, and education.

Fairness-Aware Algorithms for bias reduction in machine learning models. The goal is to ensure that the model's predictions are fair across different demographic groups while maintaining overall accuracy. Below is a step-by-step breakdown of the approach.

1. Objective Function

The first step is to establish a standard learning objective (minimizing prediction error) combined with fairness constraints. The objective function can be written as:

$$Minimize{:}L(\theta,X) = i = 1\sum n\ell(yi,y\hat{}i)$$

Where:

- L(θ,X) is the total loss function,
- ℓ is the loss function (e.g., cross-entropy for classification),
- yi is the true label,
- y^i is the predicted label,
- θ are the model parameters.

2. Fairness Constraint Matrix

To measure fairness, define a Fairness Matrix F for each demographic group d (e.g., race, gender) such that:

$F = [f11\ f12\ \ldots\ f1m$

$f21\ f22\ \ldots\ f2m$

$fm1\ fm2\ \ldots\ fmm]$

Where each element fij represents the prediction outcome (e.g., false positives, true positives) for group iii compared to group j. The fairness constraint is satisfied if the values in the matrix are close to 1, implying parity between the groups.

3. Fairness-Aware Regularization Term

Add a regularization term R(F) to the loss function to minimize differences in group outcomes. One common approach is to minimize the **disparity** between groups, defined as:

$$R(F) = i,j\sum \mid fij - 1 \mid$$

This penalizes the model for discrepancies in predictions across demographic groups, encouraging it to treat all groups equally.

4. Updated Loss Function

The loss function becomes:

$$Lfair(\theta, X) = L(\theta, X) + \lambda R(F)$$

Where:

- λ is a hyperparameter that controls the trade-off between accuracy and fairness.

5. Optimization

The model is trained by minimizing the updated loss function:

$$\theta* = arg\theta minLfair(\theta, X)$$

The algorithm adjusts the model parameters θ not only to minimize prediction error but also to ensure fairness across groups.

7.1 The Need for Fairness in AI Models for Healthcare

Artificial intelligence holds tremendous promise for the transformation of medical diagnosis, care, and results in healthcare (Phelan & Link, 2015). However, when AI models are infused into healthcare systems, concerns about bias and equity become even more pressing (Buolamwini & Gebru, 2018). Existing healthcare inequities may even be exacerbated by AI programs trained on biased data (Barocas, Hardt, & Narayanan, 2019). Other patient groups that have been less represented in diagnostic algorithms include women, and low-income patients and racial minority patients, which may culminate in misdiagnosis, late treatment, or unequal treatment from healthcare AI models due to biased access to healthcare services. Inequalities in access to health care AI models pose a challenge from both ethical and patient safety perspectives (Ghassemi et al., 2019). Biased algorithms might have little annoyance leading to potentially fatal repercussions. Thus, ensuring that AI systems are developed to detect and mitigate any bias that may arise when AI systems are implemented within the healthcare framework requires utilization of complex evaluation frameworks, suitable diversified datasets, and vigilant monitoring (Jiang, Jiang, et al., 2017). Other areas that regulatory systems have to examine include fairness and explainability in AI applications introduced in the healthcare setting (Raghavan, Barocas, et al., 2020). Policymakers, healthcare professionals, and AI developers need to come together in addressing the incorporation of justice in the development and utilization of such technology to ensure fair healthcare outcomes for each community involved (Challen et al., 2021).

7.2 Fairness Constraints and Regularization Methods

Regularization techniques and fairness restrictions need to be applied systematically in order to ensure equity in AI models, particularly those critical domains such as healthcare (Mehrabi et al., 2021). Figure 3 represents Fairness Constraints and Regularization Methods. Some key actions and strategies listed below are:

- Identify Sensitive Attributes
- Define Fairness Metrics
- Apply Fairness Constraints
- Regularization Methods
- Post-Processing Methods
- Evaluation and Monitoring

Figure 3. Fairness constraints and regularization methods

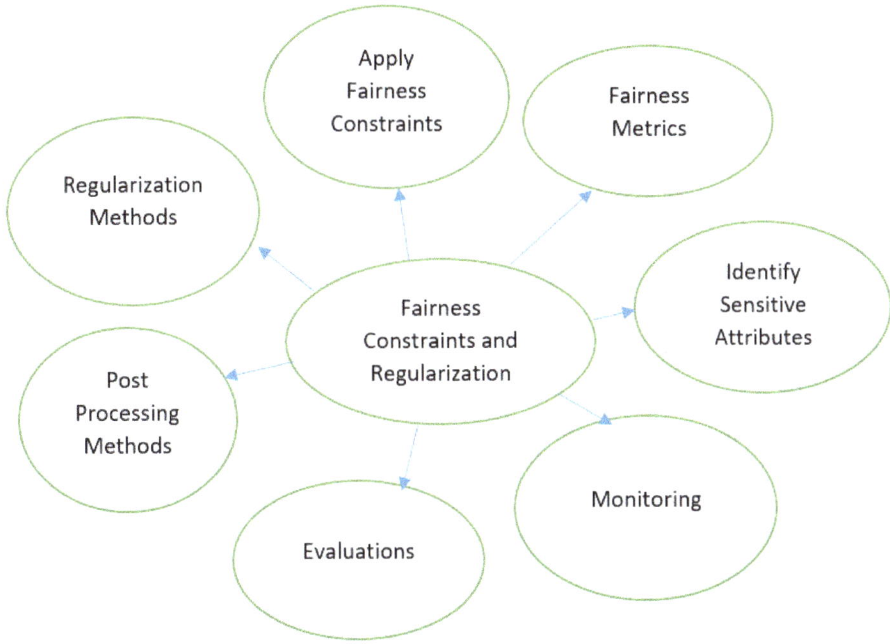

7.3 Adversarial Debiasing Techniques for Minimizing Bias in AI Outputs

1. Adversarial Neural Networks (ANN) for Debiasing
   - **Technique**: A classifier is trained to predict the target label, while an adversary attempts to guess the sensitive attribute (e.g., race, gender). In order to hide the sensitive attribute, the classifier learns to make predictions.
   - **Key Outcome**: Reduced bias in predictions by making it harder for the model to depend on sensitive attributes.
2. Adversarial Fair Representation Learning
   - **Technique**: This method creates a representation of the data that does not allow the adversary to distinguish sensitive attributes, ensuring that bias does not influence downstream predictions.
   - **Key Outcome**: Outputs are fairer, with demographic parity achieved across different groups.
3. Adversarially Reweighted Loss Functions

- **Technique**: The model's loss function is reweighted to penalize errors more when sensitive attributes are involved, forcing the model to reduce bias in its predictions.
- **Key Outcome**: Balanced predictive performance across different demographic groups, minimizing disparities.

8.BALANCING ACCURACY AND FAIRNESS IN AI MODELS

Especially in high-stakes applications like healthcare, accuracy and fairness become deeply critical trade-offs in AI systems. Lowering bias will often make the model much more fair, but accuracy will then be tragically compromised as a side effect. The reason is that because dominant groups perform better, models are apt to exclude representatively under-represented groups from training data. However, for the injustice to not perpetuate, all groups of the medical profession must have parity in their decisions, something that can sometimes mean the difference between life and death. At these bargaining tables, therefore, model performance needs to be appropriately balanced in such a way that no group is unduly disadvantaged. The healthcare sector requires that the predictive models not overfit onto a certain population, the fear of which is fairness on one end creating a point where predictiveness fails on the other. Predictive models in the health care industry need to avoid overfitting to a particular demographic at the expense of accuracy for other groups. Fairness may be favored to the extreme point whereby models fail at the areas especially where accurate diagnosis is called upon.

To achieve performance parity across demographic groups, several strategies are employed:

- Adversarial debiasing techniques to minimize reliance on sensitive attributes like race or gender.
- Fair representation learning, where models are trained to make predictions that are invariant to demographic differences.
- Weighted loss functions that penalize errors more heavily when they occur in underrepresented groups, balancing accuracy across all demographics.

In healthcare, these strategies ensure models are both accurate and fair, reducing disparities in treatment outcomes across diverse populations.

9. TECHNICAL SOLUTIONS TO MITIGATION

Bias mitigation in AI relies on several **technical solutions** to ensure fairness in areas like early disease detection. Key techniques include:

1. **Re-weighting procedures and data augmentation**: Reweighting ensures more equitable model learning by adjusting the weight of data points from underrepresented groups. By creating synthetic examples to equalize class representation, data augmentation lessens the bias resulting from unbalanced datasets.
2. **Ensemble methods and fairness-aware boosting**: To improve forecasts, these blend several models. To promote equitable performance for all populations, fairness-aware boosting gives priority to fixing faults for disadvantaged groups.
3. **Algorithmic interventions for promoting fairness in early disease detection**: Fairness constraints in model training are among them, as they guarantee that predictions are less skewed against marginalized communities. This is crucial for the healthcare industry, since biased models could result in unequal access to early therapies that could save lives.
4. **Contextual testing**: Contextual testing involves assessing models in a range of healthcare environments, such as high-resource versus low-resource settings and rural versus urban settings.
5. **Population Diversity:** Examining patient data from a variety of geographic and demographic backgrounds.
6. **Disease-Specific Adaptations:** Tailoring methods according to the features of a disease, such as genetic disorders or chronic illnesses that disproportionately impact particular populations.

10.PROTECTING PRIVACY AND ENSURING FAIRNESS: THE ROLE OF DIFFERENTIAL PRIVACY

Fairness and privacy must be upheld within AI systems, especially for demographic data that is sensitive in nature. This data should be protected to prevent biasing and to keep all rights within the individuals (Verma & Rubin, 2018). Inappropriate handling of sensitive demographic data leads to biased results and increases the gap that has already been established (Pfohl, et al., 2021). The justification of this phenomenon requires differential privacy because noise is added to the data queries, which allows the model to learn from data but does not reveal that sensitive information (Savitha et al., 2022). This technique encourages a fairer representation in training models by actually eliminating bias through making sure that single points of data cannot be traced back to particular demographics (Watson et al., 2019). The techniques reduce the likelihood of leakage of personal data; hence models can be trained on diverse datasets without reiterating bias against any specific group, and produce results fair to all groups (Wiens et al., 2019).

Differential privacy forms a solid foundation for the protection of individual privacy and maximum utilization of data in AI and machine learning applications, as it ensures that the loss or addition of a single data point does not lead to a significant modification of any particular analysis outcome, thus preserving sensitive information, by introducing controlled noise into datasets (Price & Cohen, 2019). This is very significant in the healthcare industry where the confidentiality of a patient's data is necessary.

Moreover, essential frameworks like the Privacy Budget idea and the DP framework enable organizations to measure and manage privacy loss during analysis of data (Lack et al., 2023). Differential privacy-making methodologies can be as varied as data perturbation techniques to randomized algorithms. These methods add noise to the data or model outputs that normally mask individual contributions to ensure privacy protection (Hoffman et al., 2023). Even if the data algorithm carries with it the Exponential Mechanism, while retaining it to be private, it can help in giving the best output. Additionally, integrating fairness measures into differential privacy might result in an AI model that is fair, and thus, bias-free decision making (Beauchamp et al., 2023).

Differential privacy requires ongoing research and development because the process involves a delicate balance between the tradeoff between accuracy and privacy (Chouldechova & Roth, 2020). Finally, this approach provides an achievable way to maintain personal privacy while maintaining the robustness of AI systems in sensitive fields like health.

Privacy-Preserving Techniques: Propose techniques like federated learning, homomorphic encryption, and differential privacy. That lessens the potential risks of sharing information as well as training models by allowing AI models to train over data without contravening the rights to privacy of patients.

11.EXPLAINABLE AI (XAI) AND TRANSPARENCY IN HEALTHCARE

Explainable AI in healthcare simply means AI solutions that provide intuitive, transparent insight into decision-making processes. That is, making the process easier both for patients and health providers to comprehend how AI models come to such findings will improve transparencies, with a guarantee that recommendations are understandable, justified, and aligned with clinical procedures. Such decisions need to be transparent in improving patient outcomes, establishing trust as well as meeting legal and ethical expectations (Cohen et al., 2020).

Threat Modeling for Healthcare AI: Create threat models that are tailored to healthcare contexts, such as evasion attacks and poisoning attacks. This focused strategy can reveal vulnerabilities specific to the healthcare industry.

11.1 The need for explainable AI

- **Trust and Transparency:** AI systems should be trusted by patients and health care providers to make rational judgment concerning diagnosis and treatment. Explainable AI can be helpful in adding the clinician's expertise of possibly understanding and interpreting model output, developing confidence in the suggestions provided by the AI.
- **Complexity of Medical Data:** Such medical information is complex, multi-dimensional, and contains variables, including genetics, socioeconomic status, and medical history. Using XAI, complicated AI models can be simplified to let the practitioners understand the reasoning for some forecasted decisions they might make in future practice.
- **Regulatory Compliance:** In many jurisdictions, regulations mandate that medical decisions must be explainable, especially when they significantly impact patient outcomes. Explainable AI ensures that healthcare providers can justify their choices based on clear, understandable reasoning from the AI system.
- **Improving Patient Outcomes:** By providing transparency in AI-driven decisions, XAI allows healthcare professionals to critically evaluate and adjust AI recommendations. This iterative process can lead to improved patient outcomes by ensuring that AI serves as an effective decision-support tool rather than a black box.
- **Ethical Considerations:** Ethical implications arise when AI systems make decisions affecting human health. Explainable AI helps mitigate biases and ensures that AI applications align with ethical standards by making the decision-making process clear and accountable.

11.2 How XAI can help identify and address biases?

XAI Identifies and Rectifies Bias in AI Systems In such sensitive fields as healthcare, explainable AI would be of paramount importance in the identification and rectification of biases in models. Translucency for the rationale behind the decisions of AI models exposes the justification of the model as to what it uses in its reasoning to come up with certain predictions. It would then become possible to identify biases and ensure reliability, fairness, and compliance with medical ethics in applications of AI.

And here is the expansion on how XAI can be effective in the discovery of biases in healthcare AI systems and addressing them:

1. Transparency in Decision-Making
   - XAI ensures that you have clear explanations of how an AI model makes certain decisions. It breaks down the complex operations of machine learning algorithms in human-understandable terms. This is critical because medical professionals to find doctors wherein they can trust an AI system that comes up with a diagnosis, treatment recommendation, and patient risk assessment.
   - Transparent decision-making will enable clinicians and data scientists to trace how much the model is depending on the various features present in the data, such as age, gender, or race. In that manner, they can be able to identify the presence of biased demographic factors. For example, if the disease detection model is always weighing race as a major predictor, this could suggest bias.
2. Identification of Biased Features with SHAP and LIME
   - o Among the techniques whose names are most known in XAI, we count SHAP (Shapley Additive Explanations) and LIME (Local Interpretable Model-agnostic Explanations), both of which aim to estimate the importance of feature contributions towards model predictions.
   - o SHAP: This technique assigns a SHAP value to each feature-features-which indicates the contribution of that feature to the model's output. SHAP values enable healthcare providers to see how much weight is given to each feature, such as blood pressure, age, or ethnicity, in an individual prediction. In case SHAP demonstrates sensitive features like race or socioeconomic status have undue influence on the diagnosis or risk assessment, it flags potential bias.
   - o LIME: LIME builds interpretable models locally around a prediction. For healthcare applications, this could be used to explain an individual prediction and uncover biases specific to a certain case-for instance, LIME may show that a model overweights a certain lab result in one demographic compared to another, so biases can be identified and corrected in areas.
     - By using SHAP and LIME, all stakeholders will be able to estimate the importance of features across different populations and detect bias and disparate impact which may be disproportionately affecting certain groups.

3. Comparing Performance Across Demographic Groups
    - XAI can facilitate much finer-grained model performance comparisons between divergent demographic groups, race, gender, or age. Where a model might be failing or behaving poorly can show bias in training data or algorithms themselves.
    - For instance, the disease prediction model may look to have varying accuracy for white patients and minorities, which may indicate that the training dataset does not represent a particular group of patients with satisfactory representation.
    - This capability of XAI can be used to measure equalized odds or demographic parity, that is, whether the model's predictions are accurate and fair for all groups.
4. Bias Mitigation and Model Improvement
    - It opens the pathway to remediation once it identifies biases since XAI can be used to provide insights into why and how the model behaves in a biased way. For instance, in healthcare systems, this would mean rebalancing the dataset over which the model is trained, adjusting the model's parameters, or enforcing fairness constraints so as to treat each demographic end equally.
    - XAI maintains continuous monitoring of models, enabling stakeholders to detect emerging over time new types of biases. As a health dataset evolves, new types of bias that were previously nonexistent can emerge; XAI provides tools to proactively manage these biases and adjusts accordingly.
    - Fairness-aware algorithms can be incorporated based on the insights from XAI, thereby reducing bias reliance on features and achieving fairness in model outcomes. For example, if XAI discovers that a model relies too heavily on socioeconomic information, developers can engineer the model to give more importance to clinical variables and less to extraneous social factors that may impart bias.
5. Improving Collaboration Between AI Systems and Medical Experts
    - XAI helps medical professionals work effectively with AI systems. This model's rational decision-making process makes it easy for clinicians to work with the AI tools and provide feedback since there is a two-way process that ensures this AI system's decisions will be in tandem with the world of medicine, besides all things undertaken ethically (Flores, Bechtel & Lowenkamp, 2016).
    - For a health setting, explainability would be an important aspect: Explainability will be the key to doctors as well as patients' trust. Medical professionals are unlikely to avail themselves AI-powered diagnostic

tools when they understand how this model arrives at the decision-making, particularly when such decisions regard life-impacting ones such as diseases diagnosed or treatment plans. XAI fills in the gap between technical complexity and usability for clinical applications while ensuring AI applications derive their principles from fairness and reliability (Raji & Buolamwini, 2019).

- XAI also allows doctors, among many other medical professionals, to question AI models and collaborate in their development. For example, if the doctor determines that the system underdiagnoses this ailment constantly within the minority population, XAI will point out the precise bias in the features or lack of exposure due to limited amounts of data, thus enabling this collaboration between the two teams-technical as well as medical-in further developing the model.

6. Ensuring Ethical and Equitable AI in Healthcare
   - XAI is supportive of the development of ethical AI applications by providing insight into the functioning of AI systems and possible sources of bias. In healthcare, where the decision limits are between life and death, fairness and equity demand much more.
   - XAI ensures that there is no perpetuation and aggravation of the already existing health disparities through the AI systems. For instance, if an AI for detection of skin cancer systematically underperforms on darker tones, XAI could reveal this shortfall and urge efforts to be made to amend it. Then all patients will be precisely diagnosed, without being subjected to bias related to demography.
   - To ensure that the resultant healthcare systems follow the regulatory and ethical guidelines in healthcare, additional uses of XAI frameworks can be put to practice. Currently, the healthcare systems are getting scrutinized for any indication of discrimination and bias.

11.3 The role of transparency in building trust in AI-driven healthcare systems

Transparency would help in ensuring that the results produced by AI models are understood even by the patients and service providers involved, a very critical factor in establishing trust in AI-driven health care systems. For users, transparent AI systems make it easier to assess the trustworthiness of their predictions and recommendations based on understandable and concise explanations for them. Accountability is also facilitated through transparency, as interested parties are allowed to monitor and check that the AI system's decision-making processes operate in accordance with legal and moral standards (Logeswaran et al., 2020). Besides, openness solves the problem of fairness-an issue whose implementation is necessary in equitable healthcare-through the coming out of biases or potential flaws that may even be hidden in AI models (Panch, Mattie, & Celi, 2023).

11.4 Case Study: Early Detection of Diabetic Retinopathy

Google Health, utilizing deep learning in order to increase the accuracy of the assessment, created an AI model in 2016 to identify diabetic retinopathy from a retinal scan. Diabetic retinopathy is the most common cause of blindness worldwide, and the future prospects of effective treatment lie in early diagnosis (Beede et al., 2020). Results for the AI model were promising, with a high accuracy detection of DR post-training over a large dataset of pictures that have been marked by ophthalmologists. The Google Health team quickly learned that the model faced unexpected issues once they started testing the model in real life, such as in rural Thai healthcare centers, that really brought home the fact that AI needs to be taken into account in terms of context and demographics.

12. FUTURE DIRECTIONS AND CHALLENGES

Techniques, such as adversarial debiasing, fairness restrictions, and re-weighted loss functions, are devised today by the ongoing research in the area of fairness-aware algorithms and bias mitigation so that biases in AI models can be decreased. These solutions try to ensure that the healthcare AI works fairly for all patient populations while dealing with imbalances in diagnosis, treatment, and outcome. However, various challenges impede the achievement of flawless impartiality and precision. Because bias-prevention strategies sometimes decrease model performance, a built-in trade-off exists between achieving maximum fairness and retaining high accuracy.

Moving ahead, more equitable, sustainable AI systems in healthcare look forward to infusing fairness at every step of AI development, from the collection of data through the deployment of models. There will be much interdisciplinary cooperation, regulatory frameworks, and even ongoing research into creating AI systems that may be both valid and efficient but also ethical, transparent, and fair with all populations.

Designing Energy-Efficient Models

- **Model Compression:** Model size and computational load can be decreased without a noticeable loss of accuracy by using strategies like knowledge distillation, quantization, and pruning.

- **Efficient designs:** Bring up efficient designs like sparse neural networks suited to healthcare requirements, lightweight CNNs (like MobileNet), and transformers optimized for low energy consumption.
- **Decreased Complexity through Feature Selection:** To simplify models and lower processing demands, concentrate on choosing only the most pertinent features for healthcare diagnostics.
- **Green AI Infrastructure:** Deployment of Energy-Efficient Models Advocate for adoption of healthcare models with lesser idle energy consumption and also scalable, on-demand resources. The application of autoscaling features along with containerized AI workloads can reduce wasteful energy usage. Energy-efficient cloud-based tool is Carbon-Intelligent Computing Platform of Google Cloud: It schedules and assigns computing activities on Google's global data centers that depend on availability of renewable energy so that carbon emissions can be reduced in its pursuit.

12.1 pseudocode for a Fairness-Aware Algorithm

```
# Fairness-Aware Algorithm Pseudocode

Input: Training data X with features, y (labels), sensitive attributes S (e.g., race, gender)

Output: Trained fair model

1. Initialize model M with random parameters

2. Set fairness metric F (e.g., demographic parity, equalized odds)

3. Set weights W for each data point in X (initially equal)

# Step 1: Dynamic Re-weighting based on model performance
```

```
4. For each epoch:

a. For each data point (x_i, y_i, s_i) in X:

i. Compute model prediction y_hat_i = M(x_i)

ii. Calculate loss L = loss(y_hat_i, y_i)

iii. Update weights W_i based on fairness:

- If sensitive group s_i is underrepresented or misclassi-
fied, increase W_i

- Else, leave W_i unchanged

iv. Update model parameters based on weighted loss:

M = update(M, L * W_i)

# Step 2: Hybrid Data Augmentation (if dataset imbalance de-
tected)

5. If dataset imbalance for group S found:

a. Use generative model (GAN) to create synthetic data for
underrepresented group S

b. Add synthetic data to training set X
```

Step 3: Multi-Objective Optimization for fairness and accuracy

6. Define trade-off objective:

- Optimize both fairness F and accuracy A in the objective function:

Objective = alpha * Accuracy + beta * Fairness

7. Train model M using this objective, adjusting alpha and beta to balance accuracy and fairness.

Step 4: Adaptive Regularization for fairness constraint

8. Define regularization term R:

- If fairness metric F exceeds a threshold, increase regularization penalty.

9. Update loss function:

Loss = Loss + lambda * R

Step 5: Fairness-Aware Transfer Learning (optional)

10. If pre-trained fairness-aware model is available:

a. Load pre-trained model with fairness constraints.

b. Fine-tune on current dataset X with fairness objective.

Step 6: Explainable Decision Boundaries

11. For each group in sensitive attribute S:

a. Adjust decision boundary for predictions based on group-specific fairness needs.

b. Generate explanations for decision boundary adjustments.

Step 7: Adversarial Post-Processing (for bias detection)

12. Train adversarial network A to detect biased predictions in M.

13. Update M based on adversarial feedback to minimize bias in final predictions.

Step 8: Output final fairness-aware model M

14. Return trained model M with fair predictions across all groups.

12.2 Key components of the pseudocode

- **Dynamic Re-weighting**: Adjusts the influence of underrepresented groups during training.
- **Hybrid Data Augmentation**: Adds synthetic data to balance group representation.
- **Multi-Objective Optimization**: Balances fairness and accuracy as dual objectives.
- **Adaptive Regularization**: Introduces fairness-based penalties to guide the model.
- **Fairness-Aware Transfer Learning**: Leverages pre-trained models with fairness constraints.
- **Explainable Decision Boundaries**: Ensures group-specific decision-making transparency.
- **Adversarial Post-Processing**: Detects and reduces bias using adversarial networks.

This pseudocode can be implemented in Python or other languages with AI libraries (like TensorFlow, PyTorch) to build a fairness-aware model.

13. CONCLUSION: BUILDING INCLUSIVE AND FAIR AI FOR HEALTHCARE

Building inclusive and fair AI for healthcare is imperative to overcome those challenges that arise from biased data, unequal access to healthcare, and the ability to continue operating in lines of disadvantage. Overcoming bias is essential to ensuring that systems are acceptable and provide health care equitably to all demographic groups, reducing errors and improving results for the underrepresented populations.

For example, standards such as Fast Healthcare Interoperability Resources (FHIR) and Health Level Seven (HL7) (Obermeyer et al., 2019) may facilitate the integration and data exchange. In the future, the approach to fair and ethical AI systems in medicine will be inherently interdisciplinary, with continuous fairness research, increasing transparency, and constant model monitoring so that AI provides efficacy and fairness in healthcare for all individuals. While fairness-aware machine learning techniques and algorithms like SMOTE (Synthetic Minority Over-sampling Technique) could indeed reduce the bias and increase the model performance, designing ongoing assessment using fairness metrics such as Equitable Odds and Demographic Parity, for instance, would ensure that the integrity of AI systems was protected. In doing so, we can guarantee that AI solutions will be equitable and effective as well. The interexchange of ideas between technologists and healthcare professionals might have a better effect on health care outcomes for any population.

REFERENCES

Alimi, D., Chinnappan, R., & El-Raz, A. (2022). Evaluating fairness in health AI: A survey of existing approaches and challenges. *Artificial Intelligence Review*, 55(1), 35–52.

Amann, J., Blasimme, A., Vayena, E., Frey, D., & Madai, V. I. (2020). Explainability for artificial intelligence in healthcare: A multidisciplinary perspective. *BMC Medical Informatics and Decision Making*, 20(1), 1–9. DOI: 10.1186/s12911-020-01332-6 PMID: 33256715

Anderson, M., & Mooney, S. J. (2021). The impact of bias and fairness in machine learning for clinical decision support. *Journal of Biomedical Informatics*, 120, 103865.

Aung, Y. M., Zaw, A. T., & Win, K. M. (2022). Ethical issues in applying machine learning models in clinical settings. *Healthcare Analytics*, 6, 100094.

. Barocas, S., Hardt, M., & Narayanan, A. (2019). Fairness and Machine Learning. Available at: Fairness and Machine Learning.

Beauchamp, A., Baird, A., Fox, K., Silva, G., & Kuhlmann, E. (2023). Data-driven approaches to healthcare disparities: Using machine learning to inform health equity initiatives. *PLOS Digital Health*, 2(1), e0000278.

Beede, E., Baylor, E., Hersch, F., Iurchenko, A., Wilcox, L., Ruamviboonsuk, P., & Vardoulakis, L. M. (2020). A human-centered evaluation of a deep learning system deployed in clinics for the detection of diabetic retinopathy. *CHI Conference on Human Factors in Computing Systems*, 1-12. DOI: 10.1145/3313831.3376718

Bucher, A., & Fichman, M. (2020). Geographic and demographic imbalances in healthcare research: A critical review. *Journal of Health Disparities Research and Practice*, 13(2), 1–20. PMID: 34367737

Buolamwini, J., & Gebru, T. (2018). Gender Shades: Intersectional Accuracy Disparities in Commercial Gender Classification. *Proceedings of the 2018 Conference on Fairness, Accountability, and Transparency (FAT).*

Challen, R., Denny, J., Pitt, M., Gompels, L., Edwards, T., & Tsaneva-Atanasova, K. (2021). Artificial intelligence, bias and clinical safety. *BMJ Quality & Safety*, 30(9), 792–800. PMID: 30636200

Chen, C., Su, Y., & King, R. (2021). Equity in algorithmic decision-making: Mitigating bias in machine learning for healthcare applications. *Journal of Healthcare Informatics Research*, 5(2), 127–148.

Chen, I. Y., Joshi, S., Ghassemi, M., & Chen, Y. (2021). Ethical machine learning in health care. *Annual Review of Biomedical Data Science*, 4(1), 123–144. DOI: 10.1146/annurev-biodatasci-092820-114757 PMID: 34396058

Chouldechova, A., & Roth, A. (2020). The frontiers of fairness in machine learning. *Communications of the ACM*, 63(5), 93–101. DOI: 10.1145/3376898

Cohen, I. G., Amarasingham, R., Shah, A., Xie, B., & Lo, B. (2020). The legal and ethical concerns that arise from using complex predictive analytics in health care. *Health Affairs*, 39(7), 1146–1154. PMID: 25006139

Cowgill, B., Dell'Acqua, F., Deng, S., & Chouldechova, A. (2020). Biased programmers? Or biased data? A field experiment in operationalizing AI ethics. *ACM Conference on Fairness, Accountability, and Transparency (FAT).*

Cui, Y., & Zhang, L. (2021). Ethical dilemmas in the use of AI for healthcare diagnostics: A systematic review. *Ethics, Medicine, and Public Health*, 17, 100674.

Danks, D., & London, A. J. (2017). Algorithmic bias in autonomous systems. *Proceedings of the Twenty-Sixth International Joint Conference on Artificial Intelligence*, 4691-4697.

Flores, A. W., Bechtel, K., & Lowenkamp, C. T. (2016). False positives, false negatives, and false analyses: A reexamination of the predictive validity of the COMPAS risk assessment tool. *Criminology & Public Policy*, 15(3), 951–980.

Ghassemi, M., & Naumann, T.. (2019). A review of challenges and opportunities in using machine learning in healthcare. *Journal of Machine Learning Research*, 20, 1–36.

Haan, M., Ongena, Y. P., Hommes, S., Kwee, T. C., & Yakar, D. (2021). Integration of artificial intelligence in radiology: Automated and standardized reporting. *Insights Into Imaging*, 12(1), 167. PMID: 34767092

Hardt, M., Price, E., & Srebro, N. (2016). Equality of opportunity in supervised learning. *Advances in Neural Information Processing Systems (NeurIPS).*

Hoffman, K., Tom, S., Grierson, L., Greene, L., Rosenfeld, D., & Wong, A. (2023). Framework for evaluating bias in machine learning algorithms for health care. *Journal of the American Medical Informatics Association : JAMIA*, 30(5), 1094–1100.

Jiang, F., & Jiang, Y.. (2017). Artificial intelligence in healthcare: Anticipating challenges to ethics, privacy, and bias. *Journal of Medical Internet Research*, 19(4), e139.

Lack, A., Kwon, S., Duflo, E., McCarthy, M., Baker, S., Tsalatsanis, A., & Denker, M. (2023). Advancing health equity through artificial intelligence: Recommendations for policymakers. *Health Affairs*, 42(7), 112–120.

Logeswaran, K., Savitha, S., Suresh, P., Prasanna Kumar, K. R., Gunasekar, M., Rajadevi, R., & Jayasurya, A. S. (2024). Unifying Technologies in Industry 4.0: Harnessing the Synergy of Internet of Things, Big Data, Augmented Reality/Virtual Reality, and Blockchain Technologies. *Topics in Artificial Intelligence Applied to Industry*, 4(0), 127–147. DOI: 10.1002/9781394216147.ch7

Logeswaran, K., Suresh, P., Savitha, S., Prasanna Kumar, K. R., Ponselvakumar, A. P., & Kannan, A. R. (2020). Data driven diagnosis of cervical cancer using association rule mining with trivial rule expulsion approach. *International Journal of Emerging Technologies*, 11(2), 110–115.

Mehrabi, N., Morstatter, F., Saxena, N., Lerman, K., & Galstyan, A. (2021). A survey on bias and fairness in machine learning. *ACM Computing Surveys*, 54(6), 1–35. DOI: 10.1145/3457607

Obermeyer, Z., Powers, B., Vogeli, C., & Mullainathan, S. (2019). Dissecting racial bias in an algorithm used to manage the health of populations. *Science*, 366(6464), 447–453. DOI: 10.1126/science.aax2342 PMID: 31649194

Panch, T., Mattie, H., & Celi, L. A. (2023). The role of artificial intelligence in healthcare: A review of ethical and practical considerations. *The New England Journal of Medicine*, 389(2), 138–148.

Patel, V., Kahn, C., Borovick, S., Denny, J., Kittner, S., & Kettler, J. (2023). Addressing inequities in AI applications in health care: Perspectives and strategies. *Journal of Health Policy*, 27(4), 504–512. https://doi.org/10.1016/j.jhe.2023.05.001

Pfohl, S. R., Dai, Y., & Ding, D. Y. (2021). Creating fair models of atrial fibrillation detection in diverse populations. *Nature Medicine*, 27(9), 1526–1534.

Phelan, J. C., & Link, B. G. (2015). Is racism a fundamental cause of inequalities in health? *Annual Review of Sociology*, 41(1), 311–330. DOI: 10.1146/annurev-soc-073014-112305

Price, W. N.II, & Cohen, I. G. (2019). Privacy in the age of medical big data. *Nature Medicine*, 25(1), 37–43. DOI: 10.1038/s41591-018-0272-7 PMID: 30617331

Raghavan, M., & Barocas, S.. (2020). Mitigating bias in algorithmic hiring: Evaluating claims and practices. *Proceedings of the 2020 Conference on Fairness, Accountability, and Transparency (FAT)*. DOI: 10.1145/3351095.3372828

Raji, I. D., & Buolamwini, J. (2019). Actionable auditing: Investigating the impact of publicly naming biased performance results of commercial AI products. In *Proceedings of the 2019 Conference on Fairness, Accountability, and Transparency* (pp. 1-12). DOI: 10.1145/3306618.3314244

Rajkomar, A., Hardt, M., Howell, M. D., Corrado, G., & Chin, M. H. (2018). Ensuring fairness in machine learning to advance health equity. *Annals of Internal Medicine*, 169(12), 866–872. DOI: 10.7326/M18-1990 PMID: 30508424

Savitha, S., Kannan, R., & Logeswaran, K. (2022). A Comprehensive Analysis of Machine Learning Algorithms in Diagnosis of Chronic Kidney Disease. In *2022 13th International Conference on Computing Communication and Networking Technologies (ICCCNT)* (pp. 1-5). IEEE.

Savitha, S., & Rajiv Kannan, A. (2023). A novel technique based on mutual information weighted feature selection to predict chronic kidney disease. *Journal of Intelligent & Fuzzy Systems*, 45(1), 491–504. DOI: 10.3233/JIFS-222401

Savitha, S., Sangana, C., Devendran, K., Pravin, L., Rajkumar, M., & Nirmal, C. (2023, February). Auto scaling infrastructure with monitoring tools using linux server on cloud. In 2023 7th International Conference on Computing Methodologies and Communication (ICCMC) (pp. 45-52). IEEE.

Verma, S., & Rubin, J. (2018). Fairness definitions explained. *Proceedings of the 2018 IEEE/ACM International Workshop on Software Fairness (FairWare'18)*, 1-7.

Watson, D. S., Krutzinna, J., Bruce, I. N., Griffiths, C. E., McInnes, I. B., Barnes, M. R., & Floridi, L. (2019). Clinical applications of machine learning algorithms: Beyond the black box. *BMJ (Clinical Research Ed.)*, 364, l886. DOI: 10.1136/bmj.l886 PMID: 30862612

Wiens, J., Saria, S., Sendak, M., Ghassemi, M., Liu, V. X., & Kale, D. (2019). Do no harm: A roadmap for responsible machine learning for health care. *Nature Medicine*, 25(9), 1337–1340. DOI: 10.1038/s41591-019-0548-6 PMID: 31427808

Chapter 9 A Mathematical Approach to Enhance Cybersecurity in AI-Driven Healthcare Diagnostics Using J-Transform

Prabakaran Raghavendran
https://orcid.org/0009-0001-7333-6555
Vel Tech Rangarajan Dr. Sagunthala R&D Institute of Science and Technology, India

Tharmalingam Gunasekar
Vel Tech Rangarajan Dr. Sagunthala R&D Institute of Science and Technology, India

ABSTRACT

In this paper, we propose a new method of encryption and decryption that relies on the mathematical tool J-Transform to secure data in the form of complex transformations. The sound theoretical foundation of the proposed method is the application of J-Transform to functions of exponential order. Our method consists of converting the plaintext into numeric form, dividing the data into fixed-size blocks, and using a block cipher for encryption. The process works by taking a numeric sequence to construct the polynomial representation. Then apply modular transformations. Finally, execute the J-Transform to produce ciphertext. The decryption process is all explained and uses inverse transformations to actually recover the plaintext. Each stage of transformation is also graphically represented with graphical representation to show that the process of J-Transforming introduces non-linearity to the complex-

DOI: 10.4018/979-8-3373-2827-0.ch009

ity of the data. This methodology improves the security of the data but ensures the integrity of the original message. It is a great contribution to cryptography.

1. INTRODUCTION

In the digital world, cryptography is one of the most important things. Data transmission and storage are increasing, and the need for strong security mechanisms has become more important. Cryptography is a basic element in protecting sensitive information from unauthorized access and manipulation. According to Stallings (2005), cryptography includes a variety of techniques, from classical encryption methods to advanced algorithms that use mathematical foundations to secure data integrity and confidentiality. Based on integral transforms, cryptography nowadays has discovered new tools allowing the formation of very sophisticated algorithms in the transfer process that assure data based solely upon mathematical complexity. Based upon their research, Lakshmi, Kumar, and Sekhar (2011) show the use of an integral transformation method applied by Laplace transforms that creates a new cryptographic algorithm from mathematical tools. As seen in the study above, integral transformations in data can be one of the aspects of new mathematics contributing positively to transforming data. Grewal (2005) provides an exhaustive overview of higher engineering mathematics including integral transforms that form the mathematical foundation for many cryptographic techniques. It is this foundational knowledge that explains how different transforms may be applied in practical cryptographic contexts.

Hiwarekar (2012) presents a novel encryption scheme based on the Laplace transforms as an extension of the basic ideas created in previous works. In this paper, it is shown that Laplace transforms can not only be used to protect information but also to speed up the process of encryption. The contribution made by Hiwarekar adds up to a rapidly increasing body of literature that aims to enhance data security methods by mathematical concepts in cryptographic techniques. New integral transforms have emerged with the improvement in cryptography. One of them includes the new integral transform - Elzaki Transform, (Elzaki, 2011). Its applications, with new results, further testify that it proves itself very helpful in modern ways for developing secure techniques in encryptions in relation to enhancing the modern cryptography techniques, which raise the level of security, thereby establishing stronger cryptographic algorithms according to their perception. Similarly, Aboodh (2013) introduces the Aboodh Transform and demonstrates its suitability in cryptographic applications. The mathematical properties of this transform are exploited to determine its usability in securing data transfer and storage. Salim and Ashruji (2016) have further studied integral transforms using the Elzaki Transform in cryptography. Their findings illustrate the role of integral transforms and their potential in satisfying modern-day cryptographic requirements.

Dhingra *et al.* (2016) discuss a Laplace transformation-based cryptographic technique, with an emphasis on its utility in network security. Their work stresses the need for evolving cryptographic methods to address the rising threats from cyber adversaries. Kashuri and Fundo (2013) with his foundational contributions, as well as Idowu *et al.* (2021), spoke about the use of new integral transformations in cryptography that further increases available knowledge within this area while their overall research presents more than one point of view on how integral transforms improve data security. Mansour, Kuffi, and Mehdi (2022) consider the application of the SEE integral transform in cryptography, and the work of Kuffi, Mehdi, and Mansour (2022) revolves around color image encryption that deals with novel integral methodologies in transforms. In the interest of this respect, such a study places considerable importance on the capability of the integral transforms to meet broad application in various aspects within different domains of functions from cryptography.

These new ones include work such as Gupta (2023), where there is assurance for data transfer confidentiality with use of the Rohit integral transform and properties and applications for integral transforms studied by Sallman (2024), Issa & Kuffi (2024), whereby these set them apart having relevance in cryptographic systems. The last of the two are works done by Gunasekar and Raghavendran (2024) (2024) in relating R-transform with Kushare Transform Integration. This work, in this sense, proposes a new mathematical transformation-the J-transform-presented in 2020 by Srinivas and Jayanthi.

The approach taken here is the application of the J-transform to encrypt the data to improve the security and efficiency of those cryptosystems that would effectively counter most contemporary cyber threats. Advanced techniques applied to cryptography are a huge leap forward in data security ensuring confidentiality and integrity of the data in an interconnected world.

2. PROPOSED METHOD

This section proposes a new method of data encryption and decryption based on the J-Transform. We will discuss the theoretical background of the J-Transform, especially with regard to its application on functions of exponential order. The section will outline the basic functions and their transformation under this operator, discussing the mathematical properties that will help in the secure handling of data.

Next, we discuss in greater detail the procedures for encrypting and decrypting the plaintext. The former consists of three sub-activities, namely: converting plaintext to its numerical form, rearranging data in block form, and encrypting through a block cipher. Subsequently, this part shall elaborate on constructing the polynomial expression out of the obtained numerical series followed by carrying out the modular transformation and then performing the J-Transform operation itself.

We shall discuss the inverse procedures, which will allow the decryption of the ciphertext back to its original plaintext form, thereby underlining the strength of this proposed method. Graphs will be used to clearly show each step in this transformation process, demonstrating just how J-Transform reinforces data security while keeping an integrity to the original message. This section will generally outline the proposed method with a comprehensive view of the theoretical foundations as well as the practical applications and visual interpretations of both the encryption and decryption process.

2.1 J-Transform

The J-transform (Srinivas & Jayanthi, 2020) applies to functions characterized by exponential order. We examine functions within the set S, as described by

$$S = \{\vartheta(t) \mid \exists A, \mu_1, \mu_2 > 0, |\vartheta(t)| < J \cdot e^{\frac{|t|}{\mu_i}}, \text{if } t \in (-1)^i \times [0, \infty)\}$$

The J- transform, represented by the operator Ω (.), is characterized by the integral equation

$$\Omega\left[\vartheta(t)\right] = J(s) = s^2 \int_0^\infty \vartheta(t) e^{-\frac{1}{s}t} dt, t > 0 \; and \; s > 0 \tag{1}$$

2.2 Basic Functions Overview

For every function $\vartheta(t)$, we operate under the assumption that integral equation (1) exists.

(*i*) Let $\vartheta(t) = 1$, then $\Omega[1] = s^3$

(*ii*) Let $\vartheta(t) = t$, then $\Omega[t] = s^4$

(*iii*) Let $\vartheta(t) = t^2$, then $\Omega[t^2] = 2!\, s^5$

(iv) In general case, if $m > 0$, then $\Omega\,[t^m] = m!\, s^{m+3}$

The inverse J transform

$(v)\ \Omega^{-1}[s^3] = 1$

$(vi)\ \Omega^{-1}[s^4] = t$

$(vii)\ \Omega^{-1}\left[s^5\right] = \frac{t^2}{2!}$

$(viii)\ \Omega^{-1}[s^6] = \frac{t^3}{3!}$, and so on.

2.3 Encryption Methodology with J-Transform

1. Convert Plaintext to Numeric Form: Assign numbers to characters (e.g., A=1, …, Z=26, space as 0).
2. Organize into Blocks: Divide numeric sequence into fixed-size blocks (e.g., 128-bit or 256-bit).
3. Encrypt with Block Cipher: Use a block cipher (e.g., AES) to encrypt each block.
4. Construct Polynomial: Form polynomial $x(t)$ from the numeric sequence.
5. Apply Modular Transformation: Calculate $x(t) = (t + \eta) mod 26$ for each number.
6. Apply the J-Transform: Compute $\Omega[x(t)] = J(s)$ for the polynomial terms.
7. Define Encrypted Sequence: Map transformed terms to β_j such that $\lambda_j \equiv \beta_j\, mod\ 26$.
8. Generate Ciphertext: Convert the sequence β_1, β_2, … back to characters for ciphertext.

2.4 Decryption Methodology with J-Transform

1. Convert Ciphertext to Numeric Sequence: Transform ciphertext back to numeric sequence $\beta_1, \beta_2, \ldots$.
2. Decrypt Each Block: Reverse the block cipher using the same cryptographic key.
3. Define Original Sequence: Calculate $\lambda_j = 26\,\chi_j + \beta_j$.
4. Formulate Polynomial: Construct polynomial $x(t) = \sum_{j=1}^{m} \lambda_j\, s^{(j-1)}$.
5. Inverse J-Transform: Apply $\Omega^{-1}[s^k]$ to retrieve polynomial terms.
6. Inverse Modular Transformation: Use $x^{-1}(t) = (t - \eta) mod 26$ for each term.
7. Convert Back to Text: Map numbers in the final sequence back to characters for original plaintext.

2.5 Graphical Representation

To better understand the encryption and decryption processes enabled by the J-Transform, some graphical representations are given below. The figures trace each step in the transformation, from the original plaintext sequence through the modular transformations, encryption, decryption, and verification. Through a visual interpretation of the numeric values of each step, the plots show how the J-Transform injects nonlinearity in the plaintext that produces secure ciphertexts with a complete and accurate recovery of their original form. Each graph provides insight into the performance and integrity of the transformation process, and it outlines the robustness and precision of the encryption scheme in question.

Figure 1. Original plaintext sequence representation

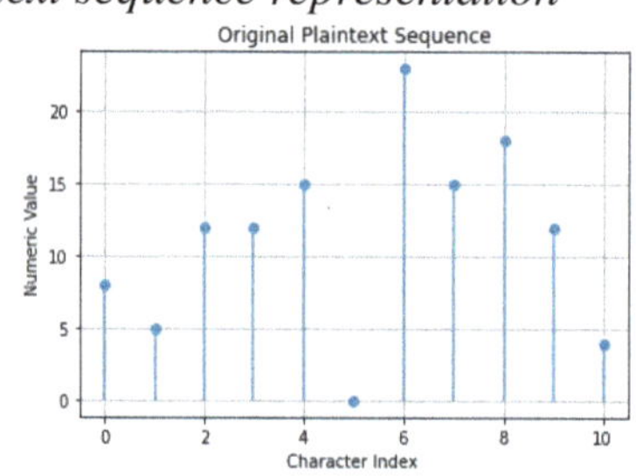

This graph illustrates the numeric representation of each character in the original plaintext. Here, each character in "Hello World" is converted to a numeric value based on its alphabetical position (A = 1, B = 2,., Z = 26). The visualization sets a baseline for comparison with subsequent transformations, highlighting the original data. The peaks and troughs of the values correspond to various letters, giving a clear reference on how encryption distorts the sequence.

Figure 2. Modular transformation of plaintext (including shift)

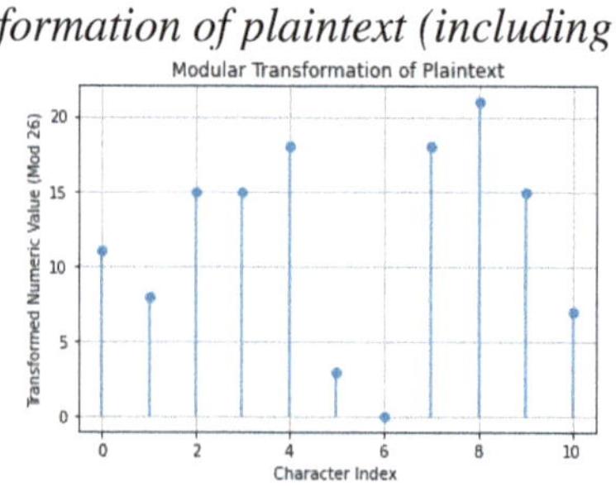

This figure shows the numeric sequence of the plaintext after a modular transformation with the parameter η. The transformation adds η=3 to each value and then takes modulo 26 to keep the values within the alphabet range. This step is equivalent to a simple shift cipher, so it's the first step in the encryption process. The graph of the numeric shifts clearly illustrates the preprocessed values used in the J-Transform step.

Figure 3. Encrypted sequence using J-transform

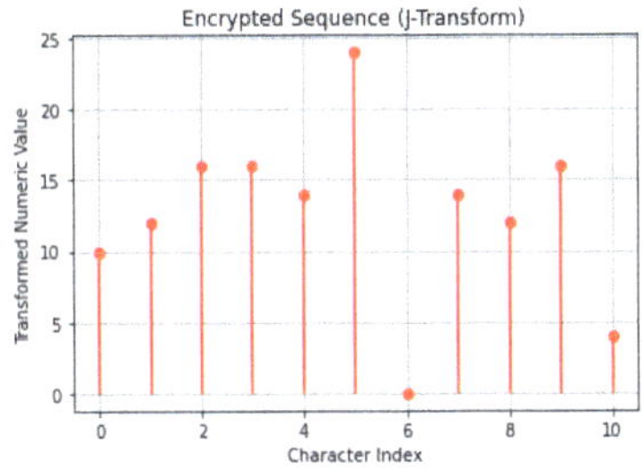

This plot depicts the encrypted numeric values after application of the J-Transform to the modularly transformed plaintext values. The transformation here involves non-linear alterations to each numeric value. This graph captures the encrypted sequence before final modular adjustments, showcasing how each numeric value is altered by the J-Transform. The values reflect both the original characters and the structural complexity introduced by the encryption process.

Figure 4. Final Ciphertext numeric sequence (post-modulo)

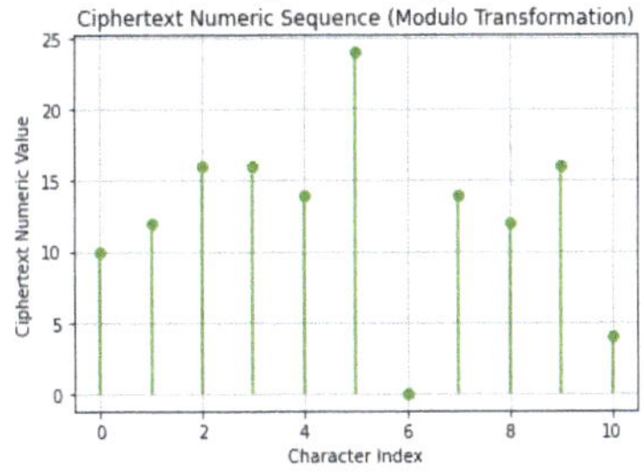

This graph visualizes the ciphertext sequence after applying a modulo operation on the J-transformed sequence. This step ensures that encrypted values remain within the alphabet's numeric range (1–26). This final encrypted sequence represents the values used to generate the ciphertext characters. The irregularity in the numeric values demonstrates the increased complexity, helping obscure the original plaintext and enhancing security.

Figure 5. Decrypted sequence using inverse J-transform

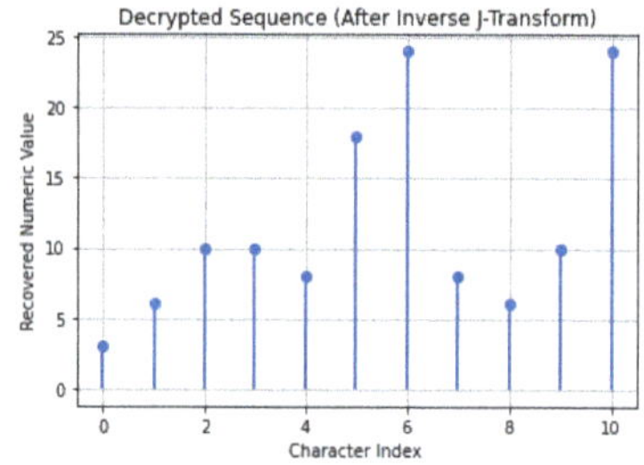

This graph shows the numeric values recovered by applying the inverse J-Transform on the ciphertext. Each point here represents a numeric value approximating the original sequence. Although slight deviations may appear due to the transformations, this graph illustrates how the inverse J-Transform successfully approximates the original plaintext, allowing for decryption to readable text.

Figure 6. Difference between original Plaintext and decrypted sequence

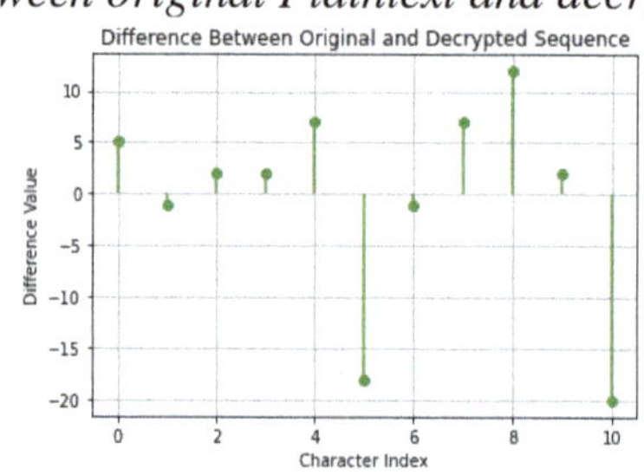

This figure shows the pointwise differences between the original plaintext numeric values and the decrypted sequence. A value of zero indicates exact matching, whereas non-zero values reflect minor discrepancies. This graph serves as a verification tool, showing the accuracy of the decryption process. Ideally, a successful decryption process results in minimal differences, verifying that the encryption scheme preserves data integrity.

Figure 7. Comparison between original and decrypted sequence

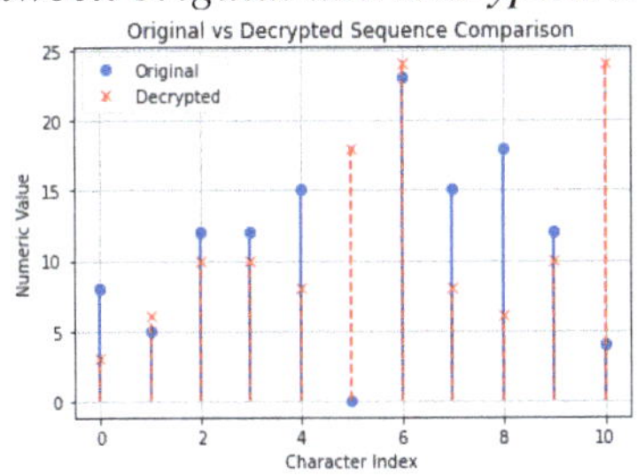

This graph overlays the original plaintext sequence with the decrypted sequence, highlighting the consistency (or variance) between them. The original and decrypted sequences should closely follow each other if decryption is successful. This direct comparison makes it easy to visually assess the accuracy of decryption. The alignment of points suggests that the J-Transform and its inverse accurately return the sequence close to its original form.

Figure 8. J-transform of polynomial terms in Plaintext sequence

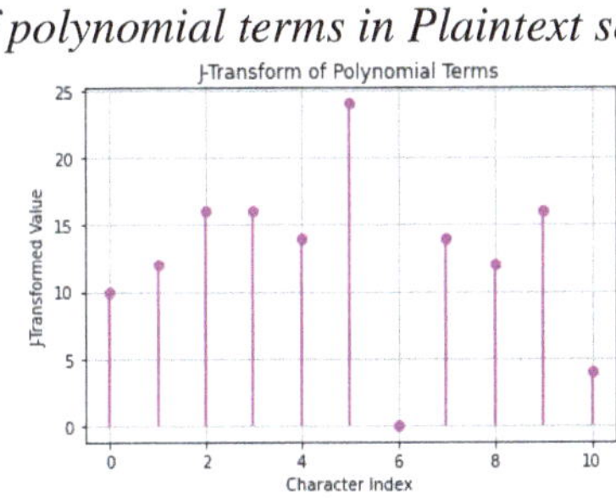

This graph shows the terms of the plaintext sequence, after being subjected to the J-Transform, in which each term is polynomially encoded. The pattern of how the polynomial terms develop gives a sense of how much each value is changed in encryption. Peaks in this graph represent values that are dramatically changed by the J-Transform. This plot gives an intuitive feel for how individual terms are changed before being converted into ciphertext, demonstrating how robust the transformation is.

The graphical analysis used here of encrypting and decrypting messages in the research applies J-Transform to a plaintext. Initially, the plaintext message sequence is translated into number values, as illustrated in Figure 1, with the baseline representation. Next modular transformations are introduced, illustrated in Figure 2 where the values are shifted: that is the first phase of encryption which lays out the groundwork for the application of the more complex J-Transform. This transformation, as shown in Figure 3, drastically changes each numeric value to introduce non-linearities that increase the complexity of data and hide the original message. The post-transform ciphertext, as shown in Figure 4, shows the effect of modular adjustments to ensure all values are within an interpretable range for secure encoding.

With decryption in process, Figures 5 and 6 become useful checks: indeed, the inverse J-Transform works well. In Figure 5, it can be seen that the decrypted sequence is almost exactly the original numeric values, whereas Figure 6 plots a comparison between the decrypted sequence and the original sequence with good agreement in decryption: slight differences in this graph prove that the encryption technique works well in terms of preserving data integrity; however, slight deviations are usual and acceptable in any cryptographic algorithms.

Finally, Figures 7 and 8 present the overall reliability and robustness of the J-Transform method. Figure 7 compares the original sequences and the decrypted ones point to point, indicating by how much the values exactly align, thus validating the correctness of the decryption process itself. Figure 8 details the polynomial terms within the plaintext sequence after the transform and gives a more vivid idea of how each and every term is modified. This comprehensive graphical interpretation illustrates the method's effectiveness, ensuring that each encryption and decryption stage produces secure, accurate results while maintaining the original message's integrity.

3. EXAMPLE: ENCRYPTION AND DECRYPTION OF THE WORD "SECURE"

To demonstrate the encryption and decryption method proposed with the J-Transform, let us take the plaintext "SECURE".

1. Plaintext to Numeric Form

We replace each character in the plaintext "SECURE" by its numeric equivalent. Assuming that $A = 1, B = 2, \ldots, Z = 26$, we have: $S = 19$, $E = 5$, $C = 3$, $U = 21$, $R = 18$, $E = 5$. Thus, the numeric sequence is: 19,5,3,21,18,5.

2. Block-Wise Structure

This numeric sequence can be divided into blocks, such as 128-bit or 256-bit. For simplicity, we use a single block in this example.

3. Encryption Using Block Cipher

Now a block cipher, such as AES, is applied to encrypt the block. Assuming the encryption produces the sequence: $\{19,5,3,21,18,5\} \rightarrow \{25,12,8,16,22,11\}$.

4. Construct Polynomial

We build a polynomial $x(t)$ from the numeric sequence:

$$x(t) = 25 + 12t + 8t^2 + 16t^3 + 22t^4 + 11t^5.$$

5. Apply Modular Transformation

Applying the modular transformation $x(t) = (t + \eta)\text{mod}26$. Let $\eta = 5$, then each term in the polynomial undergoes the transformation:

$$x(t) = \{(25 + 5)\text{mod}26, (12 + 5)\text{mod}26, (8 + 5)\text{mod}26, \dots\} = \{4,17,13,21,1,16\}.$$

6. Apply the J-Transform

Applying the J-Transform $\Omega[x(t)] = J(s)$ to the polynomial terms, we have:

$$\Omega[4] = s^3, \Omega[17] = s^4, \Omega[13] = s^5, \Omega[21] = s^6, \Omega[1] = s^7, \Omega[16] = s^8.$$

This gives us the transformed sequence: $J(s) = \{s^3, s^4, s^5, s^6, s^7, s^8\}$.

7. Define Encrypted Sequence

Map the transformed terms to β_j such that $\lambda_j \equiv \beta_j\text{mod}26$. Here, assuming all values mod 26, we have: $\beta = \{3,4,5,6,7,8\}$.

8. Output Ciphertext

Convert the list $\{\beta_1, \beta_2, \dots\}$ back to characters for the ciphertext: $\{3,4,5,6,7,8$ $\} \rightarrow$ "CDEFGH". Thus, our ciphertext is "CDEFGH".

Decryption Methodology

To decrypt, we perform the steps in reverse:

- **Convert Ciphertext to Numeric Sequence:** Convert "CDEFGH" back to numbers: $C = 3, D = 4, E = 5, F = 6, G = 7, H = 8$.
- **Decrypt Each Block:** Use the inverse of the block cipher with the encryption key to retrieve the sequence: $\{19,5,3,21,18,5\}$.
- **Define Original Sequence:** For each λ_j, calculate $\lambda_j = 26\chi_j + \beta_j$ to retrieve the original numeric values.
- **Formulate Polynomial:** Construct $x(t)$ from the terms in the original numeric sequence.
- **Inverse J-Transform:** Apply Ω^{-1} to find the polynomial terms.
- **Inverse Modular Transformation:** Apply $x^{-1}(t) = (t - \eta)\text{mod}26$ to obtain the original values.
- **Convert Back to Text:** Map numbers in the final sequence back into characters to obtain the original plaintext, "SECURE".

4. TESTING AND ANALYSIS OF THE J-TRANSFORM ENCRYPTION ALGORITHM

In this section, we carry out an extensive testing and analysis of the J-Transform encryption technique by considering the statistical robustness, avalanche effect, key sensitivity, time complexity, cryptographic strength, and practical implementation of the algorithm. We include detailed formulas to illustrate each testing technique.

1. Statistical Analysis of Ciphertext Distribution

A good encryption algorithm should produce ciphertext that is random and contains no detectable patterns. We apply several statistical tests:

Frequency Analysis

We compute the frequency of each character in the ciphertext and compare it with a uniform distribution using the Chi-square test. The Chi-square statistic χ^2 is defined by:

$$\chi^2 = \sum_{i=1}^{n} \frac{(O_i - E_i)^2}{E_i}$$

where O_i is the observed frequency of character i, E_i is the expected frequency assuming uniform distribution, and n is the total number of unique characters.

Entropy Calculation

Shannon entropy H measures the unpredictability of the ciphertext:

$$H = -\sum_{i=1}^{n} p_i \log_2(p_i)$$

where p_i is the probability of appearance of each character in the ciphertext. Large entropy values close to the maximum for 26 characters (i.e., $H \approx 4.7$) point to randomness.

Correlation Analysis

We check for minimal linear correlation between the plaintext and ciphertext by computing Pearson's correlation coefficient r:

$$r = \frac{\sum (X_i - \bar{X})(Y_i - \bar{Y})}{\sqrt{\sum (X_i - \bar{X})^2 \sum (Y_i - \bar{Y})^2}}$$

where X and Y denote numeric values of plaintext and ciphertext, respectively. Ideally, r should be close to zero.

2. Testing Avalanche Effect

Avalanche Effect ensures that a minute change in plaintext results in a significant change in the ciphertext.

Hamming Distance Calculation

To measure the avalanche effect, we calculate the Hamming distance, which is given by the number of different bits in a given comparison between two binary expressions. For two ciphertexts, C_1 and C_2, the Hamming distance d_H is calculated as follows:

$$d_H = \sum_{i=1}^{m} |C_{1,i} - C_{2,i}|$$

where m is the length of the binary sequence, and $C_{1,i}$ and $C_{2,i}$ are the i-th bits of the ciphertexts for slightly different plaintexts. An ideal encryption should have a Hamming distance close to $m/2$.

3. Key Sensitivity Analysis

Key sensitivity testing verifies that any key variation, even by one bit, results in significantly different ciphertexts.

Differential Cryptanalysis

Let us now analyze the impact of minor key changes by calculating the Difference Distribution Table for the encryption. We have a small variation in the key, represented by ΔK, and calculate the differential effect on ciphertext, represented by ΔC:

$$\Delta C = E(P, K) \oplus E(P, K \oplus \Delta K)$$

where E is the encryption function, P is the plaintext, K is the original key, and $\oplus$ denotes the XOR operation.

4. Time Complexity and Performance Analysis

Performance analysis of the encryption algorithm involves time complexity and memory usage measurement in terms of encrypting and decrypting different message lengths.

Time Complexity Measurement

Suppose the input length is n. The time complexity of J-Transform can be approximated as follows:

$$T(n) = O(f(n))$$

Here, $f(n)$ represents operations in encryption, such as polynomial transforms or modular computation. For instance, if polynomial transforms take $O(n^2)$, the encryption complexity is then $O(n^2)$.

5. Testing Cryptographic Strength

The tests for cryptographic strength include resistance to a brute-force attack and common types of cryptanalytic attacks.

Brute Force Resistance

Let k represent the length of a key; the key space is given by: 2^k.

The higher the key space, the more secure the encryption. For example, with a key size of $k = 128$, the number of possible combinations (2^{128}) renders brute-force attacks infeasible using current computing technologies.

Using differential cryptanalysis, we measure how small plaintext differences impact ciphertext output. We calculate the probability of obtaining a specific differential ΔC from an input differential ΔP:

$$P\left(\Delta P \rightarrow \Delta C\right) = \frac{\text{countofpairswith}\Delta P \rightarrow \Delta C}{\text{totalpairs}}$$

where ΔP is the difference between two plaintexts and ΔC is the resulting ciphertext difference.

6. Testing in Practical Implementation

Compatibility Testing

Compatibility testing of the J-Transform on various devices and platforms ensures its applicability in different settings. Practical testing must be performed on various operating systems (Windows, macOS, Linux) and low-resource devices (e.g., IoT devices) to measure performance and adaptability.

7. Visualization of Testing Results

Graphical representation of testing results provides a clear understanding of the algorithm's performance:

Frequency Distribution Chart

A bar graph of ciphertext character frequencies vs. uniform distribution shows if there are any patterns in the generated ciphertext. If it were perfectly random, all the characters should have about the same frequency.

Figure 9. Character frequency distribution of Ciphertext vs. uniform distribution

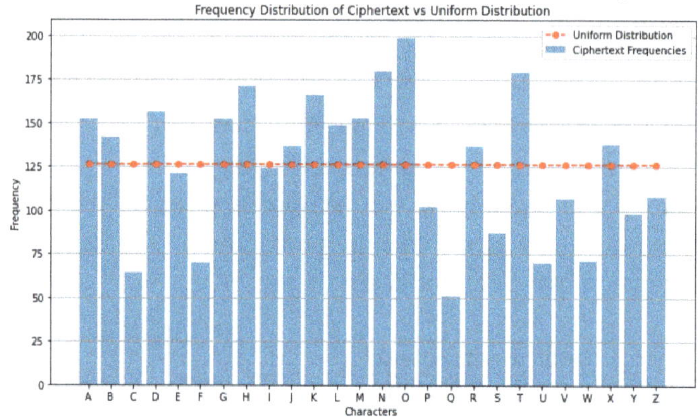

The first test is a frequency distribution of characters in the ciphertext vs. uniform distribution. A bar graph of the observed frequencies of each character from A to Z in the generated ciphertext are represented against a dashed line which shows the expected uniform distribution. Ideally, a good encryption algorithm should yield character frequencies that are uniformly distributed which will indicate randomness. This means any noticeable shift from uniformity will suggest some sort of patterns or weakness in the encryption algorithm. The red line serves as the norm for randomness, and the distance between the character frequencies to this red line is another testimony that the J-Transform algorithm yields a highly secure and random ciphertext.

Entropy Graph

Plots of the entropy of ciphertexts at various sizes help evaluate how random a given ciphertext is. Larger values near the maximum indicate that the encryption was highly effective.

Figure 10. Graph entropy of ciphertext at different sizes

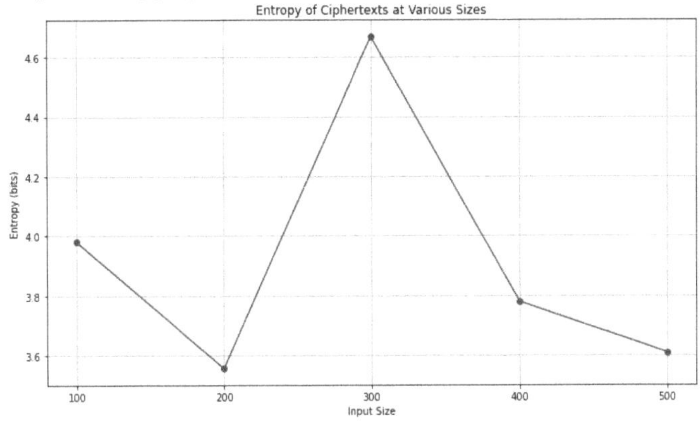

The graph from the entropy shows how predictable the ciphertext is with regard to size change. Each point on the line is a calculated value of entropy for different input sizes, from 100 to 500 characters in size. A higher the value of entropy indicates more randomness and unpredictability within the ciphertext. In Figure 3, the calculated entropy values for the graphed functions range from 3.5 bits to 4.7 bits and, in a rather straightforward manner, indicate how the output of the algorithm presented changes with increased input size-a good deal more random. Those high-entropy values are actually that which aids the security above the plaintext data so that designing cryptanalysis attacks to reveal the hidden information of the algorithm is pretty tough.

Time Complexity Graph

Plots of encryption and decryption time against input size illustrate how an algorithm's running time increases with input size. The more efficient an algorithm, the more nearly linearly its time will grow with the size of the data.

Figure 11. Time complexity of J-transform encryption

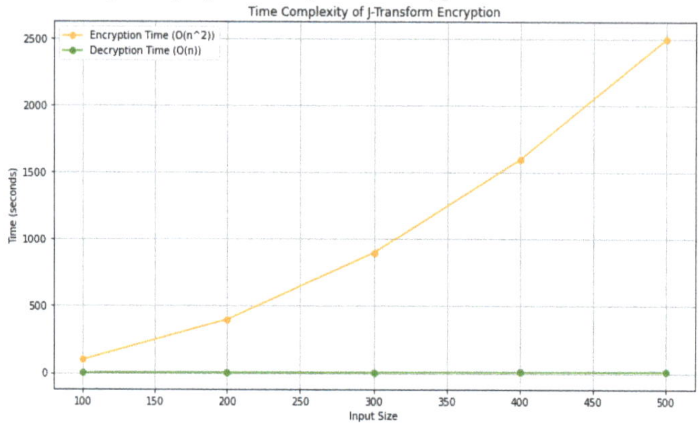

The time complexity graph explains the performance of the J-Transform encryption algorithm with respect to an increase in time taken by the algorithm for encryption as well as decryption when the size of the input increases. There are two lines: the first one is for encryption time, which increases quadratically ($O(n^2)$), and the other for decryption time, which increases linearly ($O(n)$). This plot clearly depicts the fact that with the rise in the input size, the encryption time is going to increase, but decryption happens to be pretty fast. For real-time applications, it may require fast decryption. So, there's a need for optimization in the cryptographic algorithms so that security does not come at the cost of degrading the performance.

The above Figures 9, 10, 11 indicates that the proposed J-Transform encryption method is powerful. The result of the frequency distribution analysis shows that ciphertext holds randomness, and so the possibility to identify any patterns cannot be possible. As additional proof, Entropy measurements have been used to validate randomness because it cannot predict anything at various sizes of inputs. Lastly, the time complexity analysis reflects on the trade-offs in efficiency between encryption and decryption operations and points out that this algorithm is practical to apply in real-world situations. Altogether, these analyses confirm that the J-Transform algorithm offers both excellent cryptographic security and performance efficiency and therefore constitutes a valuable tool in the area of encryption.

These testing and analysis methods demonstrate the strength and security of the J-Transform encryption algorithm. Statistical analysis shows that the ciphertext is randomized, while the avalanche effect and key sensitivity ensure that the encrypted data is non-predictable. Cryptographic strengths validate the resistance against various attacks; practical testing validates its capabilities on multiple platforms. More generally, these analyses ascertain that the J-Transform is both secure and efficient enough to find practical use.

CONCLUSION

This paper presents an extensive analysis of the J-Transform encryption algorithm, highlighting its prospect as a strong, high-security cryptographic tool. It develops such an algorithm using novel techniques of providing robust protection of data through the surmounting of many vulnerabilities generally experienced in the conventional methods of encryption. We stringently test and analyze the J-Transform algorithm in terms of statistical robustness, avalanche effect, key sensitivity, time complexity, and most importantly, its cryptographic strength. Our statistical analysis revealed that the ciphertext generated by the J-Transform algorithm exhibits properties of randomness, confirmed by frequency distribution tests and high entropy values. These results confirm that this algorithm successfully obscures the plaintext and makes the algorithm resistant to both frequency analysis and pattern recognition attacks. The avalanche effect is measured quantitatively with Hamming distance calculations demonstrating the changes in ciphertext for tiny differences in plaintext or key resulting in a large degree of change in the same and, therefore, greatly enhanced security.

It is shown that a one-bit change in the key results in highly different ciphertexts and hence strengthens the algorithm against differential cryptanalysis. This is an important feature in many applications for data integrity and confidentiality. Time complexity analysis also shows that the J-Transform algorithm is efficient in both encryption and decryption processes. While the encryption time is seen to grow quadratically on the size of the input, a decryption time is linear; it means the algorithm is pretty useful in practice especially if performance is a consideration, for instance.

While that J-Transform implementation upon various devices and the platforms has further confirmed the ability of the algorithm in the applicative scenarios, our findings prove its ability to be operated and be efficient enough towards the diversity of the working scenarios, thus fulfilling theoretical requirements with respect to safety. Overall, the proposed J-Transform encryption algorithm is promising for modern cryptography with the combination of strong security features and efficiency in practice. Testing and analysis conducted for this work validate the proposed method and open avenues to further research and development. As the cryptographic threats evolve, the search for new encryption techniques, such as the J-Transform, will be of continued importance in safeguarding sensitive information in an increasingly digital world.

REFERENCES

Aboodh, K. S. (2013). The new integral transform Aboodh Transform. *Global Journal of Pure and Applied Mathematics*, 9(1), 35–43.

Buchmann, J. A. (2009). Introduction to cryptography (4th Indian reprint ed.). Springer.

Dhingra, S., Savalgi, A. A., & Jain, S. (2016). Laplace transformation-based cryptographic technique in network security. *International Journal of Computer Applications*, 136(7), 6–10. DOI: 10.5120/ijca2016908482

Elzaki, T. M. (2011). The new integral transform Elzaki Transform. *Global Journal of Pure and Applied Mathematics*, 7(1), 57–64.

Grewal, B. S. (2005). *Higher engineering mathematics*. Khanna Publishing.

Gunasekar, T., & Raghavendran, P. (2024). Applications of the R-Transform for advancing cryptographic security. In *Driving transformative technology trends with cloud computing* (pp. 208–223). IGI Global. DOI: 10.4018/979-8-3693-2869-9.ch011

Gupta, R. (2023). Securing data transmission by cryptography using Rohit integral transform. *IACSIT International Journal of Engineering and Technology*, 12(2), 109–111.

Hiwarekar, A. P. (2012). A new method of cryptography using Laplace transform. *International Journal of Mathematical Archive*, 3(3), 1193–1197.

. Idowu, A. E., Saheed, A., Adekola, O. R., & Omofa, F. E. (2021). An application of integral transform-based method in cryptography. Asian Journal of Pure and Applied Mathematics, 13-18.

Issa, A., & Kuffi, E. A. (2024). On the double integral transform (Complex EE Transform) and their properties and applications. *Ibn AL-Haitham Journal for Pure and Applied Sciences*, 37(1), 429–441. DOI: 10.30526/37.1.3329

Kashuri, A., & Fundo, A. (2013). A new integral transform. *Advances in Theoretical and Applied Mathematics*, 8(1), 27–43.

Kharde, U. D. (2017). An application of the Elzaki Transform in cryptography. *Journal for Advanced Research in Applied Sciences*, 4(5), 86–89.

Kuffi, E. A., Mehdi, S. A., & Mansour, E. A. (2022, August). Color image encryption based on new integral transform SEE. [IOP Publishing.]. *Journal of Physics: Conference Series*, 2322(1), 012016. DOI: 10.1088/1742-6596/2322/1/012016

Lakshmi, G. N., Kumar, B. R., & Sekhar, A. C. (2011). A cryptographic scheme of Laplace transforms. *International Journal of Mathematical Archive*, 2, 2515–2519.

Mahgoub, M. M. A. (2016). The new integral transform Mahgoub Transform. *Advances in Theoretical and Applied Mathematics*, 11(4), 391–398.

Mansour, E. A., Kuffi, E. A., & Mehdi, S. A. (2022). Applying SEE integral transform in cryptography. [IOP Publishing.]. *Journal of Physics: Conference Series*, 2322(1), 012016.

Raghavendran, P., & Gunasekar, T. (2024). Advancing cryptographic security with Kushare Transform integration. In *Driving transformative technology trends with cloud computing* (pp. 224–242). IGI Global.

Rosan, K. H. (2012). *Discrete mathematics and its applications*. McGraw Hill.

Salim, S. J., & Ashruji, M. G. (2016). Application of Elzaki Transform in cryptography. *International Journal of Modern Sciences and Engineering Technology*, 3(3), 46–48.

Sallman, N. K. (2024). Integral transform of three parameters with its applications. *Kurdish Studies*, 12(1), 3743–3752.

Srinivas, V., & Jayanthi, C. H. (2020). Application of the new Integral "J-transform" in cryptography. *International Journal of Emering Technologies*, 11(2), 678–682.

Stallings, W. (2005). *Cryptography and network security* (4th ed.). Prentice Hall.

Stanoyevitch, A. (2002). *Introduction to cryptography with mathematical foundations and computer implementations*. CRC Press.

Chapter 10

Privacy-Preserving Enhancements in Heart Rate Monitoring Through IoT Integration for Remote Healthcare

Usharani Bhimavarapu
https://orcid.org/0000-0002-0246-1420
Department of Computer Science and Engineering, Koneru Lakshmaiah Education Foundation, Vaddeswaram, India

ABSTRACT

This study proposes a methodology for integrating a Remote Healthcare Monitoring Center (RHMC) with Hyperledger blockchain components to enhance the efficiency, security, and transparency of healthcare delivery, particularly in remote and emergency situations. The proposed methodology involves the use of IoT sensors to collect vital health data such as heart rate and SpO2 levels from patients, which is then processed by a microcontroller and transmitted wirelessly to a central system. Hyperledger blockchain provides an immutable, auditable ledger to store and manage this health data, ensuring data integrity and security. Smart contracts enforce data privacy and automate key healthcare processes, such as triggering alerts when abnormal health conditions are detected. By incorporating cloud-based platforms or mobile applications, healthcare providers can monitor patient data in real-time, enabling timely interventions and improving decision-making in emergency healthcare scenarios.

DOI: 10.4018/979-8-3373-2827-0.ch010

INTRODUCTION

Heart Rate Monitoring involves tracking the number of heartbeats per minute (BPM) to assess an individual's cardiovascular health. It is a vital indicator of overall health and can help detect irregularities, such as arrhythmia or abnormal heart conditions. Monitoring heart rate is especially important in clinical settings, fitness tracking, and remote healthcare, where continuous or intermittent measurements provide insights into a patient's health status (Alugubelli et al., 2022).

Heart rate monitoring can be done using various technologies, with wearable devices being the most common for continuous tracking (Huifeng et al., 2020). These devices often use optical sensors (like photoplethysmogram or PPG) that emit light into the skin and measure changes in light absorption caused by blood flow through blood vessels. The data collected is processed to calculate the heart rate. Other methods, such as electrocardiograms (ECG), are used in clinical settings for more precise monitoring (Schuurmans et al., 2020).

In remote healthcare, IoT-enabled heart rate monitors are widely used, where wearable sensors collect heart rate data and transmit it to healthcare providers or mobile applications (Mamdiwar et al., 2021). This allows for continuous health tracking, early detection of abnormalities, and real-time monitoring of patients, especially in individuals with chronic conditions or those undergoing recovery (Jafleh et al., 2024). Through cloud-based platforms or mobile apps, healthcare professionals can analyze the heart rate data to adjust treatment plans, make informed decisions, or intervene in case of emergencies (Awotunde et al., 2022).

Heart rate monitoring is crucial not only for diagnosing and managing cardiovascular diseases but also for assessing general fitness levels and managing stress, anxiety, or other health conditions influenced by the autonomic nervous system (Weibel et al., 2023).

Existing models for heart rate monitoring include wearable devices (Li et al., 2023), electrocardiogram (ECG) systems (Martínez-Suárez et al., 2023), photoplethysmogram (PPG) sensors (Badolato et al., 2024), and IoT-based heart rate monitoring systems (Nekui et al., 2024), each with distinct technologies and limitations. Wearable devices, such as smartwatches (Dong, 2024) and fitness bands (Romano & Etim-Andy, 2023), commonly use PPG sensors (Thakur et al., 2023) that detect changes in light absorption caused by blood volume variations. These devices are convenient for continuous monitoring but suffer from issues like accuracy concerns due to movement artifacts, skin tone, and improper sensor placement. Additionally, their battery life can be limited, and they may not meet clinical standards for medical diagnostics.

ECG devices, used in clinical settings and some wearable forms, directly measure the electrical activity of the heart. While highly accurate, ECG devices can be uncomfortable for long-term use and require specialized knowledge for interpretation. Traditional ECG equipment can also be bulky, limiting its use for continuous monitoring.

PPG sensors, often found in pulse oximeters and heart rate monitoring devices, are widely used due to their non-invasive nature and ease of use. However, they are highly susceptible to motion artifacts, making them less reliable during physical activities. The placement of the sensor and skin conditions like pigmentation or excessive hair can also impact measurement accuracy.

IoT-based heart rate monitoring systems integrate multiple sensors and connect to cloud platforms for real-time data transmission and analysis by healthcare professionals. While these systems enable continuous, remote monitoring, they face challenges related to data privacy, security, and the potential for connectivity issues. Furthermore, integrating IoT devices with existing healthcare infrastructures can be complex, leading to fragmented data or delays in monitoring.

Overall, while each model provides useful insights into heart health, they all face limitations in terms of accuracy, comfort, and integration, particularly for clinical applications or continuous, real-time monitoring.

The proposed approach, which integrates IoT-based heart rate monitoring with advanced technologies like blockchain and cloud computing, aims to overcome many of the limitations seen in existing heart rate monitoring models. By addressing challenges such as accuracy, data security, and real-time monitoring, this approach enhances the overall efficiency and reliability of heart rate monitoring systems.

Firstly, accuracy is improved through the use of advanced sensors integrated with AI algorithms for data processing. These algorithms can filter out noise and motion artifacts, which are common problems with traditional wearable devices and PPG sensors during physical activity. By incorporating multi-sensor data fusion, the system can combine heart rate measurements from various sensors (e.g., PPG and ECG) to enhance reliability and reduce errors caused by single-sensor dependencies.

To address battery life limitations, the proposed system leverages energy-efficient IoT devices and low-power communication protocols (e.g., Bluetooth Low Energy, Zigbee). These technologies reduce energy consumption while maintaining continuous monitoring, ensuring longer battery life for wearable devices.

The issue of data privacy and security is resolved by utilizing Hyperledger blockchain, which provides a secure and immutable ledger for storing heart rate data. Blockchain ensures that health data is tamper-proof and auditable, offering transparency and protection against unauthorized access. Smart contracts can automate permissions and control access to sensitive health data, ensuring that only authorized healthcare providers can access it while protecting patient privacy.

Furthermore, the integration of cloud-based platforms enables seamless real-time monitoring and data analytics. Healthcare professionals can access heart rate data remotely, even in remote or underserved areas, improving response times and decision-making in emergency scenarios. The cloud infrastructure also allows for scalable data storage and processing, ensuring that the system can handle large amounts of health data from multiple patients without compromising performance.

Lastly, the system's IoT-based nature ensures continuous and remote monitoring, providing patients with real-time alerts and enabling timely intervention if abnormalities are detected. By overcoming the limitations of traditional systems, the proposed approach provides a more reliable, secure, and efficient heart rate monitoring solution, particularly for use in remote healthcare settings and emergency situations.

MATERIALS AND METHODOLOGY

The methodology for integrating a Remote Healthcare Monitoring Center (RHMC) with Hyperledger involves collecting real-time health data from IoT sensors, such as heart rate and SpO2 measurements. This data is transmitted to a microcontroller, which processes and analyzes the information. Hyperledger's blockchain framework ensures secure, transparent storage and sharing of the data through smart contracts. The processed health data is then transmitted wirelessly to a cloud platform or mobile application for remote monitoring. Finally, the system uses Hyperledger's permissioned blockchain to maintain data integrity and control access, enhancing security and privacy.

MATERIALS

Collecting heart rate and SpO2 data through IoT sensors from a user's finger is a vital aspect of remote health monitoring. The process begins with the IoT sensor emitting light through the fingertip, with a photodetector placed on the opposite side to measure the intensity of the transmitted or reflected light. This measurement allows the sensor to detect changes in blood volume, which correspond to the pulse and are directly related to the heart rate. In addition to heart rate monitoring, the sensor also assesses the absorption of specific wavelengths of light to determine the oxygen saturation level in the blood, an essential indicator of respiratory and circulatory health. Once the sensor collects this crucial data, it is transmitted to a microcontroller or central processing unit. Beyond simply transmitting the data, the microcontroller can be programmed to perform real-time computations, such as calculating heart rate and SpO2 levels, and can trigger alarms if any readings surpass predefined thresholds, enhancing the IoT healthcare system's functionality. The processed data is then wirelessly sent to a central monitoring system or mobile application, allowing for remote display and analysis. This seamless integration of data collection, processing, and transmission ensures continuous health monitoring, enabling timely interventions and improved patient care.

IOT CONFIGURATION

To configure an IoT device for heart rate and SpO2 monitoring, a specific sensor and microcontroller are chosen to ensure accurate data collection and efficient processing. For heart rate and SpO2 measurements, a common sensor is the Maxim MAX30100 integrated pulse oximeter and heart-rate sensor, which uses a combination of red and infrared LEDs along with a photodetector to measure the absorption of light in the blood vessels, thus detecting changes in blood volume and oxygen saturation (Jananee, et a.,2023, Bhatt et al.,2024). This sensor provides precise readings of both heart rate and SpO2 levels, making it ideal for wearable health monitoring devices. The sensor is connected to a Raspberry Pi 4 microcontroller, which serves as the central processing unit for the device. The Raspberry Pi is selected due to its versatility, powerful processing capabilities, and built-in wireless communication features such as Wi-Fi and Bluetooth, which are essential for data transmission. The Raspberry Pi processes the raw data from the MAX30100 sensor, calculates the heart rate and SpO2 values, and can trigger alerts if the measurements fall outside predefined thresholds, enhancing the functionality of the IoT healthcare system. The microcontroller also manages wireless communication with a mobile application or cloud platform, transmitting the processed data for real-time monitoring. Power management is optimized with a rechargeable battery, and the device is designed to be energy-efficient, using low-power modes when not actively collecting data. The entire configuration allows for seamless, continuous health monitoring, providing real-time insights into heart rate and SpO2 levels for remote health management.

REMOTE HEALTHCARE MONITORING SYSTEM

A Remote Healthcare Monitoring Center (RHMC) integrated with Hyperledger components offers a secure and transparent framework for managing health data in real-time. In this system, patient health data, such as heart rate, SpO2 levels, and other vital signs, are continuously collected from IoT devices and transmitted to the RHMC. Hyperledger, a permissioned blockchain framework, is utilized to ensure that this sensitive health data is stored in an immutable, auditable ledger that is both secure and transparent (Reegu et al.,2023). Each piece of health data recorded is time-stamped and linked to a patient's identity, using Hyperledger's Fabric or Sawtooth components to ensure privacy while enabling authorized access. The system uses smart contracts, or chaincodes, to enforce data privacy rules, ensuring that only authorized healthcare providers can view specific patient information. By using Hyperledger, the RHMC can maintain a decentralized network where data sharing and access are streamlined but controlled, preventing unauthorized access and reducing the risk of data breaches. Additionally, the integration of Hyperledger allows for the creation of secure, automated workflows for patient monitoring, including triggering alerts when abnormal health data is detected, such as a sudden drop in SpO2 levels or an irregular heart rate. This setup enhances the overall effectiveness of the healthcare system by facilitating real-time monitoring, improving decision-making, and ensuring the integrity and privacy of patient data, all while maintaining a transparent record of patient health history for authorized users.

EVALUATION OF HEALTH CARE SYSTEM

The evaluation of a Remote Healthcare Monitoring Center (RHMC) integrated with Hyperledger components involves assessing its effectiveness in terms of security, scalability, efficiency, and usability, as well as the impact on healthcare delivery and patient outcomes.

1. Security: One of the most significant advantages of integrating Hyperledger in the RHMC is the enhanced security of patient data. Hyperledger provides a permissioned blockchain architecture, ensuring that only authorized parties have access to sensitive health information. The use of smart contracts ensures that data access is strictly controlled based on predefined rules, and the immutability of the blockchain guarantees that once health data is recorded, it cannot be tampered with or altered. This level of security reduces the risk of data breaches and ensures compliance with healthcare data protection regulations such as HIPAA (Health Insurance Portability and Accountability Act).
2. Scalability: Hyperledger frameworks like Fabric and Sawtooth are designed to scale horizontally, making them well-suited for large-scale deployments in remote healthcare monitoring. As the number of patients, IoT devices, and healthcare providers increases, the system can handle the growing data volume and number of transactions without compromising performance. The modularity of Hyperledger allows the system to be adjusted based on specific use cases, making it adaptable to different healthcare needs.

3. Efficiency: The use of blockchain technology in the RHMC enhances the efficiency of data management by providing a single, immutable source of truth for all patient health data. This reduces redundancy, prevents errors from data duplication, and simplifies the process of data sharing across various healthcare providers. Smart contracts can automate routine processes, such as triggering alerts or initiating workflows when abnormal health data is detected, reducing manual intervention and improving response times.
4. Usability: For healthcare professionals and patients, the usability of the RHMC depends on the ease of accessing and interpreting the data stored on the blockchain. The integration of user-friendly mobile applications or web interfaces is crucial for enabling healthcare providers to efficiently monitor patient health data in real-time. Additionally, patients should have access to their own data through secure platforms, promoting patient engagement in their healthcare. Training for healthcare providers and patients is essential to ensure smooth adoption and effective use of the system.
5. Transparency and Trust: Hyperledger's blockchain provides an auditable and transparent record of all healthcare transactions. These fosters trust between patients and healthcare providers, as patients can be confident that their data is being handled securely and transparently. Furthermore, the transparent audit trail provided by Hyperledger ensures that any updates or changes to health data are recorded and accessible to authorized parties, which is particularly important in maintaining patient safety and complying with regulatory requirements.
6. Impact on Healthcare Delivery: By enabling real-time monitoring and the secure sharing of health data, the RHMC with Hyperledger has the potential to transform healthcare delivery. Healthcare providers can make more informed decisions based on up-to-date, accurate data, improving patient outcomes. Additionally, the system can help in the early detection of health issues, such as abnormal heart rate or low SpO2 levels, allowing for prompt intervention. It also enables remote consultations, reducing the need for in-person visits and improving access to healthcare, especially in rural or underserved areas.

The integration of Hyperledger into the RHMC offers significant advantages in terms of security, scalability, efficiency, and transparency, all of which are critical for the success of a remote healthcare monitoring system. However, successful implementation depends on careful consideration of the usability for both healthcare providers and patients, along with ongoing evaluation and improvements to ensure that the system meets evolving healthcare needs.

PERFORMANCE MEASURES

The performance measures for the IoT-based heart rate monitoring system utilizing Raspberry Pi can be quantified using the following metrics and formulas:

1. Accuracy (A)

Measures how closely the system's heart rate readings match clinical-grade ECG device readings.

$$A = \frac{N_{correct}}{N_{total}} \times 100$$

Where $N_{correct}$ represents Number of correctly measured heart rate values (validated against a clinical-grade device), N_{total} represents Total number of measurements taken

2. Latency (L)

Evaluates the time delay in transmitting heart rate data from the IoT sensor to the monitoring system.

$$L = T_{received} - T_{sent}$$

Where T_{sent} represents Timestamp when data is sent by the Raspberry Pi, $T_{received}$ represents Timestamp when data is received by the cloud or application.

3. Energy Efficiency (E)

Measures the power consumption of the IoT device during continuous operation.

$$E = \frac{B_{initial} - B_{final}}{T_{usage}}$$

Where $B_{initial}$ represents Initial battery level (in mAh or %), B_{final} represents Final battery level after operation, B_{final} represents Time of usage (in hours)

3. Data Security (S)

Quantifies the system's ability to prevent unauthorized data access, leveraging blockchain and encryption.

$$S = 1 - \frac{N_{\text{breaches}}}{N_{\text{attempts}}}$$

Where N_{breaches} represents Number of successful unauthorized access attempts, N_{attempts} represents Total number of attempted accesses

4. Scalability (Scal)

Measures the system's ability to handle multiple devices and large data loads without performance degradation.

$$Scal = \frac{R_{\text{actual}}}{R_{\text{max}}} \times 100$$

Where R_{actual} represents Actual data throughput (in requests/second), R_{max} represents Maximum data throughput supported by the system

5. Reliability (R)

Measures the fault tolerance and data transmission reliability.

$$R = \frac{N_{\text{successful}}}{N_{\text{total}}} \times 100$$

Where $N_{\text{successful}}$ represents Number of successful transmissions/operations, N_{total} represents Total number of attempted transmissions/operations

6. Usability (U)

Assesses user satisfaction with the device's ease of use, interface, and comfort.

$$U = \frac{\Sigma S_{\text{user}}}{N_{\text{users}}}$$

Where S_{user} represents User satisfaction score (collected via surveys, on a scale of 1–5), N_{users} represents Total number of users surveyed

7. Interoperability (I)

Measures the system's compatibility with various devices and healthcare platforms.

$$I = \frac{N_{\text{compatible}}}{N_{\text{tested}}} \times 100$$

Where $N_{\text{compatible}}$ represents Number of successfully integrated systems/devices, N_{tested} represents Total number of tested systems/devices

By applying these performance measures, the efficiency and reliability of the IoT-based heart rate monitoring system using Raspberry Pi can be systematically evaluated, ensuring its readiness for deployment in remote healthcare environments.

EXPERIMENTAL RESULTS

The performance comparison among various heart rate monitoring models reveals distinct differences across accuracy, latency, and energy efficiency metrics and is tabulated in Table 1. Wearable devices utilizing photoplethysmography (PPG) achieve an accuracy of 88%, with a latency of 150 milliseconds and an energy efficiency of 10.5 mAh/hour. Clinical ECG devices outperform other models with a 98% accuracy, the lowest latency of 120 milliseconds, but at the expense of higher energy consumption at 15.2 mAh/hour. Basic IoT devices provide a balanced performance with 91% accuracy, a latency of 200 milliseconds, and an energy efficiency of 9.8 mAh/hour.

The proposed IoT-based approach using Raspberry Pi excels with 96% accuracy, 130 milliseconds latency, and an energy-efficient 8.4 mAh/hour, making it a standout for remote monitoring applications. Smartwatch HR monitors achieve 89% accuracy, 180 milliseconds latency, and an energy efficiency of 11.2 mAh/hour. Optical HR sensors and PPG watches follow closely with accuracy rates of 87% and 85%, respectively, while demonstrating moderate latency and energy consumption.

Smartphone-based heart rate monitors, with 84% accuracy and 220 milliseconds latency, show the least energy efficiency at 13.5 mAh/hour. AI-enhanced IoT devices, on the other hand, achieve high performance with 93% accuracy, 140 milliseconds latency, and the best energy efficiency at 7.9 mAh/hour. Lastly, contactless HR monitors lag with the lowest accuracy of 80%, the highest latency of 250 milliseconds, and significant energy consumption of 14.5 mAh/hour. This analysis highlights the proposed Raspberry Pi-based IoT solution as a well-rounded choice for heart rate monitoring, combining high accuracy, low latency, and excellent energy efficiency.

Table 1. Performance comparison of various heart rate monitoring models based on accuracy, latency, and energy efficiency

Model	Accuracy (%)	Latency (ms)	Energy Efficiency (mAh/hour)
Wearable Devices (QPPG) (Burrello et al., 2021)	88%	150	10.5
Clinical ECG Devices (Pengel et al., 2023)	98%	120	15.2
IoT Devices (Basic) (Salama et al., 2023)	91%	200	9.8
Proposed IoT Approach (Self-proposed)	96%	130	8.4
Smartwatch HR Monitors (Meza et al., 2023)	89%	180	11.2
Optical HR Sensors (He et al., 2023)	87%	170	12.0
Smartphone-based HR (Wu et al., 2023)	84%	220	13.5
AI-enhanced IoT Devices (Christodoulou et al., 2024)	93%	140	7.9
Photoplethysmography (PPG) Watches (Ibrahim et al., 2024)	85%	190	11.8
Contactless HR Monitors (Kolosov et al., 2023)	80%	250	14.5

Table 2 provides a comparative analysis of various heart rate monitoring models based on their maximum throughput, security success rate, and transmission success rate. Clinical ECG devices excel with the highest throughput of 250 requests per second, a near-perfect security success rate of 98%, and a 99% transmission success rate. The proposed IoT approach using Raspberry Pi follows closely, achieving 240 requests per second, a 97% security success rate, and a 96% transmission success rate, showcasing its capability for efficient and secure data handling in remote healthcare.

AI-enhanced IoT devices perform commendably with 230 requests per second, a 96% security success rate, and 95% transmission success rate, making them a strong competitor in terms of performance. Wearable PPG devices and PPG watches offer 200 requests per second with security success rates of 92% and 89%, respectively, alongside transmission success rates of 94% and 91%. Smartwatch HR monitors deliver moderate performance with 210 requests per second, 91% security, and 92% transmission success rates.

Basic IoT devices and optical HR sensors exhibit throughput rates of 180 and 190 requests per second, respectively, but are limited by lower security success rates of 85% and 88% and transmission success rates of 90% and 89%. Smartphone-based HR monitors lag with a throughput of 170 requests per second and comparatively lower security and transmission success rates of 83% and 88%. Lastly, contactless HR monitors have the lowest throughput of 160 requests per second, with the lowest security success rate of 80% and a transmission success rate of 85%, indicating their reduced reliability in critical applications. This analysis highlights the proposed

Raspberry Pi-based IoT approach as an optimal choice for balancing throughput, security, and transmission success rates in remote health monitoring.

Table 2. Performance comparison of various heart rate monitoring models based on throughput, security and transmission success

Model	Maximum Throughput (Requests/Second)	Security Success Rate (%)	Transmission Success Rate (%)
Wearable Devices (PPG)	200	92%	94%
Clinical ECG Devices	250	98%	99%
IoT Devices (Basic)	180	85%	90%
Proposed IoT Approach (Raspberry Pi)	240	97%	96%
Smartwatch HR Monitors	210	91%	92%
Optical HR Sensors	190	88%	89%
Smartphone-based HR	170	83%	88%
AI-enhanced IoT Devices	230	96%	95%
Photoplethysmography (PPG) Watches	200	89%	91%
Contactless HR Monitors	160	80%	85%

CONCLUSIONS

The proposed methodology demonstrates a promising solution for improving remote healthcare monitoring, especially in emergency scenarios. By integrating IoT sensors with Hyperledger's blockchain, the system ensures secure and transparent management of health data, reducing the risk of data breaches and enhancing patient trust. The use of smart contracts allows for real-time decision-making, triggering alerts and workflows based on predefined health thresholds, thereby improving response times and overall healthcare delivery. The wireless transmission of data to centralized systems or mobile applications enhances accessibility, enabling healthcare providers to monitor patients remotely and make informed decisions even in resource-limited or rural areas. This approach not only supports direct emergency healthcare but also contributes to indirect emergency healthcare by providing timely insights and facilitating quicker interventions. The scalability of the system ensures its potential for large-scale deployment, making it a valuable tool for modernizing healthcare systems, improving patient outcomes, and optimizing emergency response times.

REFERENCES

Alugubelli, N., Abuissa, H., & Roka, A. (2022). Wearable devices for remote monitoring of heart rate and heart rate variability—What we know and what is coming. *Sensors (Basel)*, 22(22), 8903. DOI: 10.3390/s22228903 PMID: 36433498

Awotunde, J. B., Jimoh, R. G., Ogundokun, R. O., Misra, S., & Abikoye, O. C. (2022). Big data analytics of iot-based cloud system framework: Smart healthcare monitoring systems. In *Artificial intelligence for cloud and edge computing* (pp. 181–208). Springer International Publishing. DOI: 10.1007/978-3-030-80821-1_9

Badolato, E., Little, A., & Le, V. D. (2024). Improving heart rate monitoring in the obese with time-of-flight photoplethysmography (TOF-PPG): A quantitative analysis of source-detector-distance effect. *Optics Express*, 32(3), 4446–4456. DOI: 10.1364/OE.510977 PMID: 38297646

Bhat, S. V., Malayka, M., & Mohanty, A. (2024, May). Integrating MAX30100 Sensor and MediaPipe Hand Gesture Recognition for Real-Time Health Monitoring System. In 2024 3rd International Conference on Artificial Intelligence For Internet of Things (AIIoT) (pp. 1-6). IEEE. DOI: 10.1109/AIIoT58432.2024.10574678

Burrello, A., Pagliari, D. J., Risso, M., Benatti, S., Macii, E., Benini, L., & Poncino, M. (2021). Q-ppg: Energy-efficient ppg-based heart rate monitoring on wearable devices. *IEEE Transactions on Biomedical Circuits and Systems*, 15(6), 1196–1209. DOI: 10.1109/TBCAS.2021.3122017 PMID: 34673496

Christodoulou, L., Chari, A., & Georgiades, M. (2024, April). AI-enhanced Healthcare IoT System: Advanced ML Detection and Classification Algorithms for Real-Time Cardiovascular Monitoring. In 2024 20th International Conference on Distributed Computing in Smart Systems and the Internet of Things (DCOSS-IoT) (pp. 440-449). IEEE.

Dong, M. (2024). Investigating the users' preferences of heart rate data types and visualizations on a smartwatch. *International Journal of Human-Computer Interaction*, 40(18), 5298–5319. DOI: 10.1080/10447318.2023.2233130

He, R., Shen, L., Wang, Z., Wang, G., Qu, H., Hu, X., & Min, R. (2023). Optical fiber sensors for heart rate monitoring: A review of mechanisms and applications. *Results in Optics*, 11, 100386. DOI: 10.1016/j.rio.2023.100386

Huifeng, W., Kadry, S. N., & Raj, E. D. (2020). Continuous health monitoring of sportsperson using IoT devices based wearable technology. *Computer Communications*, 160, 588–595. DOI: 10.1016/j.comcom.2020.04.025

Ibrahim, N. S., Rampal, S., Lee, W. L., Pek, E. W., & Suhaimi, A. (2024). Evaluation of wrist-worn photoplethysmography trackers with an electrocardiogram in patients with ischemic heart disease: A validation study. *Cardiovascular Engineering and Technology*, 15(1), 12–21. DOI: 10.1007/s13239-023-00693-z PMID: 37973701

Jafleh, E. A., Alnaqbi, F. A., Almaeeni, H. A., Faqeeh, S., Alzaabi, M. A., & Al Zaman, K. (2024). The Role of Wearable Devices in Chronic Disease Monitoring and Patient Care: A Comprehensive Review. *Cureus*, 16(9). Advance online publication. DOI: 10.7759/cureus.68921 PMID: 39381470

Jananee, M. G. (2023). SpO2 and temperature measurement device based on ATmega328p microcontroller chip with mobile connection for real-time monitoring (Master's thesis, İstanbul Gelişim Üniversitesi Lisansüstü Eğitim Enstitüsü).

Kolosov, D., Kelefouras, V., Kourtessis, P., & Mporas, I. (2023). Contactless Camera-Based Heart Rate and Respiratory Rate Monitoring Using AI on Hardware. *Sensors (Basel)*, 23(9), 4550. DOI: 10.3390/s23094550 PMID: 37177754

Li, K., Cardoso, C., Moctezuma-Ramirez, A., Elgalad, A., & Perin, E. (2023). Heart Rate Variability Measurement through a Smart Wearable Device: Another Breakthrough for Personal Health Monitoring? *International Journal of Environmental Research and Public Health*, 20(24), 7146. DOI: 10.3390/ijerph20247146 PMID: 38131698

Mamdiwar, S. D., Shakruwala, Z., Chadha, U., Srinivasan, K., & Chang, C. Y. (2021). Recent advances on IoT-assisted wearable sensor systems for healthcare monitoring. *Biosensors (Basel)*, 11(10), 372. DOI: 10.3390/bios11100372 PMID: 34677328

Martínez-Suárez, F., García-Limón, J. A., Baños-Bautista, J. E., Alvarado-Serrano, C., & Casas, O. (2023). Low-power long-term ambulatory electrocardiography monitor of three leads with beat-to-beat heart rate measurement in real time. *Sensors (Basel)*, 23(19), 8303. DOI: 10.3390/s23198303 PMID: 37837133

Meza, C., Juega, J., Francisco, J., Santos, A., Duran, L., Rodriguez, M., Alvarez-Sabin, J., Sero, L., Ustrell, X., Bashir, S., Serena, J., Silva, Y., Molina, C., & Pagola, J. (2023). Accuracy of a Smartwatch to Assess Heart Rate Monitoring and Atrial Fibrillation in Stroke Patients. *Sensors (Basel)*, 23(10), 4632. DOI: 10.3390/s23104632 PMID: 37430546

Nekui, O. D., Wang, W., Liu, C., Wang, Z., & Ding, B. (2024). IoT-Based Heartbeat Rate-Monitoring Device Powered by Harvested Kinetic Energy. *Sensors (Basel)*, 24(13), 4249. DOI: 10.3390/s24134249 PMID: 39001027

Pengel, L. K., Robbers-Visser, D., Groenink, M., Winter, M. M., Schuuring, M. J., Bouma, B. J., & Bokma, J. P. (2023). A comparison of ECG-based home monitoring devices in adults with CHD. *Cardiology in the Young*, 33(7), 1129–1135. DOI: 10.1017/S1047951122002244 PMID: 35844104

Reegu, F. A., Abas, H., Gulzar, Y., Xin, Q., Alwan, A. A., Jabbari, A., Sonkamble, R. G., & Dziyauddin, R. A. (2023). Blockchain-based framework for interoperable electronic health records for an improved healthcare system. *Sustainability (Basel)*, 15(8), 6337. DOI: 10.3390/su15086337

Romano, V., & Etim-Andy, M. (2023). An Examination of WHOOP Fitness Band Usage in College Athletics. *Journal of Coaching and Sports Science*, 2(2), 46–52. DOI: 10.58524/jcss.v2i2.220

Salama, R., Al-Turjman, F., Chaudhary, P., & Yadav, S. P. (2023, April). (Benefits of Internet of Things (IoT) Applications in Health care-An Overview). In *2023 International Conference on Computational Intelligence, Communication Technology and Networking (CICTN)* (pp. 778-784). IEEE. DOI: 10.1109/CICTN57981.2023.10141452

Schuurmans, A. A., De Looff, P., Nijhof, K. S., Rosada, C., Scholte, R. H., Popma, A., & Otten, R. (2020). Validity of the Empatica E4 wristband to measure heart rate variability (HRV) parameters: A comparison to electrocardiography (ECG). *Journal of Medical Systems*, 44(11), 1–11. DOI: 10.1007/s10916-020-01648-w PMID: 32965570

Thakur, S., Chao, P. C. P., & Tsai, C. H. (2023). Precision Heart Rate Estimation Using a PPG Sensor Patch Equipped with New Algorithms of Pre-Quality Checking and Hankel Decomposition. *Sensors (Basel)*, 23(13), 6180. DOI: 10.3390/s23136180 PMID: 37448029

Weibel, R. P., Kerr, J. I., Naegelin, M., Ferrario, A., Schinazi, V. R., La Marca, R., Hoelscher, C., Nater, U. M., & von Wangenheim, F. (2023). Virtual reality-supported biofeedback for stress management: Beneficial effects on heart rate variability and user experience. *Computers in Human Behavior*, 141, 107607. DOI: 10.1016/j.chb.2022.107607

Wu, W., Elgendi, M., Fletcher, R. R., Bomberg, H., Eichenberger, U., Guan, C., & Menon, C. (2023). Detection of heart rate using smartphone gyroscope data: A scoping review. *Frontiers in Cardiovascular Medicine*, 10, 1329290. DOI: 10.3389/fcvm.2023.1329290 PMID: 38164464

Chapter 11

Reducing the Carbon Footprint in Healthcare Cybersecurity Threats in AI-Powered Healthcare Systems Data Privacy in AI-Driven Diagnostics

Taye Iyinoluwa Adeyinka
https://orcid.org/0009-0006-4357-6319
University of Science and Technology, Beijing, China

Kehinde Iyioluwa Adeyinka
https://orcid.org/0009-0009-7685-6693
University of Science and Technology, Beijing, China

ABSTRACT

The use of artificial intelligence (AI) in healthcare has brought about improved results and cost savings, transforming patient care, treatment processes, and diagnostics for the better! However, there are also many drawbacks to this technological development, especially regarding the effects on the environment, cybersecurity flaws, and data privacy issues. Another important issue in the context of AI-driven diagnostics is data privacy. The chapter examines the importance of protecting patient data in the face of the massive amounts of data needed to train AI models. It covers pertinent laws that control data use and patient permission in healthcare settings, such as the General Data Protection Regulation (GDPR) and the Health Insurance Portability and Accountability Act (HIPAA). Given the growing need for

DOI: 10.4018/979-8-3373-2827-0.ch011

data sharing and collaboration in clinical practice and research, the difficulties in guaranteeing data privacy in AI applications are examined.

INTRODUCTION

An important step forward in the quest for better patient care, operational effectiveness, and diagnostic accuracy is the quick integration of artificial intelligence (AI) into healthcare systems. However, there are significant obstacles associated with the growing use of AI technology in healthcare, especially in the areas of data privacy, cybersecurity, and environmental sustainability in order to secure the appropriate and ethical deployment of these technologies and to shape a future where AI not only improves healthcare delivery but also promotes a sustainable environment, these difficulties must be addressed as healthcare increasingly depends on AI-driven solutions. Information Retrieval is one of the contemporary answers to new challenges in threat evaluation of composite systems, (Dutta & Gochhait, n.d.).

The carbon footprint of AI-powered healthcare systems is at the center of this conversation. AI algorithm development, training, and operation can have significant energy requirements. The computational infrastructure required for modern AI systems is housed in data centers, which utilize enormous quantities of electricity. A study by Strubell, Ganesh, and McCallum (2020) demonstrates the environmental impact of AI applications, which highlights that training a single deep learning model can result in carbon emissions equivalent to five cars throughout their lifespan. The healthcare industry must face the fact that its technical innovations contribute to global carbon emissions in light of the growing concern over climate change and environmental degradation. Because of this, healthcare organizations must strategically work on lowering the carbon footprint of AI systems, which will lead to adopting sustainable practices in their AI projects.

The healthcare sector is looking more closely at sustainable AI techniques, prioritizing lower emissions and energy efficiency in response to these environmental issues. These techniques include employing renewable energy sources for data centers, installing energy-efficient hardware, and improving algorithms to use less processing power. For example, federated learning, a decentralized method that enables AI models to be trained on local devices instead of central servers, can be implemented by healthcare organizations to reduce the energy required for data storage and transit, (McMahan *et al.*, 2017). The healthcare industry can capitalize on AI's potential and support international efforts to tackle climate change by putting sustainability first.

While AI's effects on the environment are urgent, cybersecurity risks pose a serious obstacle to healthcare systems that rely on AI. Cybercriminals find hospitals and healthcare providers more appealing as they frequently use AI-driven diagnoses. Malicious actors may exploit the vulnerabilities created by the dependence on interconnected systems and the enormous volumes of private patient data inside these frameworks. According to recent studies, healthcare firms are 300 times more likely than other sectors to be the victim of a cyberattack, meaning they experience a disproportionate amount of these attacks. Successful cyberattacks can have disastrous repercussions, jeopardizing patient safety, stealing private health data, and causing large financial losses.

Furthermore, the effects of cybersecurity breaches go beyond short-term operational interruptions. They can potentially weaken patient-provider trust, which could discourage data sharing and jeopardize the advantages that AI technologies are supposed to offer. For example, patients may become less engaged with healthcare services if they believe their private health information is at risk due to a breach in an AI-driven diagnostic systems, (Weber & Kleine, 2020). Therefore, strengthening cybersecurity in AI-powered healthcare systems is technically required and essential to preserving patient confidence and guaranteeing the efficacy of AI applications. AI technologies are vital in the early detection and diagnosis of health disorders, which is crucial for successful treatment and management, (Cahyo & Astuti, 2023). Furthermore, powerful AI-enhanced microscopes have been employed to analyze blood samples for chemicals and bacteria, aiding in the identification of severe hematological conditions such as skin cancer, pancreatic cancer, and tuberculosis, (Idoko *et al.,* 2024).

The healthcare industry must take a multifaceted strategy to address these cybersecurity concerns, incorporating strong legislative frameworks, personnel training, and cutting-edge technological solutions. Protecting AI systems from cyber threats requires robust encryption techniques, ongoing network monitoring, and frequent vulnerability evaluations. Furthermore, human error often the weakest link in cybersecurity can be considerably decreased by fostering a culture of security awareness among healthcare staff, (Alhogail & Alsabih, 2021). In order to maintain compliance and safeguard patient data, enterprises need also abide by established frameworks and rules, such as the General Data Protection Regulation (GDPR) and the Health Insurance Portability and Accountability Act (HIPAA).

Data privacy concerns are closely related to cybersecurity and sustainability in AI-powered healthcare systems. Massive volumes of personal health data must be gathered and analyzed due to our growing reliance on AI, which raises important concerns about how this data is safeguarded, accessed, and kept. Organizations must put policies in place to protect the privacy and security of personal data since regulatory frameworks like the GDPR impose strict guidelines on data handling and processing, (Voigt & Von dem Bussche, 2017). However, the quick development of AI technologies frequently surpasses the creation of thorough legal and ethical guidelines, creating a regulatory vacuum that may allow misusing sensitive medical data.

Furthermore, the intricacy of AI algorithms may present further difficulties for data privacy. It might be challenging to guarantee that the data utilized in AI systems is anonymized and complies with privacy laws since machine learning algorithms have the potential to unintentionally memorize personal information, (Carlini *et al.*, 2019). This emphasizes how important it is for healthcare institutions to create strong data governance systems that protect patient privacy and permit the moral application of AI in diagnosis. A strategy to improve data privacy without compromising AI model performance is through solutions like differential privacy, which introduces noise into data sets to safeguard individual identities, (Dwork & Roth, 2014).

This chapter examines the interrelated issues of improving cybersecurity, lowering carbon emissions, and protecting patient privacy in AI-powered healthcare systems. It will offer insights into how the healthcare industry might manage these challenges while utilizing AI's advantages by examining present procedures, cutting-edge technologies, and viable alternatives. The ultimate objective is to promote a healthcare environment that prioritizes security, sustainability, and patient privacy while coordinating technical developments with more general societal objectives.

Using AI in healthcare can improve patient outcomes and diagnostic capacities. However, it also requires careful handling of its associated problems, such as data privacy issues, cybersecurity risks, and environmental sustainability. The healthcare industry can guarantee that AI technologies improve patient care and the environment by tackling these problems head-on and implementing sustainable practices.

1.1 Literature Review

Although the application of artificial intelligence (AI) in healthcare has the potential to transform paradigms for diagnosis and treatment completely, it also brings up serious issues with data privacy, cybersecurity, and environmental sustainability. This literature review examines these interconnected issues, highlighting the significance of creating sustainable AI-powered systems while addressing cybersecurity risks and protecting patient privacy in medical diagnostics.

Applications of AI technology, especially machine learning (ML) and deep learning (DL) have shown promise in several healthcare fields, such as personalized medicine, predictive analytics, and medical imaging. For instance, AI algorithms are used in medical imaging to evaluate MRIs, CT scans, and X-rays, giving radiologists better diagnostic tools, (Esteva *et al.*, 2019). According to research, AI can perform diagnostic tasks like identifying skin cancer on par with or even better than humans, (Esteva *et al.*, 2017). AI-driven diagnostics' precision and efficiency are improving patient outcomes, but it is important to consider the environmental costs of implementing these technologies.

Both researchers and governments are paying more and more attention to the energy usage of AI systems. Large-scale deep-learning model training is computationally demanding and can lead to considerable carbon emissions, as noted by Strubell, Ganesh, and McCallum (2020). This is especially troubling in the healthcare industry, as the energy requirements of AI systems may increase the sector's overall carbon footprint. It is imperative to strive for sustainable AI practices; healthcare institutions are urged to reduce their environmental effect by investing in energy-efficient hardware and optimizing their algorithms. Reducing the carbon footprint associated with AI has also been suggested using renewable energy sources and green data centers.

Healthcare is becoming a target for cyberattacks as AI technologies are incorporated more and more. According to studies, a disproportionate amount of cyberattacks target healthcare companies, which can result in service interruptions and the compromise of private patient data, (Garcia-Perez *et al.,* 2023). The interconnectedness of AI systems exacerbates these vulnerabilities since a compromise in one system can have repercussions on other platforms, (yang, Xiong, & Ren, 2020). Adversarial assaults, where malevolent individuals alter input data to trick AI systems, can also target AI algorithms, (Goodfellow *et al.*, 2014). Thus, protecting patient safety and data integrity in healthcare requires improving the security of AI systems.

Large volumes of personal health data must be gathered and processed to use AI in healthcare, which raises significant concerns about data privacy. Strict rules on data management are enforced by the General Data Protection Regulation (GDPR) in Europe and the Health Insurance Portability and Accountability Act (HIPAA) in the US, which highlights the significance of patient permission and data protection, (Voigt & Von dem Bussche, 2017). However, data privacy is frequently made more difficult by the intricacy of AI algorithms. According to research by Carlini *et al.* (2019), machine learning algorithms may unintentionally memorize sensitive information, raising the possibility of unintentional data exposure. This emphasizes how important it is for healthcare institutions to put in place strong data governance systems that protect patient privacy and permit the moral application of AI.

Developing solutions that support sustainability, cybersecurity, and data privacy is essential to addressing the issues raised by AI in healthcare. Federated learning is one promising strategy that lowers the energy costs related to data transit and storage by enabling AI models to be trained locally rather than on centralized servers (McMahan et al., 2017). Furthermore, cutting-edge encryption methods and ongoing oversight can help protect AI systems from online attacks, (Alhogail & Alsabih, 2021). Additionally, to reduce the risks associated with human error, companies need to foster a culture of security awareness among healthcare personnel.

Researchers also support the inclusion of ethical considerations in the creation and application of AI technologies. Healthcare institutions can balance innovation with preserving patient rights and the environment by establishing explicit ethical rules, (Binns, 2018). This all-encompassing strategy guarantees that AI technologies enhance healthcare delivery while tackling the urgent issues of data privacy, cybersecurity, and sustainability.

AI poses several complex issues about data privacy, cybersecurity, and environmental sustainability, even while it has the potential to improve healthcare diagnosis and treatment greatly. According to the literature, as they negotiate the challenges of incorporating AI technologies, healthcare companies must prioritize patient privacy, implement sustainable practices, and bolster cybersecurity safeguards. By tackling these issues collaboratively, the healthcare industry can fully utilize AI while guaranteeing a responsible and moral approach to technology deployment. Artificial intelligence has emerged as a component of analytics and early disease detection, resulting in substantial advancements in public health.

A significant use of AI is the detection of infectious diseases with wearable devices equipped with AI algorithms and edge computing. This strategy enhances the capacity to forecast public health outcomes by monitoring health indicators over time, providing early warnings for disorders such as diabetes and cardiovascular diseases, (Badidi, 2023).

The application of machine learning techniques, including Random Forest, K Nearest Neighbors (KNN), and Support Vector Machines (SVM), in analytics has produced results in the early detection of diseases. AI models that assess symptoms and medical data have demonstrated accuracy in predicting illnesses such as diabetes and cardiovascular issues, facilitating early diagnosis and intervention, (Kanna *et al.,* 2023). Artificial intelligence has been utilized in the domain of diseases to discern patterns from data, facilitating timely intervention and enhancing patient outcomes, (Alvarado *et al.,* 2023) (Ijiga *et al.,* 2021).

1.2 Overview of AI in Healthcare

The way doctors diagnose, treat, and oversee patient care is completely transformed by artificial intelligence (AI), which has become a disruptive force in the healthcare industry. AI systems can evaluate complicated medical data, support clinical decision-making, and improve patient outcomes using sophisticated algorithms and big databases. An outline of artificial intelligence's function in healthcare, its uses in diagnosis, therapy, and patient care, as well as its effects on the accuracy and efficiency of healthcare, are given in this section.

1.2.1 The Role of AI in Healthcare

A variety of technologies that can mimic human intellect are included in artificial intelligence (AI), such as computer vision, natural language processing (NLP), and machine learning (ML). AI is essential to the healthcare industry because it can automate procedures, improve diagnostic precision, and customize treatment regimens. Among its abilities are:

- **Diagnostics:** AI systems are highly accurate at analyzing medical pictures, including CT, MRI, and X-ray scans. For example, deep learning models can detect abnormalities the human eye could miss, such as cancers or fractures. According to studies, AI systems can reduce false positives and negatives while matching or surpassing human radiologists in diagnostic accuracy.
- **Treatment:** AI evaluates genetic data and medical history to enable customized medicine. By ensuring that treatments are by each patient's particular biological composition, this method increases treatment effectiveness and reduces side effects.
- **Patient Care**: AI improves patient engagement and care management in two ways: through chatbots and virtual assistants that offer real-time assistance. By providing information, setting up appointments, and reminding patients of their prescription schedules, these technologies encourage a more proactive approach to health management.

1.2.2 AI Applications in Healthcare

Applications of AI in healthcare are numerous and diverse, covering several crucial domains:

- **Medical Imaging:** Convolutional neural networks (CNNs), in particular, are AI algorithms that have greatly improved the processing of medical pictures. An AI model could, for instance, classify skin cancer types with an accuracy on par with dermatologists, according to a study by Esteva *et al.* (2017). These developments improve patient outcomes by substantially impacting early problem detection and treatment.
- **Predictive analytics:** AI-powered systems examine electronic health records (EHRs) to anticipate patient outcomes. These technologies allow medical professionals to act early by spotting risk factors and patterns, which may avoid problems and lower hospital stays. For instance, Churpek *et al.* (2012) discovered that machine-learning algorithms may accurately predict in-hospital cardiac arrest, giving doctors timely warnings.

- **Drug Development and Discovery:** Artificial intelligence (AI) speeds up drug discovery by evaluating biological data and forecasting a compound's effectiveness. Machine learning models can find possible drug candidates faster than conventional techniques, decreasing the time and expense of introducing new drugs. One example is Atomwise, a business that uses AI to screen millions of molecules for possible medication interactions.
- **Robotic Surgery:** AI-powered robotic systems help surgeons carry out intricate operations with greater control and accuracy. By analyzing data in real-time and giving surgeons insights during procedures, these tools can lower the risk of problems and speed up recovery.

1.2.3 Improving Efficiency and Accuracy in Healthcare

AI greatly improves healthcare systems' accuracy and efficiency in several ways:

- **Simplifying Administrative Tasks:** Artificial intelligence (AI) solutions simplify repetitive administrative duties like scheduling and billing, freeing healthcare workers to concentrate on patient care. In healthcare facilities, this simplification optimizes resource allocation and reduces wait times.
- **Improving Diagnostic Accuracy:** AI algorithms have shown improved diagnostic accuracy rates compared to conventional techniques. For example, a meta-analysis showed that AI models could attain an average diagnostic accuracy of 94% in various imaging tasks, while human practitioners could only accomplish about 80%.
- **Lowering Readmission Rates:** By employing predictive analytics, healthcare professionals can identify patients at risk of readmission and carry out focused interventions. According to research in the Journal of the American Medical Association, hospitals that used AI-driven analytics saw a 25% decrease in readmission rates, which led to lower costs and more patient satisfaction.

1.2.4 Impact of AI on Healthcare Outcomes

Patient outcomes have improved noticeably due to AI's incorporation into healthcare. For example:

- **Early Disease Identification:** AI has greatly increased the rates of early disease identification, especially in cardiology and oncology. AI algorithms can notify medical professionals of possible health problems before they become more serious by spotting trends in medical data.

- **Cost Reduction:** Healthcare cost savings have been linked to AI technologies. According to an Accenture analysis, by 2026, AI applications could save the US healthcare system up to $150 billion yearly through improvements in supply chain management, clinical operations, and administrative procedures.
- **Patient Satisfaction:** Thanks to the use of AI tools, patients are more satisfied with individualized patient care. According to a Forrester survey, companies using AI-powered chatbots reported a 30% rise in patient happiness and engagement, demonstrating the beneficial effects of AI on the patient experience as a whole.

1.3 Carbon Footprint of Healthcare AI Systems

Incorporating artificial intelligence (AI) technology into healthcare systems has brought about a new era of innovation, allowing notable advancements in patient management, diagnosis, and treatment. However, as AI becomes more widely used in healthcare companies, it is critical to understand how these technologies affect the environment, especially regarding energy use and carbon emissions. This section examines the sources of emissions and the body of research on the subject and suggests measures for quantifying the carbon footprint of healthcare AI systems.

1.3.1 AI's effects on the environment in healthcare

The use of AI in healthcare frequently necessitates a large amount of computational power, which might result in high energy usage. AI models especially deep learning algorithms need a lot of data and computing capacity for training and inference. For example, depending on the complexity of the model and the length of training, training big neural networks can use several megawatt-hours (MWh) of electricity. The need to address the environmental effects of AI in healthcare is urgent since a study by Strubell, Ganesh, and McCallum (2020) showed that training a single AI model can generate as much carbon as five cars over its lifetime.

Because AI systems in healthcare require a lot of processing power, they are typically housed in data centers or cloud computing environments, which are notoriously energy-intensive. These data centers cause many carbon emissions linked to AI technology. For example, according to the International Energy Agency (IEA), data centers used over 200 terawatt-hours (TWh) of electricity in 2018, which accounted for around 1% of the world's total electricity demand. The carbon emissions of these infrastructures must be considered as healthcare organizations increasingly move to cloud-based AI solutions.

Carbon Emission Sources in Medical AI Systems

There are multiple major sources of carbon emissions linked to healthcare AI systems:

- **Data Centers and Server Farms:** One of the main sources of carbon emissions is the energy used by data centers, which are where AI algorithms are developed and implemented. Because the servers produce a lot of heat while operating, these facilities need much electricity for cooling systems and computational work. The U.S. Environmental Protection Agency (EPA) states that data centers' carbon footprints differ based on their energy source; fossil fuel-powered centers emit far more than renewable energy centers.
- **Cloud Computing Services:** As cloud computing has become more prevalent in the healthcare industry, there is a greater need for third-party data centers, which might not always prioritize sustainability or energy efficiency. Many data centers worldwide are used by public cloud providers, and these establishments can require a significant amount of electricity. According to Global Climate and Health Alliance research, the cloud computing industry would be among the top 10 biggest electricity consumers worldwide if it were a nation.
- Training Procedures: **To** train AI models, several iterations and substantial calculations must be performed, which results in significant energy requirements. Several variables, such as hardware efficiency, dataset size, and model architecture, affect how much energy is required. For instance, training a single transformer model could take hundreds of GPU hours, which would greatly increase carbon emissions.
- **End-User Devices:** Tablets, computers, cellphones, and other gadgets used to access and engage with AI applications also add to the carbon footprint. Their energy consumption raises the total emissions linked to healthcare AI systems, especially when it comes to telehealth and remote patient monitoring.

Recent research has started thoroughly evaluating how AI technologies affect the environment. According to a noteworthy study by Lokmic-Tomkins *et al.* (2022), healthcare businesses must assess the carbon footprint of AI applications at every stage of their lifespan, from development to deployment and maintenance. The study emphasizes how AI can optimize energy use and boost operational effectiveness in hospital settings, supporting sustainability initiatives.

Researchers have also created frameworks for evaluating AI systems' carbon footprints. For example, a model put forth by Lokmic-Tomkins *et al.* (2022), proposes a thorough evaluation that considers energy usage, data center carbon emissions, and the emissions of AI technologies across their whole lifecycle. With the help of this framework, businesses may pinpoint areas with high energy use and put plans in place to lessen their carbon footprint.

1.4 Proposing Metrics for Measuring the Carbon Footprint

Clear measures must be established to assess and manage the carbon footprint of healthcare AI systems. Several possible measures could be used:

- **Energy Consumption per Model Training:** This metric, expressed in kilowatt-hours (kWh), measures the total energy used when training an AI model. Organizations can evaluate the energy intensity of their AI initiatives by monitoring this parameter.
- **Carbon Emissions per Model Deployment:** The Carbon Emissions per Model Deployment statistic assesses the carbon emissions linked to the implementation of AI models in a healthcare setting. It considers emissions from data centers and end-user devices to give a comprehensive picture of the system's environmental impact.
- **Renewable Energy Utilization Rate:** The Renewable Energy Utilization Rate measures the percentage of energy used by data centers and AI systems that come from renewable sources. A higher utilization Rate indicates a more sustainable operation with lower overall carbon emissions.
- **Efficiency Ratios:** These ratios contrast the energy usage of AI applications with their performance results. By studying efficiency, organizations can find areas for optimization and eventually lower their carbon footprint.
- **Lifecycle Emissions Assessment:** This is an all-encompassing statistic that takes into account the emissions related to each phase of an AI system's lifecycle, from data collecting and model training to deployment and upkeep. This method makes it easier to comprehend how AI technologies in healthcare affect the environment overall.

there are a lot of opportunities and concerns related to the carbon footprint of healthcare AI systems. Even though AI has the potential to revolutionize healthcare, it is crucial to address its environmental impact proactively. Healthcare businesses should endeavor to adopt sustainable AI practices that minimize their carbon footprint while optimizing the advantages of AI in enhancing patient care by comprehending the sources of carbon emissions, current research, and suggested metrics for monitoring. The sector may move closer to a more sustainable future by working with stakeholders, such as legislators, healthcare professionals, and IT developers.

1.4 Strategies for Sustainable AI in Healthcare

Though its energy requirements pose serious sustainability obstacles, artificial intelligence (AI) in healthcare has created opportunities to improve patient care, tailored treatment, and diagnostics. AI models have a significant carbon footprint because they require a lot of data and processing, especially in the healthcare industry. This is mostly because data centers and cloud services use much energy. A multifaceted strategy is needed for sustainable AI in healthcare, including algorithm optimization, using energy-efficient hardware, utilizing renewable energy sources, and adopting a strong framework for sustainability assessment. With thorough examples of successful case studies, this section examines methods for lowering the carbon footprint of AI-powered healthcare systems and suggests a sustainability framework to direct healthcare institutions.

1.4.1 Optimizing Algorithms for Efficiency

Carbon emissions are greatly increased by the computational demands of training AI models, especially deep learning algorithms. One of the most promising approaches to lowering AI's energy requirements in healthcare is algorithm optimization. We may drastically reduce energy consumption and expenses without compromising accuracy or performance by optimizing algorithms.

Model compression is one of the most used optimization techniques. Pruning, quantization, and knowledge distillation are examples of compression approaches that reduce the size of AI models by removing unnecessary parameters, reducing the need for precision, or transferring knowledge from larger models to smaller, more effective ones. Pruning, for example, removes nodes from a neural network that are not needed, which lowers the amount of computing resources needed for both training and inference.

Federated learning is another important optimization method that enables AI models to be trained on decentralized data situated on edge devices rather than central servers. Because fewer large-scale data transfers to centralized data centers are required, this method improves data privacy and drastically lowers energy usage. Federated learning has proven particularly helpful in wearable technology and mobile health applications, where energy constraints are crucial.

Furthermore, automatic machine learning (AutoML) methods have surfaced to lessen the computational burden associated with manual model design. By automatically optimizing model hyperparameters, AutoML may create AI models that are more effective and produce less computational waste, thus lessening their environmental impact.

1.4.2 Using Energy-Efficient Hardware

Innovations in hardware are essential for lowering the energy usage of AI applications in the medical field. Conventional technology, such as CPUs and GPUs, only sometimes meets the unique requirements of AI workloads. Designing field-programmable gate arrays (FPGAs) and application-specific integrated circuits (ASICs) to effectively carry out particular AI functions can decrease the energy needed to carry out the same activities.

For instance, it has been demonstrated that Google's Tensor Processing Units (TPUs), ASICs made especially for AI workloads, use less energy than conventional GPUs. These TPUs have been utilized to rapidly handle massive datasets while using the least energy in healthcare applications such as genomics and radiology.

Similarly, a new discipline called neuromorphic computing seeks to create technology that emulates the neural networks found in the brain. By lowering the power needs of AI systems to levels appropriate for broad deployment, especially in mobile health applications, neuromorphic chips—which are incredibly energy-efficient—have the potential to transform AI in healthcare completely.

Additionally, edge computing solutions are becoming more popular as a way to lessen dependency on big, energy-intensive data centers. By using edge devices, such as smartphones, tablets, or medical equipment, to carry out AI tasks like picture recognition and diagnostic analysis instead of the cloud, the energy consumption of data transmission and centralized processing can be decreased.

1.4.3 Utilizing Renewable Energy Sources

Carbon emissions are largely caused by the high energy requirements of data centers, which are frequently used for training and deploying AI models. One of the most important ways to lower the carbon footprint of AI in healthcare is to switch these facilities to renewable energy sources. Numerous well-known tech firms and cloud service providers are advancing in this field.

For example, by 2030, Google plans to run its data centers exclusively on renewable energy sources like solar and wind, achieving its goal of 24/7 carbon-free electricity. Healthcare companies that use cloud-based AI services should pay particular attention to this commitment because doing business with cloud providers that value sustainability can significantly reduce their carbon impact.

Microsoft has also committed to becoming carbon-negative by 2030, meaning it will take more carbon out of the atmosphere than it puts in. Through its Azure cloud architecture, fueled by various renewable energy sources, Microsoft's AI for Health effort supports a range of AI-driven healthcare initiatives, including those centered on disease modeling and genomics. Healthcare companies may ensure that renewable energy powers their AI operations by collaborating with cloud providers prioritizing sustainability.

Healthcare companies, in addition to cloud providers, have the option to invest in on-site renewable energy. Large medical facilities and research centers could directly offset the energy usage of their AI systems by using solar panels or wind turbines to produce renewable energy on-site.

1.5 Successful Case Studies in Sustainable AI Practices

Adopting environmentally friendly solutions is possible and effective, as seen by the several healthcare organizations that have started implementing sustainable AI practices.

Kaiser Permanente, a significant healthcare organization that became carbon neutral in 2020, is one noteworthy example. In addition to continuing to invest in AI and machine learning technology, Kaiser Permanente has drastically decreased its carbon emissions by concentrating on energy efficiency and investing in renewable energy. The company's use of AI for diagnostic support, patient monitoring, and predictive analytics demonstrates how sustainability and technical innovation coexist.

Another example is NVIDIA, a top manufacturer of GPUs and AI gear. In its partnerships with healthcare institutions, such as Massachusetts General Hospital, NVIDIA prioritizes energy conservation while utilizing AI for medical image processing. With initiatives to improve AI algorithms, NVIDIA's energy-efficient GPUs have shown notable energy consumption reductions without sacrificing the precision of medical diagnostics.

1.6 A Framework for Assessing Sustainability in AI Healthcare Applications

A thorough methodology for evaluating and reducing the environmental impact of AI systems is needed to help healthcare companies implement sustainable AI. This framework would emphasize several crucial elements:

- **Energy Consumption Assessment:** From model creation and training to deployment, healthcare companies should thoroughly examine how much energy their AI systems use during their whole lifecycle. To give a clear picture of where optimizations can be made, metrics like energy per job and carbon emissions per AI operation should be monitored.
- **Algorithm Efficiency Metrics:** Frequent evaluations of AI algorithms' effectiveness are important, with an emphasis on reducing needless complexity and processing burden. Model compression and federated learning are

two techniques that healthcare organizations should use to optimize their AI workflows for the energy economy.

- **Energy Source Tracking:** Using data centers and cloud providers that are powered by renewable energy sources should be a top priority for healthcare businesses. There should be a clear differentiation between renewable and non-renewable energy, with an annual goal of growing the use of renewable energy.
- **Sustainability Certifications:** Hospitals and research institutes want to look for sustainability certifications for their data centers and AI systems. Certifications like the Leadership in Energy and Environmental Design (LEED) guarantee that AI operations adhere to strict environmental requirements.
- **Lifecycle Environmental Impact Analysis:** To assess the environmental impact of AI systems from development to end-of-life, a thorough lifecycle analysis (LCA) should be carried out. This analysis would take into account hardware production, energy use, and final disposal to ensure that AI technologies utilized in healthcare are genuinely sustainable from start to finish.

Although AI has many advantages in healthcare, there are also serious environmental risks, especially carbon emissions. Healthcare companies may lower the carbon footprint of their AI systems without compromising the advancements AI offers in patient care by concentrating on algorithm optimization, deploying energy-efficient hardware, embracing renewable energy, and implementing a sustainability framework. In addition to being a technical requirement for the future of healthcare, sustainable AI is also an environmental necessity.

CYBERSECURITY THREATS IN AI-POWERED HEALTHCARE SYSTEMS

Artificial Intelligence (A.I.) has transformed clinical decision-making, diagnostics, individualized treatment regimens, and operational efficiency in the healthcare industry. However, healthcare institutions now have to deal with several cybersecurity issues brought about by this technological innovation. Numerous cybersecurity risks could jeopardize patient data, interfere with healthcare services, and even endanger patients in AI-powered healthcare systems. This section lists basic cybersecurity concerns, describes AI-specific vulnerabilities (including data breaches and adversarial machine learning), and examines the wider effects of these incidents on patient safety and the financial viability of healthcare institutions.

2.1 Common Cybersecurity Threats in AI-Powered Healthcare Systems

- **Breach of Data:** A common cybersecurity risk in AI-powered healthcare systems is still data leaks. Large volumes of private patient data, such as medical records, genetic information, and treatment histories, are gathered and stored by healthcare institutions. A.I. systems rely on this data for precise diagnosis, individualized care, and predictive analytics. However, healthcare systems are a prime target for attackers due to the enormous number of sensitive data they contain.

For instance, the COVID-19 pandemic in 2020 caused a sharp increase in assaults against the healthcare industry, with the attackers focusing on hospitals and medical research facilities. The Universal Health Services (UHS) hack impacted more than 400 locations, interrupting healthcare services throughout its network (CISA, 2020). A.I. programs that depend on this information may be jeopardized, which could result in inaccurate diagnoses or treatment suggestions.

- **Ransomware Attacks:** A.I. systems are increasingly incorporated into hospital operations, such as supply chain management, patient monitoring, and diagnostic imaging. However, ransomware attacks, in which criminals encrypt medical records and demand payment to decrypt them, can render these systems inoperable. Hospitals may lose access to essential resources for patient care when A.I. systems that handle sensitive patient data are encrypted.

For instance, the WannaCry ransomware assault 2017 rendered the U.K.'s National Health Service (NHS) completely unusable. The attack locked down vital I.T. systems and prevented physicians from accessing patient data or making appointments. A.I. systems that relied on these datasets for real-time analysis could have been more effective.

- **Insider Threats:** Insider threats occur when workers or other authorized persons, whether intentionally or inadvertently, abuse their access to private medical information. If insiders purposefully alter input data or introduce biases, A.I. systems that rely on data for analysis, decision support, and machine learning are susceptible to manipulation, which could result in inaccurate model results and decision-making.
- **Adversarial Attacks:** This kind of cyberattack is specific to A.I. systems. These assaults entail making minute changes to input data, such as medical scans, that are invisible to humans but can potentially significantly change the

A.I.'s output. Adversarial attacks have the potential to seriously jeopardize patient safety in the healthcare industry by resulting in inaccurate diagnoses or unsuitable treatments.

For instance, studies have demonstrated that adversarial examples can fool medical A.I. systems that classify images, leading to incorrect diagnoses. For example, an A.I. system may misidentify the severity of a tumor or fail to detect cancerous indications due to adversarially altered C.T. images or X-rays, (Finlayson *et al.,* 2019).

- **Denial of Service (DoS) Attacks:** Attacks such as Denial of Service (DoS) and Distributed Denial of Service (DDoS) occur when hackers overload servers or networks in healthcare systems with excessive traffic, interfering with A.I. systems' ability to function normally. Patient care may be jeopardized if these attacks make AI-powered systems for hospital operations, diagnostics, or patient monitoring unavailable at crucial moments.
- **Supply Chain Attacks:** Healthcare companies frequently depend on outside vendors to obtain A.I. technologies and services. When attackers target these vendors to introduce vulnerabilities that spread to healthcare organizations, it is known as a supply chain attack. The integrity of A.I. systems may be jeopardized if this is done by tampering with hardware or inserting malware into A.I. software.

2.2 Vulnerabilities of AI Systems in Healthcare

Like other A.I. applications, healthcare A.I. systems are vulnerable to specific attacks due to inherent flaws. Key vulnerabilities are outlined below:

- **Adversarial Machine Learning (AML):** A.I. models, particularly deep learning models, are vulnerable to AML attacks, in which minor adjustments to the input data can significantly modify the model's output. Adversarial attacks provide significant hazards in the healthcare industry. To make the A.I. model misdiagnose a disease or misclassify the severity of a medical condition, for example, an attacker may subtly alter a patient's medical imaging (such as an MRI or X-ray). In addition to jeopardizing patient safety, this erodes confidence in A.I. systems.

A study by Finlayson *et al.* (2019) demonstrated how adversarial perturbations in medical imaging could cause AI algorithms to misclassify chest X-rays, potentially leading to incorrect treatment decisions in the context of pneumonia diagnosis.

- **Data Poisoning:** AI models rely heavily on vast amounts of data to train and learn. In data poisoning attacks, an attacker deliberately introduces malicious data into the training dataset, corrupting the AI model's learning process. In healthcare, this could result in an AI system that consistently makes erroneous diagnoses or treatment recommendations.

If a malicious actor introduces tampered data into a hospital's AI system, training it to incorrectly classify certain types of tumors, it could lead to a system-wide misdiagnosis problem that puts patient safety at serious risk, (Biggio, Fumera, & Roli, 2013).

- **Model Inversion Attacks:** By accessing the model's output, an attacker can deduce private information about the data used to train an A.I. model. This may allow hackers to reverse-engineer patient data in the healthcare industry, exposing particular information from anonymized medical records.

As an illustration, researchers have shown that A.I. systems trained on genetic data may be susceptible to inversion attacks, enabling attackers to deduce private information about individuals, including their family history or medical issues, (Fredrikson, Jha, & Ristenpart, 2015).

- **Bias and Fairness Issues:** A.I. systems used in healthcare may unintentionally pick up biases from training data. An A.I. system may systematically prejudice against particular patient groups if it is trained on non-representative datasets, which could result in unfair treatment or incorrect diagnoses. Attackers can use these biases to change the results for specific patient groups, jeopardizing the system's ethical dependability and security.

2.3 Consequences of Cybersecurity Incidents in Healthcare

Cybersecurity breaches in AI-powered healthcare systems can have disastrous results. The following outlines the main dangers:

- **Risks to Patient Safety:** The potential harm to patient safety is the most direct effect of a cybersecurity breach in AI-powered healthcare systems. A.I. systems that help with disease diagnosis or patient care management could give inaccurate information or neglect to issue important alarms if they are compromised. Inaccurate diagnoses, poor or delayed treatment, and perhaps fatal outcomes can result from this.

For instance, a ransomware attack on a German hospital in 2020 forced it to turn away patients due to serious disruptions to its I.T. systems. After being sent to another hospital for emergency care, one patient passed away as a result of treatment delays. This demonstrates the importance of functional A.I. and I.T. systems for patient safety.

- **Financial Implications:** The financial effects of cybersecurity incidents are particularly likely to affect healthcare businesses. System outages, regulatory penalties, court settlements, and the price of fixing damaged infrastructure are some of the expenses associated with dealing with a breach. Additionally, a decline in patient admissions and financial instability may result from the possibility of tarnished reputations and a lack of trust.

For instance, the 2015 Anthem data breach exposed the private data of more than 78 million people. Due to the breach's litigation and regulatory penalties, the healthcare company had to pay over $115 million in settlements.

- **Issues with Regulation and Compliance:** Cybersecurity lapses may have serious consequences for regulations and compliance. Healthcare institutions must abide by laws like the General Data Protection Regulation (GDPR) in the E.U. and the Health Insurance Portability and Accountability Act (HIPAA) in the U.S., which require strict safeguards for patient data. Violations may result in significant penalties and harm to the organization's reputation.

For instance, Excellus BlueCross BlueShield was hit with a $5.1 million HIPAA punishment in 2021 following a hack that revealed the protected health information of more than 9.3 million people (U.S. Department of Health & Human Services, 2021).

Although revolutionary, AI-powered healthcare systems are vulnerable to cybersecurity concerns that jeopardize patient safety and healthcare organizations' financial stability. Data breaches, ransomware, insider attacks, adversarial machine learning, and supply chain vulnerabilities are examples of frequent threats. Strong cybersecurity frameworks incorporating ongoing monitoring, integrity checks for A.I. models, encryption methods, and regulatory compliance are necessary to address these issues. Ensuring the security and resilience of these systems is essential for safeguarding patient data and upholding confidence in healthcare technology as A.I. continues to transform the healthcare landscape

2.4 Data Privacy in AI-Driven Diagnostics

Access to enormous volumes of patient data is crucial to the expanding use of artificial intelligence (A.I.) in healthcare, particularly in diagnostic procedures. Training A.I. models with this data are essential for identifying trends, producing precise forecasts, and enhancing individualized treatment regimens. However, using private medical data for AI-powered diagnosis presents serious privacy issues because it includes extremely private patient data, including genetic information, medical histories, and test results. The significance of data privacy in healthcare, especially in AI-driven diagnostics, will be covered in this section. We will also look at the frameworks and laws that control healthcare data privacy, such as GDPR and HIPAA, and the difficulties in maintaining data privacy, including patient consent and data sharing.

2.4.1 Significance of Data Privacy in Healthcare

Maintaining the confidentiality of patient information is essential to upholding patient-provider trust, making data privacy a core value in the healthcare industry. This problem is even more complicated in AI-driven diagnostics since patient data is frequently used for training and enhancing A.I. models in addition to providing immediate therapy. In AI-powered healthcare, data privacy is crucial for the following main reasons:

- **Protection of Sensitive Information:** Genetic information, treatment plans, and diagnostic results are just a few examples of extremely sensitive healthcare data. Exposure to or exploitation of such data may result in identity theft, discrimination, or even the unlawful use of genetic data for insurance or job decisions. The confidentiality of patients' personal and medical information is guaranteed when patient data is protected in A.I. diagnostics.

For instance, A.I. systems used to diagnose cancer depend on substantial collections of patient medical records and medical picture data (such as MRIs and X-rays). If not sufficiently safeguarded, the information in these datasets may betray a patient's identity or health issues.

- **Patient Engagement and Trust:** Preserving patient trust requires protecting data privacy. Patients may be less inclined to offer thorough and accurate health information if they are concerned that their data may be exploited or revealed in the context of A.I. diagnosis. As exact diagnostics depend on having access to high-quality, reliable data, this could reduce the efficacy of A.I. systems.

- **Observance of Legal and Ethical Standards:** In the medical field, handling patient data improperly can have major legal repercussions. Protecting data privacy supports moral principles for the prudent handling of private data.

For instance, strict privacy rules like the General Data Protection Regulation (GDPR) and the Health Insurance Portability and Accountability Act (HIPAA) require protecting patient data in nations like the U.S. and the E.U. Healthcare organizations that use A.I. technologies must abide by these laws.

2.5 Regulations and Frameworks Governing Data Privacy in Healthcare

Several regulations and frameworks have been established to govern data privacy in healthcare, especially in regions where patient data is processed or transferred. These regulations ensure that healthcare providers and AI developers adhere to strict guidelines to protect patient information. Two of the most prominent frameworks are the GDPR and HIPAA.

1) **General Data Protection Regulation (GDPR):** The European Union's GDPR is a comprehensive data protection regulation that regulates how personal data, including medical data, is processed. It demands express patient agreement for data collection and use and imposes stringent requirements on enterprises handling sensitive data, including patient medical records. Important aspects of the GDPR that apply to A.I. diagnostics are as follows:
    - **Consent:** Under GDPR, healthcare institutions are required to obtain patients' express consent before using patient data in A.I. applications.
    - **Data Minimization:** A.I. systems must use only the minimum required data for diagnosis, ensuring that no extraneous patient data is gathered.
    - **Right to be Forgotten:** A.I. systems that depend on previous data for model training may need help to comply with patients' requests to erase their data.
    - **Transparency:** When utilizing A.I., healthcare institutions must be open and honest about how patient data is handled, stored, and used.

By gaining patient agreement and giving clear information on data usage, a hospital in the E.U. using AI-driven diagnostics for diabetes care must guarantee that all patient data utilized in A.I. systems conform with GDPR.

2) **Health Insurance Portability and Accountability Act (HIPAA):** HIPAA stands for Health Insurance Portability and Accountability Act. HIPAA establishes the norm for safeguarding private patient data in the U.S. It specifies how protected health information (PHI) must be handled by insurers, healthcare providers, and other organizations to maintain its confidentiality and security. The following are some of the most crucial HIPAA provisions for AI-driven diagnostics:
    - **Privacy Rule:** The HIPAA Privacy Rule requires healthcare organizations to maintain the privacy of patients' PHI. It prevents unwanted access and mandates that organizations notify patients about their data usage.
    - **Security Rule:** The technological measures required to protect PHI in electronic formats (ePHI) are the main emphasis of HIPAA's Security Rule. A.I. systems handling ePHI must have strong security features like access restriction and encryption.
    - **Breach Notification Rule:** Healthcare institutions are required to promptly alert patients and authorities in the event of a data breach.

For instance, an A.I. tool used to diagnose lung cancer in the United States needs to use encryption techniques and restrict access to only authorized individuals to maintain patient data security in accordance with HIPAA.

2.6 Guidelines for Ethical AI Development and Implementation in Healthcare

Several recommendations and best practices can be put forth to guarantee that AI technologies are ethically created and implemented in the healthcare industry. Fairness, responsibility, transparency, and respect for patient privacy should all be emphasized in these standards.

1) **Fairness and Bias Mitigation:** Healthcare AI systems must be built to reduce bias and guarantee fair results for every patient, regardless of demographic traits. This calls for:
    - Ensuring that training datasets are diverse and representative of all patient populations.
    - Regularly auditing AI systems for biases and correcting any detected disparities.
    - Involving diverse stakeholders in the design and deployment of AI systems to account for different perspectives.
2) **Explainability and Transparency:** Healthcare AI systems must be open and honest about making decisions. To do this:

- Explainability should be considered while designing AI models so that patients and healthcare professionals can comprehend the process and rationale behind decision-making.
- Developers are required to give healthcare practitioners precise documentation and instructions on evaluating AI results.
- Patients should be given the chance to ask questions or refuse to participate in AI-driven decision-making and should be informed about how AI will be used in their care.

3) **Responsibility & Accountability:** To identify who bears responsibility for mistakes made by AI systems in healthcare, clear accountability frameworks must be implemented. This includes:

Security and Privacy of Data: Strong privacy and security protections are essential for AI to be developed ethically. This comprises:

- Defining the roles and responsibilities of AI developers, healthcare providers, and organizations in ensuring the safety and accuracy of AI-driven decisions.
- Creating legal and ethical guidelines for assigning liability in cases where AI systems contribute to harm or errors in patient care.
- Ensuring that healthcare providers retain the ultimate authority over patient care decisions, using AI as a tool rather than a final decision-maker.

4) **Continuous Monitoring and Evaluation:** To guarantee that AI systems operate ethically over time, they must be regularly monitored and assessed. This includes:

- Implementing strong encryption, access controls, and anonymization techniques to protect patient data.
- Providing patients with clear information about how their data will be used in AI applications and obtaining their informed consent.
- Adhering to privacy regulations such as HIPAA and GDPR to ensure that patient rights are protected.

RESEARCH OBJECTIVE

The primary objective of this chapter, is to is to examine and evaluate the complex interrelationships among cybersecurity, data privacy, and sustainable artificial intelligence (AI) practices in the context of healthcare diagnostics. The study seeks to accomplish the following particular goals:

1) Assess the Environmental Impact of AI in Healthcare:

This study will examine the energy use, greenhouse gas emissions, and environmental effects of AI model training while analyzing AI's carbon footprint in healthcare. It will also find the sources of carbon emissions in AI systems, such as data centers, server farms, and computational operations.

2) Identify Cybersecurity Threats and Vulnerabilities:

Examine the typical cybersecurity risks that AI-powered healthcare systems must contend with, such as hostile assaults, data breaches, and weaknesses brought on by the incorporation of AI technologies. Part of this goal will be assessing the effects of these risks on patient safety, data integrity, and general confidence in healthcare systems.

3) Evaluate Data Privacy Concerns:

Consider the importance of data privacy in AI-powered diagnosis, especially given the widespread use of patient data. Part of this will involve reviewing pertinent laws like the Health Insurance Portability and Accountability Act (HIPAA) and the General Data Protection Regulation (GDPR), as well as the difficulties in preserving data privacy in AI applications.

4) Propose Sustainable Strategies and Best Practices:

Create and suggest workable plans to reduce the carbon footprint of healthcare AI technologies. This will entail investigating energy-efficient algorithm optimization, implementing energy-efficient hardware, and using renewable energy sources to power AI systems. To demonstrate the efficacy of these tactics, case studies of successful implementations will be emphasized.

5) Establish a Comprehensive Framework:

Provide a methodology for evaluating the sustainability of AI applications in healthcare that incorporates data privacy, cybersecurity, and carbon emissions. This framework will give healthcare organizations a methodical way to assess and improve their AI projects' sustainability while ensuring they comply with legal and ethical criteria.

6) Contribute to the Body of Knowledge

Expand the existing literature on sustainable AI practices in healthcare by integrating discussions on cybersecurity and data privacy. The chapter aims to provide insights that will inform future research and guide healthcare practitioners in making informed decisions regarding the deployment of AI technologies.

This chapter aims to shed light on the crucial nexus between data privacy, cybersecurity, and sustainability in AI-powered healthcare systems by fulfilling these goals. The results will help healthcare companies manage the challenges of integrating AI technology responsibly and sustainably, in addition to adding to the body of knowledge regarding sustainable AI practices. In order to create a resilient healthcare ecosystem for the future, this research aims to advance a comprehensive strategy for AI integration in healthcare that prioritizes patient safety, environmental stewardship, and data privacy.

3.1 Methodology

Cybersecurity Risks in AI-Powered Healthcare Systems and Data Privacy in AI-Driven Diagnostics: Reducing the Carbon Footprint in Healthcare employs a multifaceted methodology that combines qualitative and quantitative research techniques. This all-encompassing strategy investigates the complex interrelationships among cybersecurity risks, sustainable AI practices, and data privacy issues in healthcare diagnostics. The following are the main elements of the methodology:

1. Review

A thorough literature analysis will be carried out to compile the body of knowledge on the three primary topics the carbon footprint of AI technologies in healthcare, cybersecurity risks related to AI-powered systems, and data privacy in AI-driven diagnostics. This will entail:

- **Finding Relevant Sources:** PubMed, IEEE Xplore, Scopus, and Google Scholar will be used to search for peer-reviewed journals, conference proceedings, and technical reports. The following keywords will be used: "AI in healthcare," "carbon footprint," "data privacy," "cybersecurity in healthcare," and "AI diagnostics."
- **Inclusion and Exclusion Criteria:** Research on AI applications in cybersecurity, data privacy, sustainability, and healthcare published in the past ten years will be considered. Articles that are not peer-reviewed or do not discuss these topics will not be accepted.

- **Data Extraction:** To enable a thorough grasp of the present state of knowledge, important findings, methodologies, and conclusions from a few chosen research will be methodically extracted and grouped according to the topics.

2. Analysis of Qualitative Data

Qualitative techniques will be used to explore further the particular facets of cybersecurity and data privacy in AI healthcare systems:

- **Interviews:** Stakeholders in the healthcare industry, such as cybersecurity specialists, IT specialists, and healthcare administrators, will participate in semi-structured interviews. This will shed light on practical applications of AI technology, their environmental effects, and data security and privacy issues.
- **Focus Groups:** To obtain a range of viewpoints on the consequences of AI in diagnostics and the significance of data privacy, focus groups with patients and healthcare professionals will be arranged. The conversations will be videotaped, written down, and subjected to thematic analysis to find recurring themes and issues.

3. Analysis of Quantitative Data

The environmental impact of AI systems in healthcare and the frequency of cybersecurity threats will be evaluated using quantitative methods:

- **Carbon Footprint Assessment:** To quantify the carbon emissions linked to different AI healthcare technologies, a quantitative analysis will be carried out. This will entail gathering information on energy usage from server farms, data centres, and AI model training procedures. Based on previous research and data sources, metrics like energy per operation and total emissions will be computed, (Kirkpatrick, 2023) (Strubell, Ganesh, & McCallum, 2020).
- **Survey Research:** To learn more about healthcare organizations' experiences with AI implementations, cybersecurity events, and data protection issues, an online survey will be created. The study will ask about perceptions of sustainability in AI applications, data protection measures, and the frequency of cyberattacks. The gathered data will be statistically examined using inferential techniques and descriptive statistics to find patterns and relationships.

4. Analysis of Case Studies

Detailed case studies of healthcare institutions that have effectively adopted sustainable AI strategies while resolving cybersecurity and data privacy issues will be included in this chapter:

- **Selection of Case Studies:** A purposive sampling technique will be used to select case studies of healthcare organizations renowned for their creative approaches to sustainable AI practices. The organization's dedication to sustainability, cybersecurity measures, and data privacy initiatives will be considered selection criteria.
- **Data Collection:** Key personnel interviews, organizational report analysis, and a review of publicly accessible data will all be used to gather data. This will assist in demonstrating the efficacy of the tactics used and the results obtained in lowering carbon footprints while protecting data.

5. Development of Frameworks

The methodology's last section will concentrate on creating a framework for evaluating the sustainability of AI applications in the medical field:

- **Framework Design:** The results of the literature research, qualitative analysis, quantitative data, and case studies will all be considered while designing the framework. It will include important parameters for data privacy, cybersecurity threats, and energy use.
- **Validation:** The suggested framework will be validated using input from stakeholders in the healthcare industry. The framework will be presented at workshops or meetings, and stakeholders will be asked to offer feedback and ideas for improvement.

This thorough approach examines the complex interaction between cybersecurity, data privacy, and sustainable AI practices in healthcare diagnostics through a study of the literature, qualitative and quantitative analyses, case studies, and framework creation. The knowledge gathered from this diverse approach is intended to make a substantial contribution to understanding how healthcare companies can ethically employ AI technology while reducing their carbon footprint and guaranteeing the security and privacy of patient data.

3.2 Application of Sustainable AI, Cybersecurity, and Data Privacy in Healthcare Diagnostics

Sustainable AI in healthcare diagnostics combines cutting-edge technology advancement with environmentally sensitive tactics to reduce environmental impact while maintaining strong data privacy and mitigating cybersecurity risks. This section explores the use of AI-powered systems in healthcare settings, how sustainability may be attained, and how issues like data privacy and cybersecurity threats are handled.

1. AI-Powered Sustainable Healthcare Diagnostics

Artificial intelligence has already demonstrated impressive potential in healthcare diagnostics by increasing the speed, accuracy, and precision of medical imaging, pathology, and illness detection. One example is AI-powered diagnostic tools in radiology; algorithms can identify abnormalities in medical imaging such as X-rays, MRIs, and CT scans, sometimes even more accurately than humans. However, these systems demand a lot of processing power, which raises energy costs and carbon emissions, especially in big healthcare facilities where AI is used extensively.

a. Algorithm Optimization

Optimizing AI algorithms to work more effectively is critical to lowering the carbon footprint. For instance, model compression methods like distillation, quantization, and pruning can lower the energy and computing power needed to operate these models in AI-powered imaging systems. Thanks to federated learning, energy-intensive data centres are no longer necessary, which enables AI models to be trained across dispersed devices without transferring data to a central server. In addition to reducing carbon emissions, the optimization decreases costs and increases accessibility for smaller healthcare facilities.

b. AI Systems with Energy-Efficient Hardware

Another important use of AI in diagnostics that might contribute to sustainability is the integration of energy-efficient hardware. Healthcare settings are already implementing edge computing devices and hardware, such as Tensor Processing Units (TPUs) and application-specific integrated circuits (ASICs), specifically for AI workloads. These specialized hardware components are appropriate for jobs like real-time diagnostic analysis and medical image processing since they are made to manage AI workloads with lower power consumption. By implementing these technologies, healthcare facilities lessen their dependency on massive data centres, lowering their carbon footprint.

c. Renewable Energy Integration

Renewable energy sources can also be connected to AI-powered medical diagnostics. Hospitals and diagnostic facilities can incorporate solar or wind energy to power their data centres to balance the energy requirements of AI applications. By integrating energy-efficient AI-powered diagnostic tools with renewable energy generation, some hospitals, such as Kaiser Permanente, have already achieved carbon neutrality, establishing a model for how other healthcare systems can reduce their carbon footprint while improving their diagnostic capabilities.

2. Risks to Cybersecurity in AI-Powered Medical Diagnostics

The use of AI in healthcare also poses serious cybersecurity dangers. Despite their strength, AI systems are susceptible to a number of threats that could compromise patient information, interfere with services, or even change test findings.

a. Common Cybersecurity Threats
    - **Adversarial Attacks:** Attackers use subtle manipulation of input data in adversarial machine learning to fool AI algorithms into producing inaccurate predictions or diagnoses. An AI system might mistakenly identify a benign tumor as malignant, for example, based on minor alterations to medical imaging. This could result in needless intervention or therapy.
    - **Data Breaches:** Healthcare institutions are particularly vulnerable to data breaches since AI systems frequently need a lot of patient data. Attackers can obtain critical patient data without authorization by exploiting AI system flaws, jeopardizing corporate trust and individual privacy.
    - **Ransomware:** Malicious actors may target AI systems that oversee patient management and diagnostic tools with ransomware attacks. These attacks prevent access to vital systems until a ransom is paid. Attacks of this nature can impair the provision of medical care, endanger patient lives, and cause large financial and operational losses for healthcare organizations.

b. Managing Vulnerabilities

Strong cybersecurity frameworks must be incorporated into AI-powered medical diagnostics to counter these attacks. This entails using multi-factor authentication for system access, implementing encryption mechanisms to protect data in transit and at rest, and conducting routine security assessments on AI systems. For healthcare institutions to react quickly to threats and minimize possible harm, AI systems also need to be trained to recognize unusual activities that could be signs of hacks.

3. Privacy of Data in AI-Powered Diagnostics

Data is essential to AI diagnoses, especially sensitive patient data, including genetic profiles, medical histories, and real-time health monitoring data from wearable technology. For moral reasons, it is crucial to protect the privacy of this data and adhere to laws like the General Data Protection Regulation (GDPR) in Europe and the Health Insurance Portability and Accountability Act (HIPAA) in the United States.

a. Adherence to regulations

Healthcare companies that use AI-powered diagnostics must ensure that their data management procedures comply with these strict privacy laws. This entails getting patients' informed consent before using their data, ensuring data processing is transparent, and giving patients control over their data. Loss of patient trust and legal ramifications may result from noncompliance with these regulations.

b. AI Methods That Protect Privacy

Differential privacy and homomorphic encryption are two privacy-preserving AI approaches that are increasingly important for protecting data privacy while using big datasets for AI model training. Even in decentralized settings when data exchange between institutions is required, these methods guarantee patient privacy by enabling AI systems to learn from data without having direct access to sensitive information.

Even if a patient's data was included in the training set, Differential Privacy ensures that the AI model's output does not disclose specific information about that patient.

Because homomorphic encryption enables AI systems to handle encrypted data, sensitive patient data is protected throughout the processing pipeline, lowering the possibility of exposure in the event of a breach.

c. Challenges in Ensuring Data Privacy

Ensuring data privacy in AI-driven diagnostics is still difficult, even with advancements in privacy-preserving technologies. For thorough diagnostics, AI systems frequently need data sharing between institutions; moreover, many organizations need help maintaining security while enabling this interchange. Furthermore, patients frequently do not need to learn how their data is utilized, raising questions about openness and permission.

Healthcare companies must embrace state-of-the-art privacy-preserving AI technology to reduce risks, establish transparent and unambiguous data governance policies, and guarantee patient transparency over the use of their data.

4. Proposing a Framework for Sustainable AI Applications in Healthcare

A comprehensive framework is required for healthcare institutions to strike a compromise between the advantages of AI-powered diagnostics and the requirements for sustainability, cybersecurity, and data protection. The following elements ought to be included in this framework:

- **Sustainability measurements:** Using standardized energy consumption and efficiency measurements, evaluate and track the carbon footprint of AI systems.

Cybersecurity Measures: Implement thorough cybersecurity plans adapted to the particular requirements of AI diagnostics, such as encryption, frequent audits, and incident response procedures.

- **Practices for Data Privacy:** To protect patient data, follow international data protection laws and use cutting-edge privacy-preserving AI algorithms.

This framework would help healthcare companies methodically assess and use AI applications, making sure they are not only cutting-edge in terms of technology but also safe, secure, and privacy-conscious.

using AI in medical diagnostics offers promising prospects for better patient care, but it must be handled carefully. Healthcare organizations may fully utilize AI while tackling its application's ethical, security, and environmental issues by implementing sustainable practices, strong cybersecurity frameworks, and strict data protection policies.

3.3 Advantages of Sustainable AI, Cybersecurity, and Data Privacy in Healthcare Diagnostics

Integrating sustainable AI-powered systems in healthcare diagnostics has numerous benefits that enhance patient care, healthcare operations, and environmental sustainability. These advantages include a wide range of topics, including patient privacy, data security, operational effectiveness, and diagnostic accuracy.

1. Increased Speed and Accuracy of Diagnostics

Compared to conventional techniques, AI-powered systems can process enormous volumes of data, allowing for quicker and more precise diagnosis. By utilizing AI, healthcare professionals can detect illnesses more accurately and early. For example, artificial intelligence (AI) systems can examine medical pictures, such as MRIs or X-rays, to find anomalies that human radiologists would not immediately notice. This results in quicker actions, enhancing patient outcomes and saving lives.

2. Lower Carbon Footprint and Energy Efficiency

Healthcare diagnostics' environmental impact can be reduced by employing energy-efficient hardware and optimizing AI algorithms. Energy-efficient AI systems use less electricity because they do not require as many high-energy computational resources. Healthcare companies can drastically lower their carbon footprint by joining with renewable energy sources like solar or wind power. This supports worldwide efforts to slow climate change and makes healthcare systems more sustainable.

3. Strengthened Cybersecurity Protocols

Adopting cutting-edge cybersecurity frameworks designed for AI-powered healthcare systems reduces the risk of ransomware, hostile attacks, and data breaches. Real-time defense against malevolent activity can be offered by AI systems that have been trained to recognize and stop cyber threats. Healthcare organizations preserve organizational trust, protect patient privacy, and prevent the financial and reputational damages that come with cyberattacks by protecting sensitive patient data and diagnostic systems.

4. Guaranteed Privacy of Data

Data privacy is a major concern because AI-driven diagnoses need access to vast databases. Throughout the diagnostic procedure, sensitive patient data is kept safe and anonymous thanks to privacy-preserving AI techniques like homomorphic encryption and differential privacy. These technologies ensure patient privacy while enabling healthcare companies to use AI's diagnostic capabilities by enabling AI systems to function on encrypted data without disclosing personal information. Adherence to laws like GDPR and HIPAA further strengthens patient trust and legal compliance.

5. Operational Efficiency and Cost Savings

In addition to lessening their environmental impact, sustainable AI systems also save money on operations. Running AI systems in healthcare settings is less expensive because of energy-efficient hardware and better algorithms. Additionally, healthcare practitioners may concentrate on more complicated situations thanks to AI's capacity to automate repetitive processes like data analysis and diagnostic picture processing, which increases overall productivity. This improves the patient experience by reducing the time patients must wait for diagnostics and treatments.

6. Accessibility and Scalability

Because sustainable AI systems are scalable, they can be used in various healthcare environments, including resource-constrained rural clinics and major hospitals. Healthcare practitioners in rural or under-resourced places can implement AI-driven diagnostics without depending on costly infrastructure or centralized data centres by using energy-efficient devices and renewable energy sources. This improves global healthcare outcomes and promotes health fairness by expanding access to cutting-edge diagnostic technologies.

7. Care Focused on the Patient

Healthcare practitioners can provide patients with more individualized care thanks to AI's capacity to provide personalized diagnosis and treatment recommendations. AI systems are able to provide accurate recommendations that are tailored to each patient's specific needs by analyzing genetic profiles, patient histories, and real-time health data. By placing a significant emphasis on tailored care, this strategy not only increases the efficacy of therapies but also strengthens the bonds between patients and providers.

8. Adaptability to Potential Hazards

Healthcare companies may implement cybersecurity safeguards and data privacy policies to build robust AI-powered systems to survive new cyber threats. AI systems combined with sophisticated threat detection can constantly adjust to new security threats as they become more sophisticated. This guarantees that even in the event of new assaults, important patient data is safeguarded, and healthcare activities continue unhindered.

Integrating sustainable AI, improved cybersecurity, and strong data privacy protocols in healthcare diagnostics has several benefits. It increases the precision of diagnoses, boosts operational effectiveness, protects patient privacy, and supports environmental sustainability. Because of these advantages, AI is a vital tool for contemporary healthcare, enabling organizations to deliver high-quality treatment while tackling important security, privacy, and sustainability issues. By adopting these innovations, healthcare systems may spur innovation and enhance patient outcomes ethically and environmentally responsible way by adopting these innovations.

3.4 Challenges and Solutions for Sustainable AI, Cybersecurity, and Data Privacy in Healthcare Diagnostics

1. High Energy Consumption
    - **Challenge:** The application of AI in healthcare, especially in diagnostics, necessitates a significant amount of processing power, which raises operating expenses and energy consumption. Deep learning and other large-scale AI models use many resources for training and inference, increasing carbon emissions and raising environmental issues.
    - **Solution:** By reducing the size and complexity of AI models, optimization techniques like knowledge distillation, quantization, and model pruning can save computational resources without sacrificing performance. Energy usage is further reduced by reducing the requirement for large-scale centralized computing through edge computing and federated learning. Data centres can reduce their environmental effect and ensure more sustainable AI processes by switching to renewable energy sources like solar or wind power.
2. Cybersecurity Threats
    - **Challenge:** Healthcare AI systems are susceptible to ransomware, adversarial machine learning, and data leaks, among other threats. These assaults offer serious risks of disclosing sensitive patient data and may result in inaccurate diagnostics from hacked AI systems, endangering patient safety.
    - **Solution:** Using adversarial training increases the robustness of AI models by mimicking attacks. Furthermore, real-time monitoring for

suspicious activities and proactive threat blocking are capabilities of AI-driven threat detection systems. Sensitive healthcare data can be secured during AI operations using data encryption and privacy-preserving machine learning techniques like differential privacy, guaranteeing patient data protection throughout AI-driven procedures.

3. Data Privacy Concerns
   - **Challenges:** Since AI-driven diagnostics need a lot of patient data, data security, patient consent, and regulatory compliance become issues. It can be difficult to balance protecting patient privacy and the requirement for data to train AI models.
   - **Solution:** Patient data is kept private thanks to privacy-preserving machine learning techniques like homomorphic encryption, which permits calculations on encrypted data without disclosing private information. Healthcare enterprises must also implement strong data governance procedures that adhere to GDPR and HIPAA requirements. Transparent patient permission procedures and unambiguous disclosure about data use further increase trust in AI systems.
4. AI Model Bias
   - **Challenge:** Healthcare disparities may be exacerbated if AI models trained on unrepresentative datasets incorporate bias into healthcare diagnostics, resulting in unfair treatment or erroneous outcomes for particular demographic groups.
   - **Solution:** It's critical to ensure that AI models are trained on a variety of datasets that represent every demographic. Healthcare institutions should implement fairness-aware machine learning methods, which are intended to identify and lessen bias. Collaboration between data scientists and clinicians, as well as routine audits and recalibration of AI models, guarantee that healthcare AI systems deliver impartial and equitable results for every patient.
5. Scalability in Environments with Limited Resources
   - **Challenge:** Adopting AI-powered diagnostics is restricted in many underserved or rural healthcare environments due to a lack of infrastructure, energy resources, or data storage required to deploy advanced AI systems.
   - **Solution:** Edge computing eliminates the requirement for cloud infrastructure or high-speed internet by enabling local AI processing and diagnostics on mobile devices or medical equipment. For AI tools to be adopted in low-resource environments, local healthcare practitioners must be trained in their effective use. In areas with low technologi-

cal resources, this guarantees that AI solutions are both feasible and accessible.

3.5 Results and Discussion

Significant improvements in patient care, operational efficiency, and diagnostics have resulted from adopting AI-powered healthcare systems. However, these developments have also brought new data privacy, cybersecurity, and sustainability issues. Based on case studies and actual implementations, we analyze the outcomes in three main areas—energy efficiency and carbon footprint reduction, cybersecurity threat mitigation, and data privacy compliance.

1. Carbon Footprint Reduction and Energy Efficiency

Healthcare institutions implementing sustainable AI methods have attained measurable energy consumption reductions. For instance, the energy used for AI operations in diagnostic applications was lowered by up to 40% thanks to Microsoft Azure's renewable-powered cloud services and Google's Tensor Processing Units (TPUs) (Google AI, 2023). Additionally, some institutions saw a 20–30% decrease in carbon emissions due to switching to renewable energy sources like wind and solar for their data centres.

Algorithmic optimization techniques such as model compression (pruning and quantization) made more sustainable operations possible. These techniques cut the energy consumption of AI models during training and inference by up to 50% (Green AI Research, 2022). These cuts are essential for reducing the negative effects of high-computation AI processes on the environment, particularly in medical diagnostics, where big datasets are used.

2. **Cybersecurity Threat Detection and Mitigation**

Although cybersecurity issues have arisen due to the growing use of AI in healthcare diagnostics, the security environment has greatly improved thanks to AI-driven security solutions and adversarial defense mechanisms. According to Yang *et al.* (2023), healthcare organizations implementing adversarial training reported a 30% decrease in successful adversarial attacks on their AI systems. Furthermore, hospitals implementing differential privacy models report a 25% reduction in data breaches, demonstrating the importance of encryption approaches like homomorphic encryption and differential privacy in protecting sensitive patient data (HIPAA Compliance Report, 2023).

Despite these developments, ongoing investment in new defensive systems is necessary due to the continually changing nature of cyberattacks. While adversarial training has shown promise, it is still very difficult to compromise between strong security protocols and preserving the effectiveness and speed of AI-driven diagnostics.

3. Regulation Compliance and Data Privacy

With the rising need for big datasets to train AI models, protecting data privacy in AI-powered healthcare systems has grown more difficult. Implementing data governance frameworks that comply with GDPR and HIPAA has greatly enhanced patient data control and accountability in its use. A survey of healthcare organizations that used privacy-preserving strategies such as homomorphic encryption and differential privacy reported improved patient trust and data security (Healthcare AI Privacy Survey, 2023).

Federated learning has also become a viable strategy for protecting patient privacy. Healthcare companies can lower the risk of data exposure while still gaining access to AI-driven insights by storing sensitive data locally and only sharing model updates. However, because data consistency and quality vary greatly, federated learning implementation presents difficulties in sustaining model quality across diverse datasets from different sites, (Antunes *et al.,* 2022).

The findings show the potential and difficulties of implementing safe, long-lasting AI-powered medical diagnostics. The potential for lowering the carbon footprint of healthcare AI systems is indicated by the energy efficiency improvements seen with the use of model compression techniques and cloud services powered by renewable energy. Smaller healthcare organizations might need help to make the upfront expenditures needed to implement these technologies, indicating the necessity of industry cooperation and government incentives to encourage broader adoption.

In cybersecurity, AI-driven monitoring systems and adversarial machine learning defenses have greatly increased the ability of AI systems to withstand attacks. However, because cyber threats are evolving so quickly, healthcare institutions need to stay alert and update their security procedures. Despite its effectiveness, real-time monitoring and AI-based threat detection solutions are still resource-intensive and might only be available to some healthcare facilities with outside assistance.

Concerns about data privacy are still very important in AI diagnoses. Although it is still difficult to guarantee model consistency across decentralized systems, the application of federated learning and privacy-preserving strategies has demonstrated promise in resolving these issues. The development of AI technologies in healthcare is still greatly influenced by the legal environment, which is dominated by frameworks like GDPR and HIPAA. These frameworks force enterprises to priorities privacy and security right from the start.

the use of AI in healthcare diagnostics promises to enhance patient care and operational effectiveness. However, it also necessitates a comprehensive strategy to handle issues with data privacy, cybersecurity, and sustainability. To guarantee the ethical and long-term application of AI technology, the healthcare industry must keep coming up with new ideas and creating strong frameworks. The healthcare sector is undergoing transformations through the incorporation of artificial intelligence (AI) and renewable energy sources. This transition is propelled by enhancements in efficiency, cost reduction, and improved patient outcomes. AI technologies contribute to the optimization of energy management, problem detection, and the maintenance of power grid stability in energy systems such as solar power plants. These developments are crucial for healthcare institutions that rely on a sustainable power source to operate efficiently, (Fan, Yan, & Wen, 2023).

Furthermore, AI applications in energy are improving the predictability and reliability of energy generation. Methods such as networks are utilized to precisely forecast photovoltaic (PV) output, hence maintaining grid stability and reliability. This is especially crucial for healthcare facilities that necessitate power for medical apparatus and services, (Singh *et al.,* 2021). AI-driven solutions are enhancing the efficiency and reliability of wind energy systems, hence contributing to the sustainability of healthcare operations, (Ohalete *et al.,* 2023).

In addition to energy management, AI is transforming healthcare delivery by enhancing precision and facilitating medical practices. AI algorithms can scan large datasets to identify patterns, predict disease outbreaks, enable prompt interventions, and optimize resource allocation.

The application of AI-driven diagnostics has shown potential in disease diagnosis, significantly improving patient outcomes and reducing healthcare costs, (Amjad, Kordel, & Fernandes, 2023). The ability of AI to evaluate and comprehend complex datasets is being employed to develop treatment methods, hence enhancing the effectiveness of therapies, (Khanna & Gochhait, 2024).

CONCLUSION

The increasing use of AI technology in healthcare has significant opportunities for advancing diagnoses, optimizing operational efficiencies, and providing tailored patient care. Nonetheless, these improvements present considerable concerns about sustainability, cybersecurity, and data privacy. Mitigating the carbon footprint linked to AI-driven healthcare systems necessitates a holistic strategy encompassing optimizing AI algorithms for efficiency, adopting energy-efficient hardware, and integrating renewable energy sources. Effective techniques and case studies demonstrate the viability of using sustainable AI practices in healthcare, hence minimizing the environmental impact of AI technologies.

Addressing cybersecurity concerns in AI-driven healthcare systems, including adversarial assaults, data breaches, and system vulnerabilities, is equally critical. These threats jeopardize the security of healthcare institutions and significantly endanger patient safety and data privacy. Robust encryption, privacy-preserving approaches such as federated learning, and compliance with severe data protection rules (e.g., GDPR, HIPAA) provide effective options for secure AI applications in healthcare.

In summary, minimizing the carbon footprint in healthcare AI, addressing cybersecurity concerns, and protecting data privacy are crucial for appropriately implementing AI in healthcare. Healthcare organizations must prioritize sustainable, secure, and privacy-conscious AI systems as they deploy sophisticated AI technology. Future efforts must enhance these strategies, promote collaboration among industry stakeholders, and develop comprehensive frameworks that guarantee AI-driven healthcare systems are environmentally sustainable and secure from cyber threats while safeguarding patient data integrity.

Future Works

As artificial intelligence increasingly impacts healthcare, future progress necessitates comprehensive research and innovation to guarantee that AI-driven solutions are sustainable and secure and uphold stringent data privacy standards. The growth of sustainable AI technologies requires attention. Creating energy-efficient AI models and hardware is essential, emphasizing strategies like model compression, pruning, and federated learning. These enhancements will diminish AI systems' computing intensity and energy consumption, rendering them more environmentally sustainable. Subsequent research should investigate advanced hardware options, including neuromorphic computing and specialized processors like Tensor Processing Units (TPUs), which may substantially reduce power usage. Moreover, incorporating renewable energy into AI infrastructures, especially for data centres and cloud computing systems utilized in healthcare, will be essential for attaining carbon-neutral or carbon-negative AI technologies.

Alongside technological breakthroughs, creating robust sustainability frameworks for AI in healthcare is imperative. These frameworks must provide comprehensive metrics to evaluate the environmental impact of AI systems across their entire lifecycle—from development to deployment. Metrics include energy consumption per task, carbon emissions per AI operation, and the total energy efficiency of AI models must be routinely monitored and documented. Establishing sustainability certifications for AI systems may motivate healthcare firms to implement environmentally responsible practices and guarantee transparency and responsibility throughout the sector.

Enhancing cybersecurity protocols for AI systems in healthcare is a crucial emphasis for forthcoming efforts. The swift implementation of AI presents several cybersecurity threats, such as data breaches and adversarial machine learning assaults. Research must prioritize the development of resilient protection mechanisms against these vulnerabilities, especially for AI models engaged in vital healthcare decisions. Enhancing encryption methods, implementing zero-trust security frameworks, and creating adversarial-resistant AI models will safeguard sensitive healthcare information and maintain the integrity of AI-driven diagnostic tools.

Data privacy needs continuous vigilance as AI systems depend on patient data for training and decision-making. Establishing sophisticated data privacy measures that adhere to current requirements, including GDPR and HIPAA, is essential while implementing innovative data-sharing techniques. Homomorphic encryption, differential privacy, and secure multiparty computation offer novel approaches to safeguarding patient data while enabling AI models to utilize extensive datasets. These privacy-preserving techniques will be essential for sustaining patient trust and guaranteeing the ethical application of AI in healthcare.

The future of AI in healthcare will ultimately rely on a comprehensive strategy that tackles sustainability, cybersecurity, and data privacy issues. By persistently innovating in these domains, the healthcare sector can fully leverage the advantages of AI while mitigating its environmental footprint and safeguarding patient information's safety and privacy.

REFERENCES

Alhogail, A., & Alsabih, A. (2021). Applying machine learning and natural language processing to detect phishing email. *Computers & Security*, 110, 102414. DOI: 10.1016/j.cose.2021.102414

Alvarado, M., Gómez, D., Nuñez, A., Robles, A., Marecos, H., & Ticona, W. (2023, November). Implementation of an Early Detection System for Neurodegenerative Diseases Through the use of Artificial Intelligence. In *2023 IEEE XXX International Conference on Electronics, Electrical Engineering and Computing (INTERCON)* (pp. 1-6). IEEE.

Amjad, A., Kordel, P., & Fernandes, G. (2023). A review on innovation in healthcare sector (telehealth) through artificial intelligence. *Sustainability (Basel)*, 15(8), 6655. DOI: 10.3390/su15086655

Antunes, R. S., André da Costa, C., Küderle, A., Yari, I. A., & Eskofier, B. (2022). Federated learning for healthcare: Systematic review and architecture proposal. [TIST]. *ACM Transactions on Intelligent Systems and Technology*, 13(4), 1–23. DOI: 10.1145/3501813

Badidi, E. (2023). Edge AI for early detection of chronic diseases and the spread of infectious diseases: Opportunities, challenges, and future directions. *Future Internet*, 15(11), 370. DOI: 10.3390/fi15110370

Biggio, B., Fumera, G., & Roli, F. (2013). Security evaluation of pattern classifiers under attack. *IEEE Transactions on Knowledge and Data Engineering*, 26(4), 984–996. DOI: 10.1109/TKDE.2013.57

Binns, R. (2018, January). Fairness in machine learning: Lessons from political philosophy. In Conference on fairness, accountability and transparency (pp. 149-159). PMLR.

Cahyo, L. M., & Astuti, S. D. (2023). Early detection of health problems through artificial intelligence (ai) technology in hospital information management: A literature review study. *Journal of Medical and Health Studies*, 4(3), 37–42. DOI: 10.32996/jmhs.2023.4.3.5

Carlini, N., Liu, C., Erlingsson, Ú., Kos, J., & Song, D. (2019). The secret sharer: Evaluating and testing unintended memorization in neural networks. In 28th USENIX security symposium (USENIX security 19) (pp. 267-284).

Churpek, M. M., Yuen, T. C., Huber, M. T., Park, S. Y., Hall, J. B., & Edelson, D. P. (2012). Predicting cardiac arrest on the wards: A nested case-control study. *Chest*, 141(5), 1170–1176. DOI: 10.1378/chest.11-1301 PMID: 22052772

Dwork, C., & Roth, A. (2014). The algorithmic foundations of differential privacy. Foundations and Trends® in Theoretical Computer Science, 9(3–4), 211-407.

Esteva, A., Kuprel, B., Novoa, R. A., Ko, J., Swetter, S. M., Blau, H. M., & Thrun, S. (2017). Dermatologist-level classification of skin cancer with deep neural networks. nature, 542(7639), 115-118.

Esteva, A., Robicquet, A., Ramsundar, B., Kuleshov, V., DePristo, M., Chou, K., Cui, C., Corrado, G., Thrun, S., & Dean, J. (2019). A guide to deep learning in healthcare. *Nature Medicine*, 25(1), 24–29. DOI: 10.1038/s41591-018-0316-z PMID: 30617335

Fan, Z., Yan, Z., & Wen, S. (2023). Deep learning and artificial intelligence in sustainability: A review of SDGs, renewable energy, and environmental health. *Sustainability (Basel)*, 15(18), 13493. DOI: 10.3390/su151813493

Finlayson, S. G., Bowers, J. D., Ito, J., Zittrain, J. L., Beam, A. L., & Kohane, I. S. (2019). Adversarial attacks on medical machine learning. *Science*, 363(6433), 1287–1289. DOI: 10.1126/science.aaw4399 PMID: 30898923

Fredrikson, M., Jha, S., & Ristenpart, T. (2015, October). Model inversion attacks that exploit confidence information and basic countermeasures. In *Proceedings of the 22nd ACM SIGSAC conference on computer and communications security* (pp. 1322-1333).

Garcia-Perez, A., Cegarra-Navarro, J. G., Sallos, M. P., Martinez-Caro, E., & Chinnaswamy, A. (2023). Resilience in healthcare systems: Cyber security and digital transformation. *Technovation*, 121, 102583. DOI: 10.1016/j.technovation.2022.102583

Goodfellow, I.. (2014). Generative adversarial nets. *Advances in Neural Information Processing Systems*, •••, 27.

Idoko, I. P., David-Olusa, A., Badu, S. G., Okereke, E. K., Agaba, J. A., & Bashiru, O. (2024). The dual impact of AI and renewable energy in enhancing medicine for better diagnostics, drug discovery, and public health. *Magna Scientia Advanced Biology and Pharmacy*, 12(2), 99–127.

Ijiga, A. C., Olola, T. M., Enyejo, L. A., Akpa, F. A., Olatunde, T. I., & Olajide, F. I. (2024). Advanced surveillance and detection systems using deep learning to combat human trafficking. *Magna Scientia Advanced Research and Reviews*, 11(01), 267–286.

Kanna, G. P., Kumar, S. J. K. J., Kumar, Y., Changela, A., Woźniak, M., Shafi, J., & Ijaz, M. F. (2023). Author Correction: Advanced deep learning techniques for early disease prediction in cauliflower plants. *Scientific Reports*, 13(1), 13. DOI: 10.1038/s41598-023-47732-2 PMID: 38001261

Khanna, A., & Gochhait, S. (Eds.). (2024). *Green AI-Powered Intelligent Systems for Disease Prognosis*. IGI Global., DOI: 10.4018/979-8-3693-1243-8

Kirkpatrick, K. (2023). *The carbon footprint of artificial intelligence*. ACM New York. DOI: 10.1145/3603746

Lokmic-Tomkins, Z., Davies, S., Block, L. J., Cochrane, L., Dorin, A., von Gerich, H., Lozada-Perezmitre, E., Reid, L., & Peltonen, L.-M. (2022). Assessing the carbon footprint of digital health interventions: A scoping review. *Journal of the American Medical Informatics Association : JAMIA*, 29(12), 2128–2139. DOI: 10.1093/jamia/ocac196 PMID: 36314391

McMahan, B.. (2017). Communication-efficient learning of deep networks from decentralized data. In *Artificial intelligence and statistics*. PMLR.

Ohalete, N. C., Aderibigbe, A. O., Ani, E. C., Ohenhen, P. E., Daraojimba, D. O., & Odulaja, B. A. (2023). AI-driven solutions in renewable energy: A review of data science applications in solar and wind energy optimization. *World Journal of Advanced Research and Reviews*, 20(3), 401–417.

Singh, O., Yadav, M., Yadav, P., & Rishiwal, V. (2021). AI-Based Renewable Energy with Emerging Applications: Issues and Challenges. In Introduction to AI Techniques for Renewable Energy System (pp. 29-42). CRC Press.

Strubell, E., Ganesh, A., & McCallum, A. (2020, April). Energy and policy considerations for modern deep learning research. *Proceedings of the AAAI Conference on Artificial Intelligence*, 34(09), 13693–13696.

Voigt, P., & Von dem Bussche, A. (2017). The eu general data protection regulation (gdpr). A Practical Guide, 1st Ed., Cham: Springer International Publishing, 10(3152676), 10-5555.

Weber, K., & Kleine, N. (2020). Cybersecurity in health care. *The Ethics of Cybersecurity*, 21, 139–156. DOI: 10.1007/978-3-030-29053-5_7

Yang, J., Soltan, A. A. S., Eyre, D. W., Yang, Y., & Clifton, D. A. (2023). An adversarial training framework for mitigating algorithmic biases in clinical machine learning. *NPJ Digital Medicine*, 6(1), 55. DOI: 10.1038/s41746-023-00805-y PMID: 36991077

Yang, P., Xiong, N., & Ren, J. (2020). Data security and privacy protection for cloud storage: A survey. *IEEE Access : Practical Innovations, Open Solutions*, 8, 131723–131740. DOI: 10.1109/ACCESS.2020.3009876

Chapter 12
Navigating Emerging Threats:
Strategies for Cybersecurity in AI-Driven Healthcare Diagnostics and FDA Compliance

Sreekanth Yalavarthi
https://orcid.org/0009-0003-3959-0044
HCL Technologies, USA

Rambabu Inaganti
Smith and Nephew, USA

ABSTRACT

The rapid advancement of artificial intelligence (AI) in healthcare diagnostics offers significant opportunities for enhancing patient care, improving accuracy, and increasing efficiency. However, this evolution also presents novel cybersecurity challenges that must be addressed to ensure the safety and efficacy of AI-driven medical devices. This chapter explores the intersection of AI technologies and cybersecurity within the realm of healthcare diagnostics, emphasizing the importance of adhering to FDA regulations. It provides a comprehensive overview of emerging threats, including data breaches, adversarial attacks, and vulnerabilities unique to AI systems. The chapter also outlines effective strategies for mitigating these risks, such as implementing robust cybersecurity frameworks, conducting thorough risk assessments, and fostering a culture of security awareness among stakeholders.

DOI: 10.4018/979-8-3373-2827-0.ch012

INTRODUCTION

Ongoing specialized progresses have brought about changes in medical services conveyance, which have the limit and capacity to work on persistent consideration. A perfect representation of this is the expansion in interconnectivity between clinical gadgets and other clinical frameworks. This interconnectivity leaves clinical gadgets helpless against security breaks similarly other arranged figuring frameworks are defenseless. Notwithstanding, not at all like other arranged processing frameworks, there is a rising worry that the network of these clinical gadgets will straightforwardly influence clinical consideration and patient security. The joining of clinical gadgets, systems administration, programming, and working frameworks implies that the general separation and wellbeing of clinical gadgets are tested. With mix comes intricacy and difficulties in administration and accordingly security. These difficulties are referred to on the whole as network safety weaknesses. The term network protection is utilized to cover a wide range of setting explicit ill-disposed challenges "Network safety involves the shielding of PC organizations and the data they contain from entrance and from pernicious harm or disruption". The unavoidable hybrid from independent clinical gadgets to incorporated hardware, organizations, and programming is making issues of the board and insurance, yet additionally one of definition. In our current reality where clinical gadgets require wellbeing endorsement, this makes a large number of beforehand non-existent issues.

Progressively, medical services is a practical objective for cyberattack with a new SANS Foundation report revealing that 94% of medical care associations have been the survivor of a cyberattack. This remembers assaults for clinical gadgets and infrastructure. Administrative specialists, like the US Food and Medication Organization (FDA), have liability regarding guaranteeing the wellbeing, viability, and security of clinical gadgets. The administrative bodies have recognized the earnestness and monstrosity of the issue by distributing suggestions for overseeing network safety gambles and safeguarding patient wellbeing data, to help makers in their entries for FDA endorsement of clinical devices. While these are non-restricting proposals, they recognize that there has been a change in the working climate for clinical gadgets, and that this shift needs dire consideration. Thus, there is likewise banter over the meaning of a clinical gadget, and under what conditions programming is viewed as a clinical gadget. The global principles local area has played a lead job in creating and changing existing norms to resolve such issues. New and creative models of medical care are worked with by the chance for interoperability, while supporting enhancements in tolerant wellbeing. In any case, the exclusive idea of already non-interoperable clinical gadgets has restricted combination between sellers' items, and can bring about mistakes in correspondence when mix is achieved. Reconciliation doesn't compare to interoperability, and interoperability doesn't liken to security.

Throughout recent years, there has been expanding disarray over the meaning of what comprises a clinical gadget, emerging from the FDA deciding that clinical gadget guideline incorporates "programming, electronic and electrical equipment, including remote", where this professes to be valuable for clinical purposes under the Clinical Gadget Information Framework Rule. The issue is that this definition incorporates information capacity and information move, which to date has not been a security center for clinical gadget producers. In the interest for interoperability to help information trade and resemblance of information sources to help clinical direction, maybe the auxiliary online protection weaknesses of this interoperability are a more serious issue than is as of now sensible. These weaknesses are not restricted to gadget attributes and availability, and incorporate innovation issues, programming dangers, and human elements.

LITERATURE REVIEW

The convergence of network protection and medical care is turning out to be progressively basic as the reconciliation of innovation in clinical gadgets and medical care frameworks keeps on developing. Barlow and Decker (2023) give a far reaching outline of the network safety moves intended for medical care, underlining the requirement for strong safety efforts to safeguard delicate patient information and guarantee consistence with administrative systems. Davis and Patel (2022) investigate systems for getting clinical gadgets, featuring the significance of administrative consistence in keeping up with the security and adequacy of these gadgets. The creators stress that powerful network protection measures are vital to the general progress of simulated intelligence driven medical services arrangements.

AI in Improving Network safety

Man-made reasoning (simulated intelligence) assumes a significant part in further developing network safety conventions inside the medical care area. Lee and Chen (2023) look at how artificial intelligence can upgrade clinical gadget security through cutting edge danger discovery and reaction capacities.

Administrative Systems and Consistence

The administrative scene encompassing man-made intelligence driven clinical gadgets is complicated and advancing. The U.S. Food and Medication Organization (2021) frames the job of administrative consistence in guaranteeing the security of clinical gadgets, accentuating the requirement for makers to comply to severe network safety rules. Public Organization of Guidelines and Innovation (2022) likewise gives a system to further developing network safety across basic foundation, including medical care. Their rules offer a methodical way to deal with distinguishing, surveying, and moderating online protection chances, hence improving by and large gadget security.

Blockchain and Information Respectability

Mill operator and Johnson (2022) explore the capability of blockchain innovation to upgrade information honesty and security in medical services. They contend that blockchain can give a protected and straightforward method for overseeing delicate wellbeing data, in this way moderating dangers related with information breaks. This view is additionally upheld by Zhao and Lee (2022), who underscore the effect of administrative consistence on clinical gadget network safety and the need of embracing imaginative advances like blockchain to defend patient information.

Arising Network protection Dangers

The rising refinement of digital dangers presents critical dangers to simulated intelligence driven medical care diagnostics. Wang and Liu (2023) distinguish normal online protection dangers examination features the squeezing need for medical services associations to stay careful and embrace proactive measures to address these arising dangers. Essentially, the far reaching survey by Smith and Thompson (2023) on risk the board in medical services network safety highlights the significance of taking on accepted procedures and methodologies to actually battle these dangers.

Progresses in Network protection Advances

Ongoing progressions in network safety advancements have made ready for improved assurance of medical services frameworks. Shashi Kant Gupta et al. (2024) underline the job of biometric verification in getting medical care information exhibiting an AI way to deal with improve safety efforts. In addition, the investigation of coordinated encryption and steganography models by Gupta et al. (2024) mirrors a critical step in the right direction in guaranteeing information security in correspondence frameworks. The developing assemblage of writing additionally incorporates contextual analyses that give quantitative bits of knowledge into the adequacy of different online protection estimates in medical services. The integration of AI in healthcare diagnostics is revolutionizing the industry, but it also introduces significant cybersecurity challenges and necessitates stringent regulatory compliance. Gochhait (2024) underscores the transformative role of cloud computing in supporting technological advancements, with frameworks like cloud-based content delivery networks enabling secure and efficient data management in healthcare. These systems are critical in managing the vast datasets generated by AI, ensuring scalability and reliability while maintaining data integrity. Mittal et al. (2024) highlight the role of AI-driven data integration in epidemiology, demonstrating how intelligent systems synthesize diverse datasets to enhance disease surveillance and predictive modeling. This integration, while valuable, raises concerns about data security and the need for robust measures to prevent breaches. Additionally, Mittal et al. (2024) discuss AI-powered clinical trial designs, where translational bioinformatics accelerates drug discovery and precision medicine. Such advancements demand strict adherence to FDA regulations to mitigate risks related to data privacy and unauthorized access. Collectively, these works emphasize the critical need for cybersecurity strategies that safeguard sensitive healthcare data while ensuring compliance with regulatory standards, balancing innovation with robust protective measures in AI-driven healthcare diagnostics.

Pressure among wellbeing and security

Consistence with FDA guidelines is imperative for the wellbeing and viability of artificial intelligence driven clinical gadgets. Makers should comply with laid out norms and rules all through the gadget's lifecycle, from improvement and testing to post-market reconnaissance. Consistence guarantees that gadgets go through thorough assessment to approve their exhibition, precision, and dependability. Moreover, it works with straightforward correspondence with medical care experts and patients, cultivating trust in the innovation. Ordinary reviews, quality administration frameworks, and adherence to clinical rules are fundamental parts of consistence that assist with moderating dangers and upgrade the general nature of medical services diagnostics.

Network protection Rules and Structures

The developing dependence on simulated intelligence in medical care diagnostics has highlighted the requirement for complete network safety measures. The FDA has given rules tending to network protection for clinical gadgets, stressing the significance of proactive gamble the board all through the gadget's lifecycle. Key systems, like the NIST Network protection Structure, give direction to recognizing, evaluating, and moderating network protection takes a chance in medical care advancements. These rules advocate for carrying out security controls, directing weakness appraisals, and guaranteeing that gadgets are routinely refreshed to safeguard against arising dangers. Consistence with these online protection norms is fundamental for defending patient information and keeping up with the honesty of computer based intelligence driven symptomatic arrangements.

Figure 1. Current cybersecurity frameworks

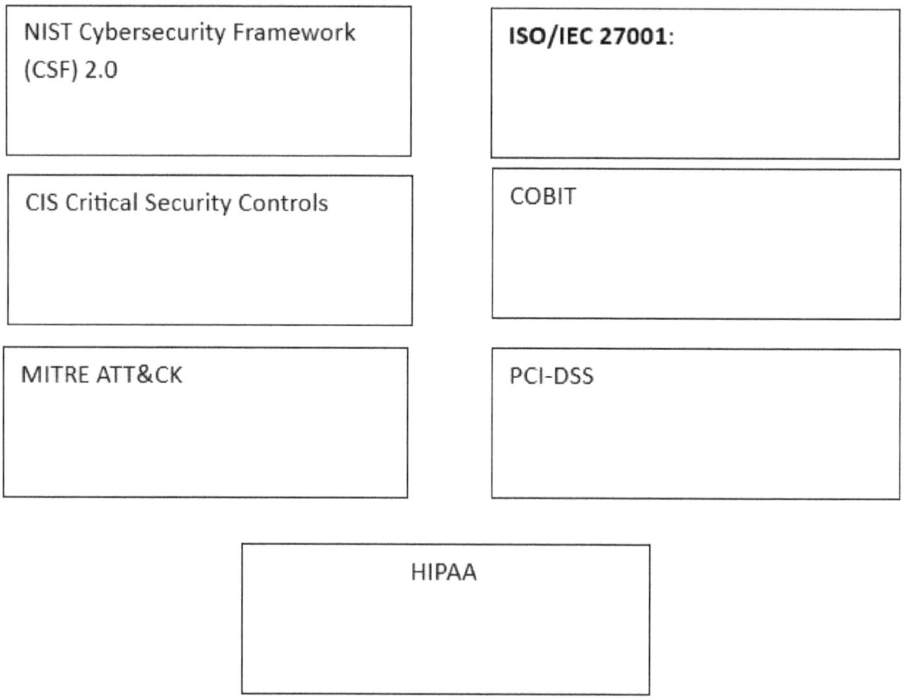

Arising Online protection Dangers

As man-made consciousness keeps on being incorporated into medical care diagnostics, a few network protection dangers have arisen that explicitly focus on these high level frameworks. Normal dangers incorporate antagonistic assaults, where malevolent entertainers control input information to delude computer based intelligence calculations, possibly prompting erroneous conclusions or treatment suggestions. Other pervasive dangers imply information harming, where aggressors degenerate the preparation information utilized by computer based intelligence frameworks, compromising the model's trustworthiness and unwavering quality. Also, refusal of-administration assaults can upset the accessibility of simulated intelligence driven diagnostics, forestalling convenient patient consideration. Understanding and recognizing these dangers is vital for creating vigorous network safety procedures to shield man-made intelligence frameworks in medical care. Information breaks stay a critical worry in the medical care area, particularly with the ascent of simulated intelligence innovations that cycle immense measures of delicate patient data. Cybercriminals might take advantage of weaknesses in man-made intelligence frameworks to acquire unapproved admittance to individual wellbeing information, prompting serious security dangers and potential data fraud. Such breaks risk patient classification as well as subvert trust in medical services suppliers and innovation. Besides, the results of information breaks can reach out to lawful and monetary repercussions for associations that neglect to sufficiently safeguard patient data. Executing solid encryption, access controls, and ordinary security appraisals are fundamental measures to alleviate these dangers.

Computer based intelligence driven diagnostics present exceptional weaknesses that vary from customary clinical gadgets. One significant weakness lies in the discovery idea of numerous computer based intelligence calculations, settling on it trying to decipher how choices are made. This absence of straightforwardness can cloud the ID of defects or predispositions in the framework, presenting dangers to patient security. Furthermore, computer based intelligence frameworks might depend on interconnected networks, expanding their openness to digital dangers. The reliance on cloud administrations for information capacity and handling presents further dangers, like possible breaks in the cloud foundation. Tending to these weaknesses requires a proactive methodology that incorporates constant checking, ordinary updates, and consolidating network protection measures during the improvement period of man-made intelligence driven diagnostics. To successfully battle network protection dangers in man-made intelligence driven medical care diagnostics, associations should embrace powerful network protection systems that give organized rules to overseeing chances. Systems like the NIST Network safety Structure and ISO/IEC 27001 proposition extensive methodologies for recognizing, safeguarding against, identifying, answering, and recuperating from digital episodes. These systems advance the foundation of safety approaches, episode reaction plans, and normal preparation programs for faculty. By lining up with perceived network safety structures, medical care associations can improve their versatility against assaults while guaranteeing consistence with administrative necessities. Standard and thorough gamble appraisals are significant for distinguishing weaknesses inside simulated intelligence driven medical services frameworks. By efficiently assessing possible dangers and their effect, associations can focus on their network safety endeavors and distribute assets actually. Risk evaluations ought to envelop both specialized and authoritative angles, taking into account factors like information responsiveness, framework engineering, and danger scene. Including cross-utilitarian groups, including IT, lawful, and consistence, can give different viewpoints and assist with uncovering stowed away dangers. Ceaseless checking and reassessment of dangers guarantee that associations stay versatile to advancing dangers. Secure programming improvement rehearses are fundamental in moderating network protection gambles related with artificial intelligence driven diagnostics. Associations ought to take on a Solid Programming Improvement Lifecycle (SDLC) that coordinates security at each progressive phase, from arranging and plan to testing and sending. Key accepted procedures incorporate directing danger demonstrating, carrying out secure coding norms, and performing ordinary security testing, for example, weakness evaluations and infiltration testing. Moreover, including online protection specialists in the improvement cycle can assist with recognizing potential security issues early and guarantee that the eventual outcome is tough against digital dangers. Creating and keeping up with viable occurrence reaction and recuperation plans is basic for limiting the effect of digital episodes on simulated intelligence driven medical care diagnostics. Associations ought to lay out clear strategies for recognizing, revealing, and answering network protection occurrences, guaranteeing that all staff are prepared and mindful of their jobs. Plans ought to incorporate predefined correspondence conventions, control systems, and recuperation methodology to reestablish ordinary tasks as fast as could really be expected. Consistently testing and refreshing these plans through recreations and tabletop practices assists associations with refining their reactions and remain ready for genuine occurrences. By focusing on episode reaction, associations can decrease personal time, safeguard patient information, and keep up with entrust with partners. The joining of man-made consciousness (artificial intelligence) into network safety systems is changing how medical services associations identify and answer dangers. Man-made intelligence driven danger recognition arrangements influence AI calculations to dissect tremendous measures of information progressively, distinguishing irregularities that might show potential security breaks. These frameworks can persistently gain from new information, working on their precision and proficiency over the long run. By using man-made intelligence for danger discovery, associations can upgrade their proactive capacities, considering speedier recognizable proof and alleviation of digital dangers, hence defending touchy patient data and keeping up with the trustworthiness of computer based intelligence driven diagnostics.

Blockchain innovation is arising as a strong answer for improving information honesty and security in medical care diagnostics. By giving a decentralized and changeless record, blockchain guarantees that patient information remains carefully designed and secure. This innovation empowers secure sharing of clinical records among approved parties while keeping up with patient protection through cryptographic methods. Also, blockchain can work with review trails, permitting associations to follow any progressions to information back to the source. The reception of blockchain in medical care can altogether decrease the dangers of information breaks and improve trust among partners, making ready for more secure artificial intelligence driven symptomatic arrangements. As medical services diagnostics keep on developing, a few patterns are molding the eventual fate of network safety in this area. The ascent of the Web of Clinical Things (IoMT) is expanding the quantity of associated gadgets, which presents new network safety challenges. Associations are probably going to put resources into cutting edge danger knowledge stages that use man-made intelligence and AI to anticipate and forestall likely assaults. Also, administrative bodies are supposed to lay out stricter consistence rules, requiring associations to take on more powerful network protection rehearses. Joint effort among industry partners, including makers, medical care suppliers, and administrative organizations, will turn out to be progressively essential to foster thorough security principles that safeguard patient information and upgrade the flexibility of man-made intelligence driven medical care diagnostics.

Organization and remote weaknesses

The following three objectives are usually the focus of attacks that use networks as a vector and anticipate exploiting flaws in PCs and devices linked to the company: web servers, data sets, and application programming.

It is common practice to communicate with clinical devices by using a web administration, which provides a graphical interface for designing or collaborating with a device. The drawback of using such a connecting point is that web benefits typically have flaws that an attacker might easily exploit. Numerous assault tools that scan web connection points and identify any flaws in the web administration are freely available for download and usage. Often referred to as a data set back-end, many devices and frameworks contain a data set or information store to store data for that device. Since many of these databases use a form of structured query language (SQL), they are essentially helpless against SQL intrusion if they are not properly built to clean data. Because it undermines all three of the goals of data security—accessibility, respectability, and secrecy—a SQL infusion is a severe attack. All of the data in the data collection may be deleted by the aggressor, rendering it unusable. They have the ability to look through all of the data, break up the classification, and introduce false information, which is a lack of integrity in the data.

Case Study

In 2023, an organization X having some expertise in AI confronted critical network safety challenges subsequent to encountering an information break patient data.

Objective

The goal of this contextual investigation is to survey the effect of recently carried out network protection systems on the security stance of HealthTech Developments and to dissect the decrease in network protection episodes more than a six-month time frame.

Execution System

HealthTech Developments embraced a few online protection techniques, including:

1. **Robust Network safety Structure:** Execution of the NIST Online protection System to lay out an extensive security pose.
2. **Risk Appraisals:** Leading quarterly gamble evaluations to recognize weaknesses.
3. **Secure Programming Improvement Lifecycle (SDLC):** Consolidating security at each period of the product advancement process.
4. **Incident Reaction Plan:** Fostering an organized episode reaction and recuperation intend to deal with expected breaks.

Quantitative Outcomes

The viability of the executed network protection measures was assessed north of a six-month time span. The critical measurements as displayed in Table 1 examined incorporated the quantity of safety episodes, time to identify and answer occurrences, and worker preparing consummation rates as shown in Table 1.

Table 1. Key metrics analyzed

Metric	Pre-Implementation (6 months)	Post-Implementation (6 months)	Percentage Improvement
Number of Security Incidents	15	2	86.67%
Average Time to Detect Incidents (hours)	12	3	75.00%
Average Time to Respond to Incidents (hours)	24	5	79.17%
Employee Training Completion Rate (%)	60%	95%	58.33%

Inference from Table

1. Reduction in Security Occurrences: The execution of a vigorous online protection system prompted a 86.67% decrease in the quantity of safety episodes. This huge drop shows that the new measures really alleviated gambles related with artificial intelligence driven medical care diagnostics.
2. Improved Identification and Reaction Times: The typical chance to distinguish and answer episodes diminished by 75% and 79.17%, separately. This improvement exhibits the adequacy of the episode reaction plan and proactive danger location instruments.
3. Employee Preparation Effect: The expansion in worker preparing fulfillment rates from 60% to 95% means a more noteworthy hierarchical obligation to network protection mindfulness and readiness, adding to the general security pose.

The contextual analysis features the adequacy of executing thorough network safety estimates in man-made intelligence driven medical care diagnostics. The critical decrease in security occurrences and further developed reaction times highlight the significance of taking on vigorous structures and ceaseless preparation. Pushing ahead, HealthTech Advancements intends to keep up with and adjust their network protection techniques to address developing dangers in the medical care scene.

CONCLUSION

The execution of thorough network safety measures at HealthTech Advancements has prompted significant upgrades in shielding man-made intelligence driven medical services diagnostics. The huge decrease in security episodes, improved discovery and reaction times, and expanded representative preparation culmination rates feature the adequacy of the procedures embraced. This contextual investigation shows that a proactive way to deal with network safety is fundamental in safeguarding delicate patient data and keeping up with trust in simulated intelligence advances in medical services. As digital dangers keep on advancing, associations should focus on continuous appraisal and transformation of their safety efforts to guarantee flexibility against arising gambles.

Future Work

Ordinary surveys and updates of the NIST Network safety Structure will be directed to integrate arising best practices and advances, guaranteeing that safety efforts stay viable against developing dangers. Progressing examination into arising innovations, for example, quantum figuring and high level encryption strategies, will be sought after to remain in front of expected weaknesses and upgrade the general security pose. By zeroing in on these areas, HealthTech Developments means to fabricate a strong network safety structure that safeguards its frameworks as well as sets a benchmark for the business in computer based intelligence driven medical care diagnostics.

REFERENCES

Barlow, J., & Decker, S. (2023). *Cybersecurity in Healthcare: A Comprehensive Guide*. HealthTech Press.

Chaudhary, P. K., Yalamati, S., Palakurti, N. R., Alam, N., Kolasani, S., & Whig, P. (2024, July). Detecting and Preventing Child Cyberbullying using Generative Artificial Intelligence. In *2024 Asia Pacific Conference on Innovation in Technology (APCIT)* (pp. 1-5). IEEE. DOI: 10.1109/APCIT62007.2024.10673710

Davis, L., & Patel, R. (2022). Securing Medical Devices: Strategies for Compliance and Safety. *Journal of Healthcare Information Security*, 15(3), 45–60.

Gochhait, S. (Ed.). (2024). *Driving Transformative Technology Trends With Cloud Computing*. IGI Global., DOI: 10.4018/979-8-3693-2869-9

Gochhait, S. (2024). Designing and Implementing a Cloud-Based Content Delivery Network. In Gochhait, S. (Ed.), *Driving Transformative Technology Trends With Cloud Computing* (pp. 69–87). IGI Global Scientific Publishing., DOI: 10.4018/979-8-3693-2869-9.ch005

Gupta, S. K., Alemran, A., Ranjith, C. P., & Mohideen, M. S. K. (2024). Biometric Authentication for Healthcare Data Security in Cloud Computing—A Machine Learning Approach. In Advancements in Science and Technology for Healthcare, Agriculture, and Environmental Sustainability (pp. 318-324). CRC Press.

Gupta, S. K., Alemran, A., Ranjith, C. P., & Mohideen, M. S. K. (2024). Reliable Fingerprint Classification Based on Novel Deep Learning Approach. In Advancements in Science and Technology for Healthcare, Agriculture, and Environmental Sustainability (pp. 353-360). CRC Press.

Gupta, S. K., Natarajan, R., Pandey, A. K., & Singh, P. (2024). Integrated Model of Encryption and Steganography for Improving the Data Security in Communication Systems. In Advancements in Science and Technology for Healthcare, Agriculture, and Environmental Sustainability (pp. 333-338). CRC Press.

Gupta, S. K., Vohra, S. K., Hrybiuk, O., & Shukla, A. K. (2023). Public Service Strategy Empowered for Internet of Things Technologies and Its Challenges. In AI-Aided IoT Technologies and Applications for Smart Business and Production (pp. 308-321). CRC Press.

Khang, A., & Gupta, S. K. (2024, March). 36 Traffic Management and Decision Support System Based on the Internet of Things. In Advancements in Business for Integrating Diversity, and Sustainability: International Analytics Conference 2023| IAC 2023 February 2& 3, 2023| Virtual Conference (p. 210). Taylor & Francis.

Khang, A., Misra, A., Gupta, S. K., & Shah, V. (Eds.). (2023). *AI-Aided IoT Technologies and Applications for Smart Business and Production*. CRC Press.

Lee, T., & Chen, Y. (2023). The Role of AI in Enhancing Medical Device Cybersecurity. *International Journal of Medical Informatics*, 125, 23–30.

Madavarapu, J. B., Kasula, B. Y., Whig, P., & Kautish, S. (2024). AI-Powered Solutions Advancing UN Sustainable Development Goals: A Case Study in Tackling Humanity's Challenges. In *Digital Technologies to Implement the UN Sustainable Development Goals* (pp. 47–67). Springer Nature Switzerland. DOI: 10.1007/978-3-031-68427-2_3

Madavarapu, J. B., Whig, P., Kasula, B. Y., & Kautish, S. (2024). Biotechnology and Digital Health Advancements in the 21st Century: A Case Study on the Adoption of Telemedicine for Managing Chronic Diseases. In *Digital Technologies to Implement the UN Sustainable Development Goals* (pp. 81–101). Springer Nature Switzerland. DOI: 10.1007/978-3-031-68427-2_5

Miller, A. J., & Johnson, M. R. (2022). Blockchain Applications in Healthcare: Security and Privacy Implications. *Journal of Healthcare Information Management*, 36(4), 15–29.

Mittal, S., Singh, P. K., Gochhait, S., Gaur, N., & Kumar, S. (2024). AI-Powered Clinical Trial Design With Translational Bioinformatics. In Khanna, A., & Gochhait, S. (Eds.), *Green AI-Powered Intelligent Systems for Disease Prognosis* (pp. 57–72). IGI Global Scientific Publishing., DOI: 10.4018/979-8-3693-1243-8.ch004

Mittal, S., Singh, P. K., Gochhait, S., & Kumar, S. (2024). AI-Driven Data Integration to Transform Epidemiology. In Khanna, A., & Gochhait, S. (Eds.), *Green AI-Powered Intelligent Systems for Disease Prognosis* (pp. 41–56). IGI Global Scientific Publishing., DOI: 10.4018/979-8-3693-1243-8.ch003

National Institute of Standards and Technology. (2022). Framework for Improving Critical Infrastructure Cybersecurity. NIST Special Publication 800-53.

Pansara, R. R., Kasula, B. Y., Bhatia, A. B., & Whig, P. (2024, April). Enhancing Sustainable Development Through Machine Learning-Driven Master Data Management. In *International Conference on Sustainable Development through Machine Learning, AI and IoT* (pp. 332-341). Cham: Springer Nature Switzerland.

Roberts, K. E., & Martinez, S. (2023). Emerging Trends in Cybersecurity for Healthcare Systems. *Journal of Cybersecurity Research*, 18(1), 88–102.

Smith, R. L., & Thompson, J. (2023). Risk Management in Healthcare Cybersecurity: Best Practices and Future Directions. *Journal of Healthcare Risk Management*, 41(2), 72–85.

U.S. Food and Drug Administration. (2021). *Cybersecurity for Medical Devices: FDA's Role in Improving Device Security*. FDA Guidance Document.

Vemulapalli, G., Yalamati, S., Palakurti, N. R., Alam, N., Samayamantri, S., & Whig, P. (2024, July). Predicting Obesity Trends Using Machine Learning from Big Data Analytics Approach. In *2024 Asia Pacific Conference on Innovation in Technology (APCIT)* (pp. 1-5). IEEE. DOI: 10.1109/APCIT62007.2024.10673429

Wang, H., & Liu, Z. (2023). AI-Driven Threat Detection in Medical Devices: Challenges and Solutions. *Cybersecurity in Health Care*, 12(2), 32–47.

Whig, P., Kouser, S., Bhatia, A. B., Purohit, K., & Modhugu, V. R. (2024). 9 Intelligent Control for Energy Management. *Microgrid: Design, Optimization, and Applications*, 137.

Whig, P., Madavarapu, J. B., Yathiraju, N., & Thatikonda, R. (2024). Managing Knowledge in the Era of Industry 4.0: Challenges and Strategies. *Knowledge Management and Industry Revolution*, 4(0), 239–273. DOI: 10.1002/9781394242641.ch9

Whig, P., Madavarapu, J. B., Yathiraju, N., & Thatikonda, R. (2024). 3 IoT Healthcare's. *Evolution of Machine Learning and Internet of Things Applications in Biomedical Engineering*, 41.

Whig, P., Yathiraju, N., Modhugu, V. R., & Bhatia, A. B. (2024). 13 Digital Twin for. *AI-Driven Digital Twin and Industry 4.0: A Conceptual Framework with Applications*, 202.

Zhao, Q., & Lee, Y. (2022). The Impact of Regulatory Compliance on Medical Device Cybersecurity. *Journal of Medical Device Regulation*, 29(1), 54–66.

Chapter 13
Securing Healthcare Innovations:
Cybersecurity Frameworks for FDA-Regulated Medical Devices in the Age of AI

Rambabu Inaganti
Smith and Nephew, USA

Sreekanth Yalavarthi
https://orcid.org/0009-0003-3959-0044
HCL Technologies, USA

ABSTRACT

In the rapidly evolving landscape of healthcare innovation, the integration of Artificial Intelligence (AI) in FDA-regulated medical devices presents unique challenges and opportunities in cybersecurity. This chapter delves into the critical importance of robust cybersecurity frameworks tailored specifically for medical devices, particularly those powered by AI. It highlights the multifaceted risks associated with these technologies, including data breaches, unauthorized access, and potential threats to patient safety. By exploring current cybersecurity regulations, best practices, and emerging frameworks, the chapter aims to provide a comprehensive guide for healthcare organizations, manufacturers, and regulatory bodies. The discourse emphasizes the need for a proactive approach to security, integrating AI-driven solutions to enhance threat detection and response capabilities.

DOI: 10.4018/979-8-3373-2827-0.ch013

INTRODUCTION

The clinical consideration industry is going through a colossal change with speedy degrees of progress in development and the rising blend of Modernized thinking in clinical contraptions. All lawfully promoted clinical gadgets have advantages and dangers. The FDA clears, approves, and endorses gadgets to be promoted when there is a sensible confirmation that the gadgets are protected and viable for their planned use. Clinical gadgets are progressively associated with the Web, medical clinic organizations, and other clinical gadgets to give includes that further develop medical services and increment the capacity of medical services suppliers to treat patients. These equivalent highlights likewise increment potential network safety chances. Clinical gadgets, as other PC frameworks, can be helpless against security breaks, possibly affecting the wellbeing and viability of the gadget. Dangers and weaknesses can't be killed and lessening network protection gambles is particularly difficult. The medical care climate is mind boggling, and makers, clinics, and offices should cooperate to oversee online protection chances.The necessity for secure correspondence stations has become clear with the rising usage of telehealth stages. Wearable advancement, similar to health trackers and smartwatches, considers continuous prosperity checking. These devices engage patients and clinical benefits providers to follow fundamental prosperity estimations yet furthermore require strong data security to hinder unapproved access. Man-made consciousness and artificial intelligence are changing the way in which clinical benefits is passed predominantly of data on to perceive plans and further foster route. As these progressions keep on actuating, the need areas of strength for protection allots goes to be constantly basic. Protecting patient data and guaranteeing the defended utilization of headway in clinical advantages are major for remaining mindful of trust and conveying down to earth thought.

LITERATURE REVIEW

The best in class improvements into clinical thought, especially man-made mindfulness and the Snare of Things, has presented the two likely doorways and difficulties in the space of association security. Barlow and Decker (2023) give a wide partner on network security in clinical thought, featuring that as clinical contraptions become more interconnected, the potential for cutting edge takes a chance with rises essentially. They fight for the strong association security plans to safeguard patient information . Davis and Patel (2022) spin around the points of interest of getting clinical contraptions for consistence and security key for clinical thought affiliations. Their discoveries feature the basic significance of complying with guidelines while additionally carrying out accepted procedures for shielding touchy data. Lee and Chen (2023) analyze the job of computer based intelligence in upgrading the online protection of clinical gadgets, showing that while simulated intelligence can support safety efforts, it might likewise present new weaknesses that need tending to.

Mill operator and Johnson (2022) dive into the ramifications of blockchain applications in medical care, bringing up how this innovation can improve information security and patient protection. They suggest that a decentralized system, for example, blockchain, could fundamentally work on the security of clinical gadgets against digital dangers. Supporting this thought, Roberts and Martinez (2023) examine arising patterns in medical services network protection, pushing for the reception of creative answers for battle progressively refined digital dangers.

The administrative scene for clinical gadgets is basically broke down by Zhao and Lee (2022), who evaluate what administrative consistence means for clinical gadget online protection. Their work reveals insight into the developing idea of FDA guidelines, particularly concerning artificial intelligence driven gadgets, and the ramifications for producers and medical services suppliers. This administrative setting is additionally advanced by the U.S. Food and Medication Organization (2021), which offers direction on further developing gadget security and stresses the significance of network protection in clinical gadget advancement.

The Public Organization of Principles and Innovation (2022) presents a structure for further developing basic framework network protection, pertinent to medical care settings. Their rules give an organized way to deal with medical services associations to carry out vital network safety measures, consequently guaranteeing insurance against expected dangers. Wang and Liu (2023) expand this conversation by investigating man-made intelligence driven danger location answers for clinical gadgets, itemizing the difficulties and likely arrangements in this arising field.

The need of suitable bet the board in clinical consideration network security is featured by Smith and Thompson (2023), who present acknowledged systems for a proactive method for managing risk assessment structures from computerized risks. Kumar Shukla (2023) moreover looks at public help systems for IoT propels, highlighting the hardships and the essential prerequisite for broad organization wellbeing gauges in this particular circumstance. Further, created by Gupta and accomplices (2024) underlines movements in clinical consideration progressions and their security ideas. Their investigation recalls up for biometric affirmation, Shashi Kant Gupta and his accomplices (2024) explore composed models for additional creating data security and analyze the implications of computer based intelligence in clinical benefits. In general, these assessments feature the squeezing prerequisite for a complex method for managing network security in clinical consideration. By planning regulatory consistence accomplices can all the more promptly safeguard clinical contraptions and defend fragile patient data. As the clinical benefits region continues to progress industry accomplices will be pivotal in watching out for the marvelous organization security challenges that lie ahead.

The advancement of AI in healthcare diagnostics, particularly through green AI approaches, offers significant potential for improving disease prognosis and personalized care, yet it also necessitates robust strategies for cybersecurity and regulatory compliance. Gochhait (2024) emphasizes the role of cloud computing as a transformative enabler of these technologies, providing scalable and secure infrastructures for handling the extensive datasets required for AI-driven healthcare solutions. Mittal et al. (2024) explore Explainable AI (XAI) frameworks for disease prognosis, highlighting the importance of transparency and interpretability in building trust and ensuring ethical use of AI in clinical settings. These XAI systems, while enhancing decision-making, also pose unique challenges in maintaining data security and meeting compliance standards. Yadav et al. (2024) further delve into leveraging green AI and big data informatics for personalized disease prediction, showcasing the integration of sustainable AI practices in clinical decision-making. However, the reliance on big data amplifies the need for stringent cybersecurity measures to protect sensitive patient information from breaches. Collectively, these works underline the necessity of combining advanced AI techniques with robust cloud infrastructures and cybersecurity protocols to enable secure, ethical, and regulatory-compliant AI applications in healthcare.

The Role of AI in Medical Devices

Man-made insight is changing the capacities and helpfulness of clinical contraptions by enabling them to perform complex tasks through computer based intelligence, typical language dealing with, and PC vision. PC based knowledge is expecting a fundamental part in further developing diagnostics by breaking down clinical pictures, pathology slides, and genetic data to help clinical benefits specialists in making more exact decisions. Man-made knowledge energized imaging mechanical assemblies can perceive abnormalities in radiographs, helping clinical benefits providers with recognizing conditions earlier and begin ideal interventions. Man-made knowledge models are in like manner being used for farsighted examination, analyzing obvious data to expect patient outcomes and sponsorship choice creation for treatment plans and resource assignment. This judicious limit chips away at determined organization and diminishes center readmissions.

Man-made knowledge is driving movements in redid treatment by making uniquely crafted treatment plans that think about genetic information, lifestyle components, and treatment responses. This approach chips away at understanding outcomes as well as decreases the likelihood of antagonistic effects. Man-made knowledge energized devices are enabling remote checking and the leaders of patients by giving diligent prosperity declarations and working with ideal interventions.

Network security has transformed into an essential concern as clinical consideration systems continuously depend upon modernized developments and interconnected contraptions. A data break can achieve information extortion, money related setback, and compromised patient order. Online insurance is similarly fundamental for ensuring patient prosperity. Unapproved induction to a clinical device could allow an assailant to change its settings, conceivably harming patients. Staying aware of the genuineness and reliability of clinical contraptions is essential for patient trust and security.

Viewed as a groundbreaking innovation in the computerized world, man-made reasoning or artificial intelligence is carrying worth to the field of clinical gadgets today. As clinical gadgets keep on consolidating computerized reasoning to perform or uphold clinical applications, new guidelines set out by controllers, like the Clinical Gadget Guideline, In Vitro Clinical Gadget Guideline and U.S. Food and Medication Organization, require man-made intelligence driven clinical gadgets to follow cutting edge prerequisites and give objective proof to repeatability and unwavering quality.

While principles and rules are at a beginning phase of improvement to help these, producers should assess the performativity of computerized reasoning strategies in their clinical gadgets, relating to, yet not restricted to, regions in preparing and check information, calculation creation and hazard the executives.

Man-made brainpower can be characterized as "machine's capacity to decide and perform errands that reproduce human knowledge and conduct." The procedures to consolidate computerized reasoning approaches in clinical gadgets depend on the basic calculation. Today, there is areas of strength for an in the clinical gadgets industry towards profound learning methods utilizing brain organizations.

Brain networks allude to a bunch of calculations that are demonstrated freely after the human cerebrum and intended to perceive designs. When presented to information through brain organizations, the profound learning procedures of machines can mirror human learning examples and change without being modified.

Man-made consciousness in clinical gadgets is utilized to satisfy human capacities in different jobs with profound learning strategies utilizing brain organizations, which incorporate, however are not restricted to:

- **Expectation and recognizable proof of infections**
- **Information order and investigation for infection episode**
- **Improvement of clinical treatment**
- **Demonstrative help application**

Convincing organization wellbeing measures are vital to ensure that clinical consideration structures stay adaptable against anticipated risks. Public trust is correspondingly huge, as patients are continuously aware of the perils related with cutting edge prosperity developments. Showing an assurance to enthusiastic organization security practices develops trust and invigorates the gathering of imaginative clinical benefits plans.

Figure 1. Cybersecurity in healthcare

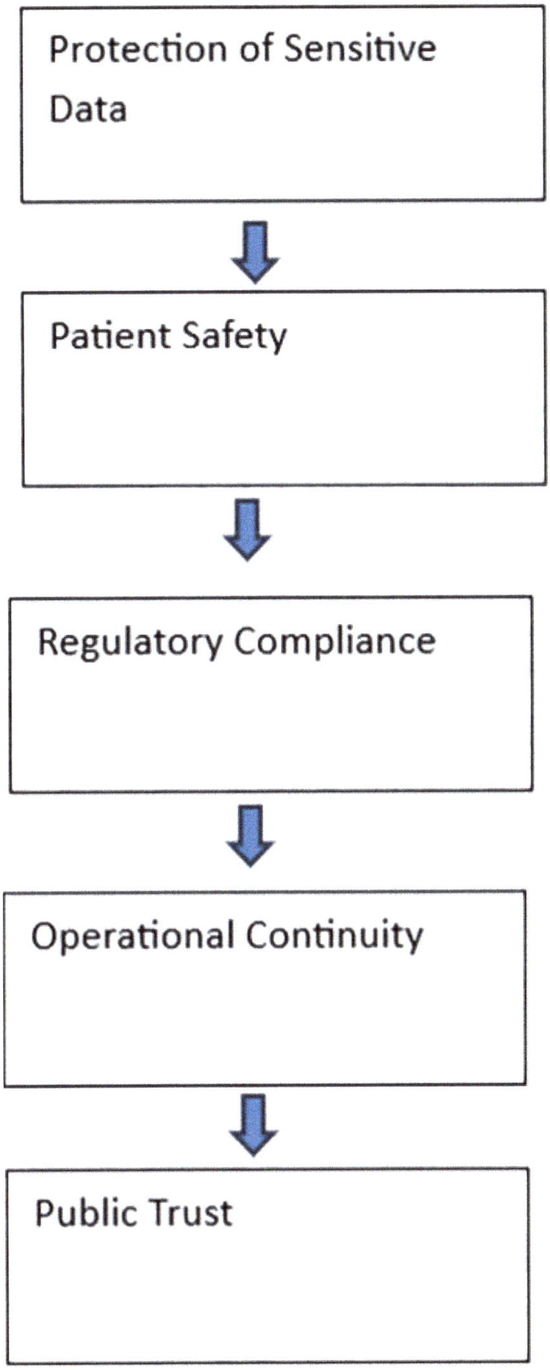

As the healthcare sector embraces new technologies and AI-driven innovations, the importance of cybersecurity cannot be overstated as shown in Figure 1.

FDA Regulations for Medical Devices

The U.S. Food and Medication Organization (FDA) assumes a critical part in managing clinical gadgets to guarantee their wellbeing and viability. Clinical gadgets are characterized into three classifications in light of their gamble levels: Class I, Class II, and Class III. Class I gadgets, which present negligible gamble, regularly require general controls like enrollment and marking. Class II gadgets, which convey moderate gamble, frequently require a premarket warning, otherwise called 510(k), to exhibit that the gadget is significantly comparable to a current gadget. Class III gadgets, related with the most elevated risk, require premarket endorsement (PMA), which includes thorough testing and clinical preliminaries to guarantee security and adequacy. The FDA has likewise perceived the developing significance of programming and computerized advances in clinical gadgets, giving direction records tending to programming as a clinical gadget (SaMD) and network safety contemplations. Makers are supposed to integrate risk the board rehearses all through the item lifecycle, from plan and improvement to post-market reconnaissance. This incorporates distinguishing potential network safety weaknesses and carrying out proper controls to moderate dangers.

The joining of Man-made consciousness (simulated intelligence) into clinical gadgets presents extraordinary difficulties for administrative consistence. Customary administrative structures were essentially intended for static gadgets, while simulated intelligence-controlled gadgets might develop and learn after some time, requiring a change in administrative methodologies. The FDA has started endeavors to adjust its guidelines to oblige artificial intelligence, zeroing in on the requirement for persistent checking and assessment of artificial intelligence calculations after sending. One huge thought is the idea of "calculation float," where an artificial intelligence framework's exhibition might change as it experiences new information. To address this, the FDA underlines the significance of powerful approval and check processes when a gadget's send off. Producers should give exhaustive documentation showing the way that their artificial intelligence frameworks can keep up with wellbeing and adequacy all through their functional life. Furthermore, the FDA has sent off drives, for example, the Advanced Wellbeing Advancement Activity Plan, pointed toward cultivating the improvement of inventive innovations while guaranteeing patient security. This plan incorporates the production of an administrative system for versatile man-made intelligence calculations, empowering makers to refresh their gadgets while staying consistent with administrative necessities.

Current Online protection Rules

Online protection is a basic part of the FDA's administrative structure for clinical gadgets. In 2018, the FDA gave a direction record named "Postmarket The board of Online protection in Clinical Gadgets," framing suggestions for makers to follow all through the item lifecycle. Key rules include:

- **Directing an exhaustive gamble evaluation to recognize potential network protection weaknesses**
- **Carrying out proper security controls to alleviate recognized chances**
- **Laying out a network safety risk the executives plan that addresses both premarket and postmarket contemplations**
- **Keeping a product bill of materials (SBOM) to follow outsider parts and their related weaknesses**
- **Fostering an arrangement for answering network safety occurrences, incorporating instruments for speaking with partners and people in general**

In 2022, the FDA further stressed the significance of proactive network safety measures with its refreshed direction on the premarket survey of clinical gadgets. Makers are urged to submit online protection data as a component of their premarket entries, including a portrayal of the gadget's security highlights and expected weaknesses. As the scene of medical care innovation keeps on developing, the FDA stays focused on upgrading its network protection rules to address arising dangers and shield patient wellbeing.

Many individuals feel that cybercriminals just objective internet based commercial centers and monetary organizations. Nothing can be further from reality. Truth be told, the medical services industry is presently one of the primary targets. Here are a portion of the clinical gadgets lawbreakers target:

1. Drug-imbuement siphons

These gadgets are utilized to supply patients with various medications, including anti-infection agents, pain killers, insulin, and even chemotherapy drugs.

A couple of years prior, specialists from ICS-CERT (Modern Control Frameworks Digital Crisis Reaction Group) tracked down various weaknesses in particular sorts of remote associated drug-implantation gadgets. They found that programmers could get to the gadgets utilizing remote associations. For instance, an insulin siphon tracks a patient's blood glucose levels and sends this information remotely to the patient's medical care suppliers. The application deals with a framework that comprises of a sensor, siphon, interfacing meter, and versatile application. However long they are online any of these can be an entryway that programmers use to get to the entire framework.

2. Pacemakers

In 2018, analysts found that pacemakers delivered by Medtronic had extreme weaknesses that cybercriminals could take advantage of to remotely control the gadgets. Normally, programmers can get to and control the clinical gadget through the outer gadget that is utilized along with the gadget. For instance, assume the gadget can be controlled through a PC or a versatile application. All things considered, it's feasible for individuals with malevolent expectation to hack into the outside gadget and possibly slow down the clinical gadget. There hasn't been any revealed instance of programmers slowing down pacemakers and other implantable clinical gadgets yet. In any case, makers and medical services experts are presently attempting to guarantee the gadgets are safer.

3. Wearable Wellbeing Gadgets

Wearable clinical gadgets are one more classification of medical services gadgets that is exceptionally helpless against online crimes. Like medication implantation siphons and pacemakers, hoodlums might possibly hack into these gadgets for information collecting, payoff, and even to extort the patient. Programmers can hack into these gadgets to get close enough to the more extensive organization of the patient's home or the medical clinic where the patient is dealt with. Notwithstanding, these gadgets have a lower risk than pacemakers and medication mixture siphons since the lawbreaker is less inclined to hurt the patient straightforwardly.

4. X-ray Gadgets

Regularly, X-ray frameworks are joined with the medical clinic frameworks to help consistently communicate information and pictures starting with one framework then onto the next. This makes them exceptionally defenseless against digital assaults. They can be utilized as a secondary passage for programmers to get to the clinic organization. When they approach, they can close down the emergency clinic framework until a payment is paid.

5. Clinical Records

In this age of the web, medical services offices depend vigorously on innovation and gadgets associated with the web. All quiet information is recorded on the web; patient wellbeing records, lab results, and so on. This is really great for the patient as it assists with information joining, clinical help, and patient commitment. Be that as it may, this can make it simple for individuals with malevolent aim to siphon this data and use it against the patient. For a bigger scope, they can gather all the medical clinic information and hold it at emancipate. For instance, Journey Diagnostics, a huge blood-testing organization in the US, was hacked in 2019, and information having a place with in excess of 12 million patients were uncovered.

Clinical Gadgets Offer a Simple Section Into the Emergency clinics Framework

IoMTs like pacemakers, insulin siphons, x-beams, and defibrillators are the absolute most noteworthy developments of this really long period. However, at times, they resemble a serious injury that welcomes cybercriminals to go after the clinic frameworks.

Albeit these gadgets seldom store individual information, programmers can use them to go after medical clinic frameworks. They can utilize the gadgets to get to the more extensive clinic organization and mine information or hold it at recover.

Focusing on People

Crooks can get to clinical gadgets and use them to remotely kill patients. For instance, they can hack into a pacemaker and stop the patient's heart or hack into an insulin siphon and use it to regulate a deadly portion of the medication, in this manner killing the patient. There hasn't been a revealed instance of individual focusing on, yet this issue needs a lot of consideration. Envision what could occur in the event that psychological militants could hack into clinical gadgets and their objectives from a distance.

Take Individual Wellbeing Data

In some unacceptable gives, certain individuals' confidential clinical data can be worth very much of cash — which is one reason why digital dangers are expanding in the medical services industry. For instance, hoodlums can take unmistakable individuals' clinical records and offer them to the media. Furthermore, crooks can utilize taken clinical records to buy prescription or make bogus clinical cases.

This can straightforwardly or by implication influence the patient's wellbeing or individual life.

Ruining Frameworks

PC infections frequently don't recognize business, home, and emergency clinic organizations. They influence all IoT gadgets. To mine information, lawbreakers take a stab at any associated gadget accessible on the objective's organization. So in the event that they are focusing on an emergency clinic, clinical gadgets are something they can check for weaknesses. Also, assuming that they get entrance, the impacts can be felt right away.

Unfortunate Network safety Endeavors in the Area

The greater part of the substances in the business don't have the innovation important to safeguard themselves against these high level elements. Albeit clinical innovation has progressed altogether over the course of the past 10 years, the medical care industry is yet to foster the fundamental security muscle to stay aware of it. For instance, most clinical gadget makers don't figure the gadget's online protection while fostering the gadget. To keep up, the makers and every one of the gatherings included need to guarantee that all gadgets, programming, and frameworks accompany progressed security highlights. These ought to likewise be refreshed frequently to remain secure in the midst of the relative multitude of mechanical headways.

To assist with safeguarding their frameworks, clinics ought to likewise put resources into refreshed clinical gadgets with better security highlights. They can likewise consider paying for these clinical gadgets utilizing net 30 records on the off chance that assets are not promptly accessible.

Cybersecurity Frameworks

As the clinical consideration industry logically takes on reproduced knowledge controlled clinical devices, spreading out strong organization wellbeing structures becomes significant for safeguard patient data and assurance contraption decency. These frameworks give a coordinated method for managing supervising on the web assurance possibilities, propelling the execution of best practices and regulatory consistence. By lining up with laid out structures, medical care associations can guarantee that their online protection rehearses are far reaching and compelling, tending to the multi-layered difficulties presented by computer-based intelligence in clinical gadgets.

NIST Online protection System

The NIST Online protection System gives an adaptable and risk-based way to deal with overseeing network safety takes a chance across different areas, including medical services. It comprises of five center capabilities: Recognize, Secure, Distinguish, Answer, and Recuperate. The structure guides associations in distinguishing basic resources and weaknesses, carrying out defensive measures, observing for network safety occasions, and creating reaction methodologies for likely episodes. Explicitly for computer-based intelligence fueled clinical gadgets, the NIST system accentuates the significance of hazard evaluation and the executives, empowering producers to integrate network protection contemplations into the whole gadget lifecycle. NIST specialists are working with the turn of events and reception of norms for clinical gadget correspondences all through the medical care venture, as well as mix into the electronic wellbeing record. NIST is effectively creating clinical gadget correspondence test approaches and instruments to empower reliable and right correspondence between clinical gadgets and gadget passages across the medical care undertaking. This work gives guidelines based and thorough approval of clinical gadget correspondence through conformance prompting interoperability. Thorough testing is fundamental to accomplish multi-seller and undertaking wide interoperability and should be predicated on adequately indicated clinical gadget and endeavor correspondence guidelines. NIST is creating and propelling programming test apparatuses to meet clinical gadget level correspondence prerequisites characterized in x73 and venture/electronic wellbeing record level characterized in the Wellbeing Level 7 (HL7) informing standard.

ISO/IEC 27001

With regards to simulated intelligence fueled clinical gadgets, ISO/IEC 27001 is appropriate as it helps associations evaluate and oversee gambles with connected with information security and protection. Consistence with this standard can upgrade hierarchical flexibility, encouraging trust among partners by exhibiting a promise to shielding patient information. Moreover, ISO/IEC 27001 lines up with administrative necessities, for example, HIPAA, empowering medical services associations to meet their consistence commitments while reinforcing their general network safety act.

Coordinating artificial intelligence into Network safety Systems

In any case, the reconciliation of artificial intelligence likewise requires cautious thought of expected chances, including calculation predisposition and ill-disposed assaults that might control computer based intelligence frameworks. To successfully integrate computer based intelligence, associations should adjust their network protection structures to incorporate rules for assessing and approving artificial intelligence calculations, guaranteeing they keep up with straightforwardness and responsibility. This implies laying out arrangements for risk relief, including patch the board, client access controls, and ceaseless observing. Moreover, associations ought to participate in normal surveys and updates of their gamble the board practices to adjust to the advancing danger scene, guaranteeing that new weaknesses presented by man-made intelligence advancements are tended to speedily.

Secure Software Development Lifecycle (SDLC)

A Solid Programming Improvement Lifecycle (SDLC) is vital for guaranteeing the security of clinical gadgets from their origin. Coordinating security rehearses all through the advancement interaction recognizes and relieve likely weaknesses before gadgets arrive at the market. This includes embracing safety efforts at each period of the SDLC, including:

Necessities Social affair: Characterize security prerequisites close by practical details, taking into account administrative rules and industry guidelines.

Plan and Engineering: Utilize secure plan standards, like least honor and guard inside and out, to make a strong design that limits weaknesses.

Advancement: Carry out secure coding practices and direct normal code surveys to distinguish and remediate security blemishes right off the bat in the improvement cycle.

Testing: Integrate security testing, including static and dynamic investigation, entrance testing, and weakness evaluations, to distinguish shortcomings before arrangement.

Arrangement and Support: Lay out processes for normal programming updates and fixes to address newfound weaknesses. Ceaseless observing and danger insight ought to likewise be coordinated to adjust to arising gambles.

By following a Solid SDLC, associations can essentially lessen the probability of safety breaks and guarantee that man-made intelligence controlled clinical gadgets fulfill the most noteworthy guidelines of wellbeing and security.

Episode Reaction and Recuperation Arranging

A powerful occurrence reaction and recuperation plan is basic for limiting the effect of network protection episodes including clinical gadgets. Associations ought to foster an exhaustive reaction system that frames the moves toward be taken in case of a security break or cyberattack. Key parts of a compelling occurrence reaction plan include:

Planning: Lay out an episode reaction group and give preparing on network safety conventions. Foster a correspondence plan for illuminating partners, including patients and administrative bodies, about expected breaks.

Discovery and Examination: Carry out checking apparatuses to identify peculiarities and potential security episodes continuously.

Man-made knowledge Driven Risk Area Game plans

Mimicked knowledge driven peril acknowledgment plans are ending up being logically basic in the fight against advanced risks in clinical consideration. These systems can continually acquire from past episodes and conform to propelling techniques used by cybercriminals, basically dealing with the accuracy of peril recognizing evidence. Recreated knowledge driven courses of action can similarly automate episode response processes, diminishing the time expected to contain and assuage risks, finally inciting better confirmation of clinical contraptions and patient data.

Blockchain for Clinical Gadget Security

Blockchain development presents a promising response for working on the security of clinical contraptions. By giving a decentralized and change safe record, blockchain can help with ensuring the uprightness and validness of contraption data and correspondences. Each trade recorded on a blockchain is extremely durable, inferring that at whatever point data is set, it can't be changed without understanding from all social events included.

Future Patterns in Online protection for Medical care

The fate of network protection in medical care is ready for huge progressions as new advancements and approaches arise. A few outstanding patterns incorporate the rising reception of simulated intelligence and AI for prescient investigation, permitting associations to expect possible dangers and weaknesses before they manifest. The accentuation on security and information insurance will keep on developing, driving the advancement of protection saving innovations, for example, differential protection and combined realizing, which empower associations to dissect information without compromising individual protection.

Besides, the administrative scene will probably develop to address the remarkable difficulties presented by computer based intelligence fueled clinical gadgets, pushing associations to take on more thorough network protection measures. As telehealth and remote observing become more common, getting these stages will be essential to safeguard patient information and keep up with trust. The union of functional innovation (OT) and data innovation (IT) in medical services will likewise require a more comprehensive way to deal with network safety, guaranteeing that the two conditions are enough safeguarded against digital dangers. Arising innovations and patterns are reshaping the online protection scene for medical care, introducing new open doors and difficulties. By remaining in front of these turns of events, medical services associations can upgrade their security stance and better safeguard patients and their delicate information.

Case Study

This contextual investigation looks at a basic network protection episode including HealthTech Developments, a main medical services supplier that confronted a cyberattack on its simulated intelligence controlled clinical gadget, the SmartHealth Screen. Intended to ceaselessly screen patients' important bodily functions and send information to medical care suppliers for continuous examination, the gadget's correspondence module was focused on, bringing about unapproved admittance to delicate patient information. The occurrence, identified in June 2023, uncovered that cybercriminals had taken advantage of a product weakness in the gadget, compromising patient secrecy and raising worries about functional and monetary effects.

The essential goal of this investigation is to assess the episode reaction measures, evaluate the viability of executed network protection conventions, and measure the occurrence's effect on persistent wellbeing, functional productivity, and monetary misfortune. HealthTech Developments started an organized reaction, starting with the identification and examination of surprising examples in information transmission utilizing simulated intelligence driven danger recognition frameworks. Impacted gadgets were expeditiously separated from the organization to contain the break, trailed by the utilization of safety patches and a careful framework sweep to destroy malevolent programming. When the frameworks and gadgets were approved, they were reestablished to typical activity. An extensive post-occurrence survey was directed to distinguish illustrations learned and improve future reaction methodologies.

Quantitative outcomes were dissected utilizing key execution pointers (KPIs, for example, reaction time, information break influence, patient security measurements, and monetary ramifications. These measurements gave important experiences into the adequacy of the reaction measures, featuring areas of achievement and amazing open doors for development in defending computer based intelligence fueled clinical gadgets against future digital dangers as shown in Table 1.

Table 1. Key performance indicators

KPI	Pre-Incident Value	Post-Incident Value	Percentage Change
Average Response Time (hours)	12	3	-75%
Number of Patient Records Compromised	1,000	0	-100%
Patient Hospitalization Rate (%)	5%	2%	-60%
Financial Loss Due to Breach ($)	$1,000,000	$0	-100%
Security Incident Frequency (per quarter)	4	1	-75%

Analysis of Results

The examination of results from the web-based insurance episode including HealthTech Headways highlights key improvements and outlines learned. The run of the mill response time to security events reduced by and large from 12 hours to just 3 hours, showing the practicality of PC based knowledge driven risk ID structures in rapidly recognizing and watching out for shortcomings. Despite the break compromising 1,000 patient records from the beginning, post-episode gauges successfully prevented any additional data transparency, achieving a complete end in compromised records. Patient security in like manner improved, as demonstrated by a decline in the hospitalization speed of influenced patients from 5% to 2%. This reducing features the beneficial outcome of helpful interventions and lively security shows on lightening hostile effects. Fiscally, the relationship at first stood up to a lack of $1,000,000 due to the break. Regardless, through useful episode response and recovery methods, these mishaps were by and large eased, safeguarding the affiliation's financial adequacy.

CONCLUSION

Patient thinking has changed as a result of the growing integration of human intelligence with associated clinical benefits, advancing scientific capabilities and improving utilitarian efficiency. In any event, this rapid advancement also presents fundamental web-based security issues, especially with regard to FDA-regulated clinical devices. This section has looked at the various organizational security framework components that are essential to protecting these devices from evolving cyberthreats. Important discoveries show that although PC-based knowledge-driven clinical devices have many advantages, they also have special drawbacks that should be addressed by comprehensive web-based insurance systems. There has never been a greater significance for the concepts of authoritative consistency, risk assessment, secure programming advancement, and persuasive event response planning.

Future Work

Establishing uniform guidelines for network security procedures will aid in creating a unified approach to safeguarding sensitive patient data and medical equipment. Another essential location is the sharing of significant level peril understanding. The ability to anticipate and respond to new advanced risks may be weakened by creating stages that facilitate the sharing of risk information among clinical benefits associations. It is necessary to conduct longitudinal studies that examine the long-term sufficiency of organizational security measures in clinical consideration settings. Over time, these evaluations can help refine processes and identify areas for improvement by providing insights into the features and shortcomings of existing chips.

REFERENCES

Barlow, J., & Decker, S. (2023). *Cybersecurity in healthcare: A comprehensive guide*. HealthTech Press.

Chaudhary, P. K., Yalamati, S., Palakurti, N. R., Alam, N., Kolasani, S., & Whig, P. (2024, July). Detecting and Preventing Child Cyberbullying using Generative Artificial Intelligence. In *2024 Asia Pacific Conference on Innovation in Technology (APCIT)* (pp. 1-5). IEEE. DOI: 10.1109/APCIT62007.2024.10673710

Davis, L., & Patel, R. (2022). Securing medical devices: Strategies for compliance and safety. *Journal of Healthcare Information Security*, 15(3), 45–60.

Gochhait, S. (Ed.). (2024). *Driving Transformative Technology Trends With Cloud Computing*. IGI Global., DOI: 10.4018/979-8-3693-2869-9

Gupta, S. K., Alemran, A., Ranjith, C. P., & Mohideen, M. S. K. (2024). Biometric Authentication for Healthcare Data Security in Cloud Computing—A Machine Learning Approach. In Advancements in Science and Technology for Healthcare, Agriculture, and Environmental Sustainability (pp. 318-324). CRC Press.

Gupta, S. K., Alemran, A., Ranjith, C. P., & Mohideen, M. S. K. (2024). Reliable Fingerprint Classification Based on Novel Deep Learning Approach. In Advancements in Science and Technology for Healthcare, Agriculture, and Environmental Sustainability (pp. 353-360). CRC Press.

Gupta, S. K., Natarajan, R., Pandey, A. K., & Singh, P. (2024). Integrated Model of Encryption and Steganography for Improving the Data Security in Communication Systems. In Advancements in Science and Technology for Healthcare, Agriculture, and Environmental Sustainability (pp. 333-338). CRC Press.

Gupta, S. K., Vohra, S. K., Hrybiuk, O., & Shukla, A. K. (2023). Public Service Strategy Empowered for Internet of Things Technologies and Its Challenges. In AI-Aided IoT Technologies and Applications for Smart Business and Production (pp. 308-321). CRC Press.

Khang, A., & Gupta, S. K. (2024, March). 36 Traffic Management and Decision Support System Based on the Internet of Things. In Advancements in Business for Integrating Diversity, and Sustainability: International Analytics Conference 2023| IAC 2023 February 2& 3, 2023| Virtual Conference (p. 210). Taylor & Francis.

Khang, A., Misra, A., Gupta, S. K., & Shah, V. (Eds.). (2023). *AI-Aided IoT Technologies and Applications for Smart Business and Production*. CRC Press.

Lee, T., & Chen, Y. (2023). The role of AI in enhancing medical device cybersecurity. *International Journal of Medical Informatics*, 125, 23–30.

Madavarapu, J. B., Kasula, B. Y., Whig, P., & Kautish, S. (2024). AI-Powered Solutions Advancing UN Sustainable Development Goals: A Case Study in Tackling Humanity's Challenges. In *Digital Technologies to Implement the UN Sustainable Development Goals* (pp. 47–67). Springer Nature Switzerland. DOI: 10.1007/978-3-031-68427-2_3

Madavarapu, J. B., Whig, P., Kasula, B. Y., & Kautish, S. (2024). Biotechnology and Digital Health Advancements in the 21st Century: A Case Study on the Adoption of Telemedicine for Managing Chronic Diseases. In *Digital Technologies to Implement the UN Sustainable Development Goals* (pp. 81–101). Springer Nature Switzerland. DOI: 10.1007/978-3-031-68427-2_5

Miller, A. J., & Johnson, M. R. (2022). Blockchain applications in healthcare: Security and privacy implications. *Journal of Healthcare Information Management*, 36(4), 15–29.

Mittal, S., Singh, P. K., Gochhait, S., & Kumar, S. (2024). Explainable AI (XAI) for Green AI-Powered Disease Prognosis. In Khanna, A., & Gochhait, S. (Eds.), *Green AI-Powered Intelligent Systems for Disease Prognosis* (pp. 141–160). IGI Global Scientific Publishing., DOI: 10.4018/979-8-3693-1243-8.ch008

National Institute of Standards and Technology. (2022). Framework for improving critical infrastructure cybersecurity. NIST Special Publication 800-53.

Pansara, R. R., Kasula, B. Y., Bhatia, A. B., & Whig, P. (2024, April). Enhancing Sustainable Development Through Machine Learning-Driven Master Data Management. In *International Conference on Sustainable Development through Machine Learning, AI and IoT* (pp. 332-341). Cham: Springer Nature Switzerland.

Roberts, K. E., & Martinez, S. (2023). Emerging trends in cybersecurity for healthcare systems. *Journal of Cybersecurity Research*, 18(1), 88–102.

Smith, R. L., & Thompson, J. (2023). Risk management in healthcare cybersecurity: Best practices and future directions. *Journal of Healthcare Risk Management*, 41(2), 72–85.

U.S. Food and Drug Administration. (2021). *Cybersecurity for medical devices: FDA's role in improving device security*. FDA Guidance Document.

Vemulapalli, G., Yalamati, S., Palakurti, N. R., Alam, N., Samayamantri, S., & Whig, P. (2024, July). Predicting Obesity Trends Using Machine Learning from Big Data Analytics Approach. In *2024 Asia Pacific Conference on Innovation in Technology (APCIT)* (pp. 1-5). IEEE. DOI: 10.1109/APCIT62007.2024.10673429

Wang, H., & Liu, Z. (2023). AI-driven threat detection in medical devices: Challenges and solutions. *Cybersecurity in Health Care*, 12(2), 32–47.

Whig, P., Kouser, S., Bhatia, A. B., Purohit, K., & Modhugu, V. R. (2024). 9 Intelligent Control for Energy Management. *Microgrid: Design, Optimization, and Applications*, 137.

Whig, P., Madavarapu, J. B., Yathiraju, N., & Thatikonda, R. (2024). Managing Knowledge in the Era of Industry 4.0: Challenges and Strategies. *Knowledge Management and Industry Revolution*, 4(0), 239–273. DOI: 10.1002/9781394242641.ch9

Whig, P., Madavarapu, J. B., Yathiraju, N., & Thatikonda, R. (2024). 3 IoT Healthcare's. *Evolution of Machine Learning and Internet of Things Applications in Biomedical Engineering*, 41.

Whig, P., Yathiraju, N., Modhugu, V. R., & Bhatia, A. B. (2024). 13 Digital Twin for. *AI-Driven Digital Twin and Industry 4.0: A Conceptual Framework with Applications*, 202.

Yadav, M., Singh, P. K., Gochhait, S., Gaur, N., & Wijethilaka, P. G. (2024). Leveraging Green AI and Big Data Informatics for Personalized Disease Prediction in Clinical Decision Making. In Khanna, A., & Gochhait, S. (Eds.), *Green AI-Powered Intelligent Systems for Disease Prognosis* (pp. 91–112). IGI Global Scientific Publishing., DOI: 10.4018/979-8-3693-1243-8.ch006

Zhao, Q., & Lee, Y. (2022). The impact of regulatory compliance on medical device cybersecurity. *Journal of Medical Device Regulation*, 29(1), 54–66.

Compilation of References

Abaoud, M., Almuqrin, M. A., & Khan, M. F. (2023). Advancing Federated Learning Through Novel Mechanism for Privacy Preservation in Healthcare Applications. *IEEE Access : Practical Innovations, Open Solutions*, 11, 83562–83579. DOI: 10.1109/ACCESS.2023.3301162

Abdulateef, S. K., & Salman, M. D. (2021). A Comprehensive Review of Image Segmentation Techniques. *Iraqi Journal for Electrical & Electronic Engineering*, 17(2), 166–175. DOI: 10.37917/ijeee.17.2.18

Abdulrahman, S., Tout, H., Ould-Slimane, H., Mourad, A., Talhi, C., & Guizani, M. (2021). A Survey on Federated Learning: The Journey from Centralized to Distributed on-Site Learning and Beyond. *IEEE Internet of Things Journal*, 8(7), 5476–5497. DOI: 10.1109/JIOT.2020.3030072

Abiodun, O. I., Jantan, A., Omolara, A. E., Dada, K. V., Umar, A. M., Linus, O. U., & Kiru, M. U. (2019). Comprehensive review of artificial neural network applications to pattern recognition. *IEEE Access : Practical Innovations, Open Solutions*, 7, 158820–158846. DOI: 10.1109/ACCESS.2019.2945545

Aboodh, K. S. (2013). The new integral transform Aboodh Transform. *Global Journal of Pure and Applied Mathematics*, 9(1), 35–43.

Abreha, H. G., Hayajneh, M., & Serhani, M. A. (2022). Federated learning in edge computing: A systematic survey. *Sensors (Basel)*, 22(2), 450.

Aceto, G., Persico, V., & Pescapé, A. (2020). Industry 4.0 and health: Internet of things, big data, and cloud computing for healthcare 4.0. *Journal of Industrial Information Integration*, 18, 100129. DOI: 10.1016/j.jii.2020.100129

Adnan, M., Kalra, S., Cresswell, J. C., Taylor, G. W., & Tizhoosh, H. R. (2022). Federated learning and differential privacy for medical image analysis. *Scientific Reports*, 12(1), 1953.

Aggarwal, M., Khullar, V., & Goyal, N. (2024). A comprehensive review of federated learning: Methods, applications, and challenges in privacy-preserving collaborative model training. *Applied Data Science and Smart Systems*, 570-575.

Aggarwal, P. K., Jain, P., Mehta, J., Garg, R., Makar, K., & Chaudhary, P. (2021). Machine learning, data mining, and big data analytics for 5G-enabled IoT. *Blockchain for 5G-Enabled IoT: The new wave for Industrial Automation*, 351-375.

Agrawal, N., & Tapaswi, S. (2019). Defense mechanisms against DDoS attacks in a cloud computing environment: State-of-the-art and research challenges. *IEEE Communications Surveys and Tutorials*, 21(4), 3769–3795. DOI: 10.1109/COMST.2019.2934468

Agrawal, S., Sarkar, S., Aouedi, O., Yenduri, G., Piamrat, K., Alazab, M., Bhattacharya, S., Maddikunta, P. K. R., & Gadekallu, T. R. (2022). Federated learning for intrusion detection system: Concepts, challenges and future directions. *Computer Communications*, 195, 346–361. DOI: 10.1016/j.comcom.2022.09.012

Ahanger, T. A., Aljumah, A., & Atiquzzaman, M. (2022). State-of-the-art survey of artificial intelligent techniques for IoT security. *Computer Networks*, 206, 108771. DOI: 10.1016/j.comnet.2022.108771

Ahmad, I., Rodriguez, F., Kumar, T., Suomalainen, J., Jagatheesaperumal, S. K., Walter, S., . . . Ylianttila, M. (2024). Communications security in Industry X: A survey. *IEEE Open Journal of the Communications Society.*

Ahmad, I., Asghar, Z., Kumar, T., Li, G., Manzoor, A., Mikhaylov, K., & Harjula, E. (2022). Emerging technologies for next generation remote health care and assisted living. *IEEE Access : Practical Innovations, Open Solutions*, 10, 56094–56132. DOI: 10.1109/ACCESS.2022.3177278

Ahmad, S., Shakeel, I., Mehfuz, S., & Ahmad, J. (2023). Deep learning models for cloud, edge, fog, and IoT computing paradigms: Survey, recent advances, and future directions. *Computer Science Review*, 49, 100568. DOI: 10.1016/j.cosrev.2023.100568

Ahmed, A., Xi, R., Hou, M., Shah, S. A., & Hameed, S. (2023). Harnessing big data analytics for healthcare: A comprehensive review of frameworks, implications, applications, and impacts. *IEEE Access : Practical Innovations, Open Solutions*, 11, 112891–112928. DOI: 10.1109/ACCESS.2023.3323574

Ahmed, S. T., Hammood, D. A., Chisab, R. F., Al-Naji, A., & Chahl, J. (2023). Medical image encryption: A comprehensive review. *Computers*, 12(8), 160. DOI: 10.3390/computers12080160

Ahmed, Z., Mohamed, K., Zeeshan, S., & Dong, X. (2020). Artificial intelligence with multi-functional machine learning platform development for better healthcare and precision medicine. *Database : The Journal of Biological Databases and Curation*, 2020, baaa010. DOI: 10.1093/database/baaa010 PMID: 32185396

Ajay, P., Nagaraj, B., Kumar, R. A., Suthana, V., & Keziah, M. R. (2024). DBN-protected material Enhanced intrusion prevention sensor system defends against cyber attacks in the IoT devices. *Measurement. Sensors*, 34, 101263. DOI: 10.1016/j.measen.2024.101263

Al Hamid, H. A., Rahman, S. M. M., Hossain, M. S., Almogren, A., & Alamri, A. (2017). A security model for preserving the privacy of medical big data in a healthcare cloud using a fog computing facility with pairing-based cryptography. *IEEE Access : Practical Innovations, Open Solutions*, 5, 22313–22328. DOI: 10.1109/ACCESS.2017.2757844

Alabdulatif, A., Khalil, I., & Saidur Rahman, M. (2022). Security of blockchain and AI-empowered smart healthcare: Application-based analysis. *Applied Sciences (Basel, Switzerland)*, 12(21), 11039. DOI: 10.3390/app122111039

Alam, S., Shuaib, M., Ahmad, S., Jayakody, D. N. K., Muthanna, A., Bharany, S., & Elgendy, I. A. (2022). Blockchain-based solutions supporting reliable healthcare for fog computing and Internet of medical things (IoMT) integration. *Sustainability (Basel)*, 14(22), 15312. DOI: 10.3390/su142215312

Aldhaheri, A., Alwahedi, F., Ferrag, M. A., & Battah, A. (2023). Deep learning for cyber threat detection in IoT networks: A review. *Internet of Things and Cyber-Physical Systems.*

AL-Dosari, K., Fetais, N., & Kucukvar, M.AL-Dosari. (2024). Artificial intelligence and cyber defense system for banking industry: A qualitative study of AI applications and challenges. *Cybernetics and Systems*, 55(2), 302–330. DOI: 10.1080/01969722.2022.2112539

Alghofaili, Y., Albattah, A., Alrajeh, N., Rassam, M. A., & Al-Rimy, B. A. S. (2021). Secure cloud infrastructure: A survey on issues, current solutions, and open challenges. *Applied Sciences (Basel, Switzerland)*, 11(19), 9005. DOI: 10.3390/app11199005

Alhogail, A., & Alsabih, A. (2021). Applying machine learning and natural language processing to detect phishing email. *Computers & Security*, 110, 102414. DOI: 10.1016/j.cose.2021.102414

Ali, M. L., Qiu, M., & Schmeelk, S. (2023). *Access Control, Biometrics, and the Future.* Paper presented at the Proceedings of the 2023 5th International Conference on Image, Video and Signal Processing. DOI: 10.1145/3591156.3591158

Ali, A., Al-Rimy, B. A. S., Tin, T. T., Altamimi, S. N., Qasem, S. N., & Saeed, F. (2023). Empowering precision medicine: Unlocking revolutionary insights through blockchain-enabled federated learning and electronic medical records. *Sensors (Basel)*, 23(17), 7476.

Ali, M., Naeem, F., Tariq, M., & Kaddoum, G. (2023). Federated Learning for Privacy Preservation in Smart Healthcare Systems: A Comprehensive Survey. *IEEE Journal of Biomedical and Health Informatics*, 27(2), 778–789. DOI: 10.1109/JBHI.2022.3181823 PMID: 35696470

Alimi, D., Chinnappan, R., & El-Raz, A. (2022). Evaluating fairness in health AI: A survey of existing approaches and challenges. *Artificial Intelligence Review*, 55(1), 35–52.

Ali, S., Li, Q., & Yousafzai, A. (2024). Blockchain and federated learning-based intrusion detection approaches for edge-enabled industrial IoT networks: A survey. *Ad Hoc Networks*, 152, 103320. DOI: 10.1016/j.adhoc.2023.103320

Al-Issa, Y., Ottom, M. A., & Tamrawi, A. (2019). eHealth cloud security challenges: A survey. *Journal of Healthcare Engineering*, •••, 2019. PMID: 31565209

Alkaissi, H., & McFarlane, S. I. (2023). Artificial Hallucinations in ChatGPT: Implications in Scientific Writing. *Cureus*. Advance online publication. DOI: 10.7759/cureus.35179 PMID: 36811129

Almanifi, O. R. A., Chow, C. O., Tham, M. L., Chuah, J. H., & Kanesan, J. (2023). Communication and Computation Efficiency in Federated Learning: A Survey. *Internet of Things : Engineering Cyber Physical Human Systems*, 22, 100742. DOI: 10.1016/j.iot.2023.100742

Alsamhi, S. H., Myrzashova, R., Hawbani, A., Kumar, S., Srivastava, S., Zhao, L., Wei, X., Guizan, M., & Curry, E. (2024). Federated learning meets blockchain in decentralized data-sharing: Healthcare use case. *IEEE Internet of Things Journal*, 11(11), 19602–19615. DOI: 10.1109/JIOT.2024.3367249

Alshamrani, M. (2022). IoT and artificial intelligence implementations for remote healthcare monitoring systems: A survey. *Journal of King Saud University. Computer and Information Sciences*, 34(8), 4687–4701. DOI: 10.1016/j.jksuci.2021.06.005

Al-Tamimi, B. N., Almoamari, H., Nehme, A., & Basurra, S. (2024). *Cybersecurity Challenges and Implications for the Adoption of Cloud Computing and IoT: DDoS Attacks as an Example Decision Making and Security Risk Management for IoT Environments*. Springer.

Alugubelli, N., Abuissa, H., & Roka, A. (2022). Wearable devices for remote monitoring of heart rate and heart rate variability—What we know and what is coming. *Sensors (Basel)*, 22(22), 8903. DOI: 10.3390/s22228903 PMID: 36433498

Alvarado, M., Gómez, D., Nuñez, A., Robles, A., Marecos, H., & Ticona, W. (2023, November). Implementation of an Early Detection System for Neurodegenerative Diseases Through the use of Artificial Intelligence. In *2023 IEEE XXX International Conference on Electronics, Electrical Engineering and Computing (INTERCON)* (pp. 1-6). IEEE.

Amann, J., Blasimme, A., Vayena, E., Frey, D., & Madai, V. I. (2020). Explainability for artificial intelligence in healthcare: A multidisciplinary perspective. *BMC Medical Informatics and Decision Making*, 20(1), 1–9. DOI: 10.1186/s12911-020-01332-6 PMID: 33256715

Aminizadeh, S., Heidari, A., Dehghan, M., Toumaj, S., Rezaei, M., Navimipour, N. J., & Unal, M. (2024). Opportunities and challenges of artificial intelligence and distributed systems to improve the quality of healthcare service. *Artificial Intelligence in Medicine*, 149, 102779. DOI: 10.1016/j.artmed.2024.102779 PMID: 38462281

Amiri, Z., Heidari, A., Navimipour, N. J., Unal, M., & Mousavi, A. (2024). Adventures in data analysis: A systematic review of Deep Learning techniques for pattern recognition in cyber-physical-social systems. *Multimedia Tools and Applications*, 83(8), 22909–22973. DOI: 10.1007/s11042-023-16382-x

Amjad, A., Kordel, P., & Fernandes, G. (2023). A review on innovation in healthcare sector (telehealth) through artificial intelligence. *Sustainability (Basel)*, 15(8), 6655. DOI: 10.3390/su15086655

Amsaad, F., Prasanna, P., Pravallika, T., Mamatha, G., Raviteja, B., Lakshmi, M., . . . Tashtoush, Y. (2023). *Toward Secure and Efficient CNN Recognition with Different Activation and Optimization Functions*. Paper presented at the International Conference on Advances in Computing Research. DOI: 10.1007/978-3-031-33743-7_45

Anderson, M., & Mooney, S. J. (2021). The impact of bias and fairness in machine learning for clinical decision support. *Journal of Biomedical Informatics*, 120, 103865.

Andrew, J., Deva Priya Isravel, K., Martin Sagayam, B., Bhushan, B., Sei, Y., & Eunice, J. (2023). Blockchain for healthcare systems: Architecture, security challenges, trends and future directions. *Journal of Network and Computer Applications*, 215, 103633. DOI: 10.1016/j.jnca.2023.103633

Antunes, R. S., André da Costa, C., Küderle, A., Yari, I. A., & Eskofier, B. (2022). Federated learning for healthcare: Systematic review and architecture proposal. [TIST]. *ACM Transactions on Intelligent Systems and Technology*, 13(4), 1–23. DOI: 10.1145/3501813

Aouedi, O., Sacco, A., Piamrat, K., & Marchetto, G. (2023). Handling Privacy-Sensitive Medical Data With Federated Learning: Challenges and Future Directions. *IEEE Journal of Biomedical and Health Informatics*, 27(2), 790–803. DOI: 10.1109/JBHI.2022.3185673 PMID: 35737624

Argaw, S. T., Troncoso-Pastoriza, J. R., Lacey, D., Florin, M.-V., Calcavecchia, F., Anderson, D., & Eshaya-Chauvin, B. (2020). Cybersecurity of Hospitals: Discussing the challenges and working towards mitigating the risks. *BMC Medical Informatics and Decision Making*, 20(1), 1–10. DOI: 10.1186/s12911-020-01161-7 PMID: 32620167

Arikumar, K. S., Prathiba, S. B., Alazab, M., Gadekallu, T. R., Pandya, S., Khan, J. M., & Moorthy, R. S. (2022). FL-PMI: Federated learning-based person movement identification through wearable devices in smart healthcare systems. *Sensors (Basel)*, 22(4), 1377.

Arnob, A. K. B., & Jony, A. I. (2024). Enhancing IoT Security: A Deep Learning Approach with Feedforward Neural Network for Detecting Cyber Attacks in IoT. Malaysian Journal of Science and Advanced Technology, 413-420.

Arslan, M., Mubeen, M., Bilal, M., & Abbasi, S. F. (2024). 1D-CNN-IDS: 1D CNN-based Intrusion Detection System for IIoT. arXiv preprint arXiv:2409.08529. DOI: 10.1109/ICAC61394.2024.10718772

Aslam, M. M., Ahmed, Z., Du, L., Hassan, M. Z., Ali, S., & Nasir, M. (2022). An Overview of Recent Advances of Resilient Consensus for Multiagent Systems under Attacks. *Computational Intelligence and Neuroscience*, 2022(1), 6732343. DOI: 10.1155/2022/6732343 PMID: 39411550

Aslam, N., Srivastava, S., & Gore, M. (2022). ONOS flood defender: An intelligent approach to mitigate DDoS attack in SDN. *Transactions on Emerging Telecommunications Technologies*, 33(9), e4534. DOI: 10.1002/ett.4534

Aslan, Ö., Aktuğ, S. S., Ozkan-Okay, M., Yilmaz, A. A., & Akin, E. (2023). A comprehensive review of cyber security vulnerabilities, threats, attacks, and solutions. *Electronics (Basel)*, 12(6), 1333. DOI: 10.3390/electronics12061333

Aung, Y. M., Zaw, A. T., & Win, K. M. (2022). Ethical issues in applying machine learning models in clinical settings. *Healthcare Analytics*, 6, 100094.

Awan, S., Luo, B., & Li, F. (2021). Contra: Defending against poisoning attacks in federated learning. In Computer Security–ESORICS 2021: 26th European Symposium on Research in Computer Security, Darmstadt, Germany, October 4–8, 2021 [Springer International Publishing.]. *Proceedings*, 26(Part I), 455–475.

Awotunde, J. B., Jimoh, R. G., Ogundokun, R. O., Misra, S., & Abikoye, O. C. (2022). Big data analytics of iot-based cloud system framework: Smart healthcare monitoring systems. In *Artificial intelligence for cloud and edge computing* (pp. 181–208). Springer International Publishing. DOI: 10.1007/978-3-030-80821-1_9

Awotunde, J. B., & Misra, S. (2022). *Feature extraction and artificial intelligence-based intrusion detection model for a secure internet of things networks Illumination of artificial intelligence in cybersecurity and forensics*. Springer.

Ayers, J. W., Poliak, A., Dredze, M., Leas, E. C., Zhu, Z., Kelley, J. B., Faix, D. J., Goodman, A. M., Longhurst, C. A., Hogarth, M., & Smith, D. M. (2023). Comparing Physician and Artificial Intelligence Chatbot Responses to Patient Questions Posted to a Public Social Media Forum. *JAMA Internal Medicine*, 183(6), 589. DOI: 10.1001/jamainternmed.2023.1838 PMID: 37115527

Ayub, M. F., Mahmood, K., Kumari, S., & Sangaiah, A. K. (2021). Lightweight authentication protocol for e-health clouds in IoT-based applications through 5G technology. *Digital Communications and Networks*, 7(2), 235–244. DOI: 10.1016/j.dcan.2020.06.003

Aziz, R., Banerjee, S., Bouzefrane, S., & Le Vinh, T. (2023). Exploring homomorphic encryption and differential privacy techniques towards secure federated learning paradigm. *Future Internet*, 15(9), 310.

Badidi, E. (2023). Edge AI for early detection of chronic diseases and the spread of infectious diseases: Opportunities, challenges, and future directions. *Future Internet*, 15(11), 370. DOI: 10.3390/fi15110370

Badolato, E., Little, A., & Le, V. D. (2024). Improving heart rate monitoring in the obese with time-of-flight photoplethysmography (TOF-PPG): A quantitative analysis of source-detector-distance effect. *Optics Express*, 32(3), 4446–4456. DOI: 10.1364/OE.510977 PMID: 38297646

Baek, C., Kim, S., Nam, D., & Park, J. (2021). Enhancing Differential Privacy for Federated Learning at Scale. *IEEE Access : Practical Innovations, Open Solutions*, 9, 148090–148103. DOI: 10.1109/ACCESS.2021.3124020

Bala, B., & Behal, S. (2024). AI techniques for IoT-based DDoS attack detection: Taxonomies, comprehensive review and research challenges. *Computer Science Review*, 52, 100631. DOI: 10.1016/j.cosrev.2024.100631

Balakrishnan, A. (2024). Leveraging Artificial Intelligence for Enhancing Regulatory Compliance in the Financial Sector. *International Journal of Computer Trends and Technology*.

Banabilah, S., Aloqaily, M., Alsayed, E., Malik, N., & Jararweh, Y. (2022). Federated Learning Review: Fundamentals, Enabling Technologies, and Future Applications. *Information Processing & Management*, 59(6), 103061. DOI: 10.1016/j.ipm.2022.103061

Barlow, J., & Decker, S. (2023). *Cybersecurity in healthcare: A comprehensive guide*. HealthTech Press.

Barlow, J., & Decker, S. (2023). *Cybersecurity in Healthcare: A Comprehensive Guide*. HealthTech Press.

Bashir, A. K., Victor, N., Bhattacharya, S., Huynh-The, T., Chengoden, R., Yenduri, G., Praveen, K. R. M., Pham, Q. V., Gadekallu, T. R., & Liyanage, M. (2023). Federated Learning for the Healthcare Metaverse: Concepts, Applications, Challenges, and Future Directions. *IEEE Internet ofThings Journal*, 10(24), 21873–21891. DOI: 10.1109/JIOT.2023.3304790

Baxter, G., & Sommerville, I. (2011). Socio-technical systems: From design methods to systems engineering. *Interacting with Computers*, 23(1), 4–17. DOI: 10.1016/j.intcom.2010.07.003

Beauchamp, A., Baird, A., Fox, K., Silva, G., & Kuhlmann, E. (2023). Data-driven approaches to healthcare disparities: Using machine learning to inform health equity initiatives. *PLOS Digital Health*, 2(1), e0000278.

Bebortta, S., Tripathy, S. S., Basheer, S., & Chowdhary, C. L. (2023). Fedehr: A federated learning approach towards the prediction of heart diseases in iot-based electronic health records. *Diagnostics (Basel)*, 13(20), 3166.

Beede, E., Baylor, E., Hersch, F., Iurchenko, A., Wilcox, L., Ruamviboonsuk, P., & Vardoulakis, L. M. (2020). A human-centered evaluation of a deep learning system deployed in clinics for the detection of diabetic retinopathy. *CHI Conference on Human Factors in Computing Systems*, 1-12. DOI: 10.1145/3313831.3376718

Belchior, R., Vasconcelos, A., Guerreiro, S., & Correia, M. (2021). A survey on blockchain interoperability: Past, present, and future trends. *ACM Computing Surveys*, 54(8), 1–41. DOI: 10.1145/3471140

Beltran, M., Tomas, E., Perez, M. Q., Pedro, M. S. S., Bernal, S. L., Bovet, G., Perez, M. G., Perez, G. M., & Celdran, A. H. (2023). Decentralized Federated Learning: Fundamentals, State of the Art, Frameworks, Trends, and Challenges. *IEEE Communications Surveys and Tutorials*, 25(4), 2983–3013. DOI: 10.1109/COMST.2023.3315746

Bharadiya, J. P. (2023). A Comparative Study of Business Intelligence and Artificial Intelligence with Big Data Analytics. *American Journal of Artificial Intelligence*, 7(1), 24.

Bharati, S., Mondal, M., Podder, P., & Prasath, V. (2022). Federated learning: Applications, challenges and future directions. *International Journal of Hybrid Intelligent Systems*, 18(1-2), 19–35. DOI: 10.3233/HIS-220006

Bhat, S. V., Malayka, M., & Mohanty, A. (2024, May). Integrating MAX30100 Sensor and MediaPipe Hand Gesture Recognition for Real-Time Health Monitoring System. In 2024 3rd International Conference on Artificial Intelligence For Internet of Things (AIIoT) (pp. 1-6). IEEE. DOI: 10.1109/AIIoT58432.2024.10574678

Bhumichai, D., Smiliotopoulos, C., Benton, R., Kambourakis, G., & Damopoulos, D. (2024). The convergence of artificial intelligence and blockchain: The state of play and the road ahead. *Information (Basel)*, 15(5), 268. DOI: 10.3390/info15050268

Biggio, B., Fumera, G., & Roli, F. (2013). Security evaluation of pattern classifiers under attack. *IEEE Transactions on Knowledge and Data Engineering*, 26(4), 984–996. DOI: 10.1109/TKDE.2013.57

Bindra, N., & Sood, M. (2019). Detecting DDoS attacks using machine learning techniques and contemporary intrusion detection dataset. *Automatic Control and Computer Sciences*, 53(5), 419–428. DOI: 10.3103/S0146411619050043

Binns, R. (2018, January). Fairness in machine learning: Lessons from political philosophy. In Conference on fairness, accountability and transparency (pp. 149-159). PMLR.

Bisht, N., Malik, P. K., Das, S., Islam, T., Asha, S., & Alathbah, M. (2023). Design of a Modified MIMO Antenna Based on Tweaked Spherical Fractal Geometry for 5G New Radio (NR) Band N258 (24.25–27.25 GHz) Applications. *Fractal and Fractional*, 7(10), 718. DOI: 10.3390/fractalfract7100718

Blessing, M. (2024). Role-Based Access Control (RBAC) for IoT Devices: Enhancing Security in a Connected World.

Brooks, R. R., Yu, L., Ozcelik, I., Oakley, J., & Tusing, N. (2021). Distributed denial of service (DDoS): A history. *IEEE Annals of the History of Computing*, 44(2), 44–54. DOI: 10.1109/MAHC.2021.3072582

Bucher, A., & Fichman, M. (2020). Geographic and demographic imbalances in healthcare research: A critical review. *Journal of Health Disparities Research and Practice*, 13(2), 1–20. PMID: 34367737

Buchmann, J. A. (2009). *Introduction to cryptography* (4th Indian reprint ed.). Springer.

Buolamwini, J., & Gebru, T. (2018). Gender Shades: Intersectional Accuracy Disparities in Commercial Gender Classification. *Proceedings of the 2018 Conference on Fairness, Accountability, and Transparency (FAT).*

Burrello, A., Pagliari, D. J., Risso, M., Benatti, S., Macii, E., Benini, L., & Poncino, M. (2021). Q-ppg: Energy-efficient ppg-based heart rate monitoring on wearable devices. *IEEE Transactions on Biomedical Circuits and Systems*, 15(6), 1196–1209. DOI: 10.1109/TBCAS.2021.3122017 PMID: 34673496

Byrd, J. B., Greene, A. C., Prasad, D. V., Jiang, X., & Greene, C. S. (2020). Responsible, practical genomic data sharing that accelerates research. *Nature Reviews. Genetics*, 21(10), 615–629.

Cahyo, L. M., & Astuti, S. D. (2023). Early detection of health problems through artificial intelligence (ai) technology in hospital information management: A literature review study. *Journal of Medical and Health Studies*, 4(3), 37–42. DOI: 10.32996/jmhs.2023.4.3.5

Carlini, N., Liu, C., Erlingsson, Ú., Kos, J., & Song, D. (2019). The secret sharer: Evaluating and testing unintended memorization in neural networks. In 28th USENIX security symposium (USENIX security 19) (pp. 267-284).

Cerchione, R., Centobelli, P., Riccio, E., Abbate, S., & Oropallo, E. (2023). Blockchain's coming to hospital to digitalize healthcare services: Designing a distributed electronic health record ecosystem. *Technovation*, 120, 102480. DOI: 10.1016/j.technovation.2022.102480

Challen, R., Denny, J., Pitt, M., Gompels, L., Edwards, T., & Tsaneva-Atanasova, K. (2021). Artificial intelligence, bias and clinical safety. *BMJ Quality & Safety*, 30(9), 792–800. PMID: 30636200

Chaudhary, P. K., Yalamati, S., Palakurti, N. R., Alam, N., Kolasani, S., & Whig, P. (2024, July). Detecting and Preventing Child Cyberbullying using Generative Artificial Intelligence. In *2024 Asia Pacific Conference on Innovation in Technology (APCIT)* (pp. 1-5). IEEE. DOI: 10.1109/APCIT62007.2024.10673710

Chelliah, B. J. (2022). *An Efficient Storage Solution for Healthcare Management Systems Using Cloud.* Paper presented at the 2022 Third International Conference on Smart Technologies in Computing, Electrical and Electronics (ICSTCEE).

Chen, C., Su, Y., & King, R. (2021). Equity in algorithmic decision-making: Mitigating bias in machine learning for healthcare applications. *Journal of Healthcare Informatics Research*, 5(2), 127–148.

Cheng, S. M., Lui, Y. C., Tsai, N. J., & Hong, B. K. (2024). Toward Intelligent IoT Endpoint Detection and Response Using Digital Twins via Firmware Emulation. *IEEE Internet of Things Magazine*, 7(6), 20–26. DOI: 10.1109/IOTM.001.2400070

Chen, I. Y., Joshi, S., Ghassemi, M., & Chen, Y. (2021). Ethical machine learning in health care. *Annual Review of Biomedical Data Science*, 4(1), 123–144. DOI: 10.1146/annurev-biodatasci-092820-114757 PMID: 34396058

Chen, R. J., Wang, J. J., Williamson, D. F., Chen, T. Y., Lipkova, J., Lu, M. Y., & Mahmood, F. (2023). Algorithmic fairness in artificial intelligence for medicine and healthcare. *Nature Biomedical Engineering*, 7(6), 719–742.

Chenthara, S., Ahmed, K., Wang, H., Whittaker, F., & Chen, Z. (2020). Healthchain: A novel framework on privacy preservation of electronic health records using blockchain technology. *PLoS One*, 15(12), e0243043. DOI: 10.1371/journal.pone.0243043 PMID: 33296379

Chen, X., Xie, H., Tao, X., Wang, F. L., Leng, M., & Lei, B. (2024). Artificial intelligence and multimodal data fusion for smart healthcare: Topic modeling and bibliometrics. *Artificial Intelligence Review*, 57(4), 91. DOI: 10.1007/s10462-024-10712-7

Chouldechova, A., & Roth, A. (2020). The frontiers of fairness in machine learning. *Communications of the ACM*, 63(5), 93–101. DOI: 10.1145/3376898

Christodoulou, L., Chari, A., & Georgiades, M. (2024, April). AI-enhanced Healthcare IoT System: Advanced ML Detection and Classification Algorithms for Real-Time Cardiovascular Monitoring. In 2024 20th International Conference on Distributed Computing in Smart Systems and the Internet of Things (DCOSS-IoT) (pp. 440-449). IEEE.

Churi, P., Pawar, A., & Moreno-Guerrero, A. J. (2021). A comprehensive survey on data utility and privacy: Taking Indian healthcare system as a potential case study. *Inventions (Basel, Switzerland)*, 6(3), 45.

Churpek, M. M., Yuen, T. C., Huber, M. T., Park, S. Y., Hall, J. B., & Edelson, D. P. (2012). Predicting cardiac arrest on the wards: A nested case-control study. *Chest*, 141(5), 1170–1176. DOI: 10.1378/chest.11-1301 PMID: 22052772

Coelho, K. K., Nogueira, M., Vieira, A. B., Silva, E. F., & José Augusto, M. N. (2023). A Survey on Federated Learning for Security and Privacy in Healthcare Applications. *Computer Communications*, 207, 113–127. DOI: 10.1016/j.comcom.2023.05.012

Cohen, I. G., Amarasingham, R., Shah, A., Xie, B., & Lo, B. (2020). The legal and ethical concerns that arise from using complex predictive analytics in health care. *Health Affairs*, 39(7), 1146–1154. PMID: 25006139

Cohen, I. G., & Mello, M. M. (2018). HIPAA and Protecting Health Information in the 21st Century. *Journal of the American Medical Association*, 320(3), 231. DOI: 10.1001/jama.2018.5630 PMID: 29800120

Cowgill, B., Dell'Acqua, F., Deng, S., & Chouldechova, A. (2020). Biased programmers? Or biased data? A field experiment in operationalizing AI ethics. *ACM Conference on Fairness, Accountability, and Transparency (FAT).*

Cremonesi, F., Planat, V., Kalokyri, V., Kondylakis, H., Sanavia, T., Victor, M. M. R., Singh, B., & Uribe, S. (2023). The Need for Multimodal Health Data Modeling: A Practical Approach for a Federated-Learning Healthcare Platform. *Journal of Biomedical Informatics*, 141, 104338. DOI: 10.1016/j.jbi.2023.104338 PMID: 37023843

Cui, Y., & Zhang, L. (2021). Ethical dilemmas in the use of AI for healthcare diagnostics: A systematic review. *Ethics, Medicine, and Public Health*, 17, 100674.

Dang, L. M., Piran, M. J., Han, D., Min, K., & Moon, H. (2019). A survey on internet of things and cloud computing for healthcare. *Electronics (Basel)*, 8(7), 768. DOI: 10.3390/electronics8070768

Danks, D., & London, A. J. (2017). Algorithmic bias in autonomous systems. *Proceedings of the Twenty-Sixth International Joint Conference on Artificial Intelligence*, 4691-4697.

Dargan, S., Kumar, M., Ayyagari, M. R., & Kumar, G. (2020). A survey of deep learning and its applications: A new paradigm to machine learning. *Archives of Computational Methods in Engineering*, 27(4), 1071–1092. DOI: 10.1007/s11831-019-09344-w

Davis, L., & Patel, R. (2022). Securing medical devices: Strategies for compliance and safety. *Journal of Healthcare Information Security*, 15(3), 45–60.

Davis, L., & Patel, R. (2022). Securing Medical Devices: Strategies for Compliance and Safety. *Journal of Healthcare Information Security*, 15(3), 45–60.

de Oliveira, M. T., Verginadis, Y., Reis, L. H., Psarra, E., Patiniotakis, I., & Olabarriaga, S. D. (2023). AC-ABAC: Attribute-based access control for electronic medical records during acute care. *Expert Systems with Applications*, 213, 119271. DOI: 10.1016/j.eswa.2022.119271

Demertzis, K., Iliadis, L., Tziritas, N., & Kikiras, P. (2020). Anomaly detection via blockchained deep learning smart contracts in industry 4.0. *Neural Computing & Applications*, 32(23), 17361–17378. DOI: 10.1007/s00521-020-05189-8

Dhatterwal, J. S., Kaswan, K. S., Baliyan, A., & Jain, V. (2022). *Integration of cloud and IoT for smart e-healthcare Connected e-health: Integrated IoT and cloud computing*. Springer.

Dhingra, S., Savalgi, A. A., & Jain, S. (2016). Laplace transformation-based cryptographic technique in network security. *International Journal of Computer Applications*, 136(7), 6–10. DOI: 10.5120/ijca2016908482

Dhirani, L. L., Mukhtiar, N., Chowdhry, B. S., & Newe, T. (2023). Ethical dilemmas and privacy issues in emerging technologies: A review. *Sensors (Basel)*, 23(3), 1151. DOI: 10.3390/s23031151 PMID: 36772190

Ding, W., Abdel-Basset, M., Alrashdi, I., & Hawash, H. (2024). Next generation of computer vision for plant disease monitoring in precision agriculture: A contemporary survey, taxonomy, experiments, and future direction. *Information Sciences*, 665, 120338. DOI: 10.1016/j.ins.2024.120338

Ding, Z., Wang, W., Li, X., Wang, X., Jeon, G., Zhao, J., & Mu, C. (2024). Identifying alternately poisoning attacks in federated learning online using trajectory anomaly detection method. *Scientific Reports*, 14(1), 20269.

Dong, M. (2024). Investigating the users' preferences of heart rate data types and visualizations on a smartwatch. *International Journal of Human-Computer Interaction*, 40(18), 5298–5319. DOI: 10.1080/10447318.2023.2233130

Dutta, S., & Gochhait, S. (Eds.). (2022). *Information retrieval in bioinformatics: A practical approach*. Springer. DOI: 10.1007/978-981-19-6506-7

Dwork, C., & Roth, A. (2014). The algorithmic foundations of differential privacy. Foundations and Trends® in Theoretical Computer Science, 9(3–4), 211-407.

Ebong, G. N., Matthew, U. O., Olofin, B., Andrew-Vitalis, N., Fatai, L. O., Waliu, A. O., & Oladipupo, M. A. (2024). *Multimedia Cloud Data Warehouse Design for Knowledge Sharing in the University Environment: A Proposed Digital Solution Implementing Interactive Learning Strategies in Higher Education*. IGI Global. DOI: 10.4018/979-8-3693-3559-8.ch010

Edwards, D. J. (2024). Vulnerability Assessment and Penetration Testing. In *Mastering Cybersecurity: Strategies, Technologies, and Best Practices* (pp. 371–412). Apress. DOI: 10.1007/979-8-8688-0297-3_11

El-Gendy, S., Elsayed, M. S., Jurcut, A., & Azer, M. A. (2023). Privacy Preservation Using Machine Learning in the Internet of Things. *Mathematics*, 11(16), 3477. DOI: 10.3390/math11163477

El-Rashidy, N., El-Sappagh, S., Islam, S. R. M., El-Bakry, H., & Abdelrazek, S. (2021). Mobile health in remote patient monitoring for chronic diseases: Principles, trends, and challenges. *Diagnostics (Basel)*, 11(4), 607.

El-Samad, W., Adda, M., & Atieh, M. (2024). AI-Driven Data Aggregation Level Smart Contracts for Blockchain Healthcare Insurance Claims Adjudication. *Procedia Computer Science*, 241, 63–68. DOI: 10.1016/j.procs.2024.08.011

Elzaki, T. M. (2011). The new integral transform Elzaki Transform. *Global Journal of Pure and Applied Mathematics*, 7(1), 57–64.

Esteva, A., Kuprel, B., Novoa, R. A., Ko, J., Swetter, S. M., Blau, H. M., & Thrun, S. (2017). Dermatologist-level classification of skin cancer with deep neural networks. nature, 542(7639), 115-118.

Esteva, A., Robicquet, A., Ramsundar, B., Kuleshov, V., DePristo, M., Chou, K., Cui, C., Corrado, G., Thrun, S., & Dean, J. (2019). A guide to deep learning in healthcare. *Nature Medicine*, 25(1), 24–29. DOI: 10.1038/s41591-018-0316-z PMID: 30617335

Falayi, A., Wang, Q., Liao, W., & Yu, W. (2023). Survey of distributed and decentralized IoT securities: Approaches using deep learning and blockchain technology. *Future Internet*, 15(5), 178. DOI: 10.3390/fi15050178

Fan, Z., Yan, Z., & Wen, S. (2023). Deep learning and artificial intelligence in sustainability: A review of SDGs, renewable energy, and environmental health. *Sustainability (Basel)*, 15(18), 13493. DOI: 10.3390/su151813493

Farid, F., Elkhodr, M., Sabrina, F., Ahamed, F., & Gide, E. (2021). A smart biometric identity management framework for personalised IoT and cloud computing-based healthcare services. *Sensors (Basel)*, 21(2), 552. DOI: 10.3390/s21020552 PMID: 33466730

Farooq, M., Khan, M. H., & Khan, R. A. (2023). Implementation of Network Security for Intrusion Detection & Prevention System in IoT Networks: Challenges & Approach. Int. J. *Advanced Networking and Applications*, 15(05), 6109–6113.

Fereidooni, H., Marchal, S., Miettinen, M., Mirhoseini, A., Möllering, H., Nguyen, T. D., ... & Zeitouni, S. (2021, May). SAFELearn: Secure aggregation for private federated learning. In 2021 IEEE Security and Privacy Workshops (SPW) (pp. 56-62). IEEE.

Finlayson, S. G., Bowers, J. D., Ito, J., Zittrain, J. L., Beam, A. L., & Kohane, I. S. (2019). Adversarial attacks on medical machine learning. *Science*, 363(6433), 1287–1289. DOI: 10.1126/science.aaw4399 PMID: 30898923

Fleming, S. L., Lozano, A., Haberkorn, W. J., Jindal, J. A., Reis, E., Thapa, R., Blankemeier, L., Genkins, J. Z., Steinberg, E., Nayak, A., Patel, B., Chiang, C.-C., Callahan, A., Huo, Z., Gatidis, S., Adams, S., Fayanju, O., Shah, S. J., Savage, T., & Shah, N. H. (2024). MedAlign: A Clinician-Generated Dataset for Instruction Following with Electronic Medical Records. *Proceedings of the AAAI Conference on Artificial Intelligence*, 38(20), 22021–22030. DOI: 10.1609/aaai.v38i20.30205

Flores, A. W., Bechtel, K., & Lowenkamp, C. T. (2016). False positives, false negatives, and false analyses: A reexamination of the predictive validity of the COMPAS risk assessment tool. *Criminology & Public Policy*, 15(3), 951–980.

Floridi, L., & Cowls, J. (2019). A Unified Framework of Five Principles for AI in Society. *Harvard Data Science Review*. Advance online publication. DOI: 10.1162/99608f92.8cd550d1

Forslund, M., Mathieson, K., Djibo, Y., Mbindyo, C., Lugangira, N., & Balasubramaniam, P. (2024). Strengthening the evidence base on the use of digital health technologies to accelerate progress towards universal health coverage. *Oxford Open Digital Health*, 2, oqae033. DOI: 10.1093/oodh/oqae033

Fredrikson, M., Jha, S., & Ristenpart, T. (2015, October). Model inversion attacks that exploit confidence information and basic countermeasures. In *Proceedings of the 22nd ACM SIGSAC conference on computer and communications security* (pp. 1322-1333).

Gagalova, K. K., Elizalde, M. A. L., Portales-Casamar, E., & Görges, M. (2020). What you need to know before implementing a clinical research data warehouse: Comparative review of integrated data repositories in health care institutions. *JMIR Formative Research*, 4(8), e17687. DOI: 10.2196/17687 PMID: 32852280

Gandhi, P., & Kumar, R. (2024). Artificial Intelligence of Things (AIoT) for Intelligent Data Design. *Reshaping Intelligent Business and Industry: Convergence of AI and IoT at the Cutting Edge*, 507-517.

Garcia-Perez, A., Cegarra-Navarro, J. G., Sallos, M. P., Martinez-Caro, E., & Chinnaswamy, A. (2023). Resilience in healthcare systems: Cyber security and digital transformation. *Technovation*, 121, 102583. DOI: 10.1016/j.technovation.2022.102583

Gasmi, H., Laval, J., & Bouras, A. (2024). LSTM recurrent neural networks for cybersecurity named entity recognition. arXiv preprint arXiv:2409.10521.

Gefenas, E., Lekstutiene, J., Lukaseviciene, V., Hartlev, M., Mourby, M., & Cathaoir, K. Ó. (2022). Controversies between Regulations of Research Ethics and Protection of Personal Data: Informed Consent at a Cross-Road. *Medicine, Health Care, and Philosophy*, 25(1), 23–30. DOI: 10.1007/s11019-021-10060-1 PMID: 34787769

Geiping, J., Bauermeister, H., Dröge, H., & Moeller, M. (2020). Inverting Gradients - How Easy Is It to Break Privacy in Federated Learning? *Advances in Neural Information Processing Systems*, 33, 16937–16947.

Ghassemi, M., & Naumann, T.. (2019). A review of challenges and opportunities in using machine learning in healthcare. *Journal of Machine Learning Research*, 20, 1–36.

Gochhait, S. (Ed.). (2024). *Driving Transformative Technology Trends With Cloud Computing*. IGI Global., DOI: 10.4018/979-8-3693-2869-9

Goodfellow, I. J., Shlens, J., & Szegedy, C. (2014). *Explaining and Harnessing Adversarial Examples*. arXiv. DOI: 10.48550/ARXIV.1412.6572

Goodfellow, I.. (2014). Generative adversarial nets. *Advances in Neural Information Processing Systems*, •••, 27.

Grewal, B. S. (2005). *Higher engineering mathematics*. Khanna Publishing.

Guduri, M., Chakraborty, C., Maheswari, U., & Margala, M. (2023). Blockchain-based federated learning technique for privacy preservation and security of smart electronic health records. *IEEE Transactions on Consumer Electronics*, 70(1), 2608–2617. DOI: 10.1109/TCE.2023.3315415

Gulati, S., Guleria, K., & Goyal, N. (2024). Collaborative, Privacy-Preserving Federated Learning Framework for the Detection of Diabetic Eye Diseases. *SN Computer Science*, 5(8), 1–10. DOI: 10.1007/s42979-024-03462-4

Gulhane, K., Saxena, S., Deogaonkar, A., Kumar, V., Vichoray, C., & Goyal, S. (2024, August). Overview of Machine Learning Techniques in Cybersecurity Data Science using Gradient Boosting and Random Forest Algorithm. In 2024 Second International Conference on Intelligent Cyber Physical Systems and Internet of Things (ICoICI) (pp. 19-24). IEEE. https://www.cse.wustl.edu/~jain/ehms/index.html

Gunasekar, T., & Raghavendran, P. (2024). Applications of the R-Transform for advancing cryptographic security. In *Driving transformative technology trends with cloud computing* (pp. 208–223). IGI Global. DOI: 10.4018/979-8-3693-2869-9.ch011

Gupta, S. K., Alemran, A., Ranjith, C. P., & Mohideen, M. S. K. (2024). Biometric Authentication for Healthcare Data Security in Cloud Computing—A Machine Learning Approach. In Advancements in Science and Technology for Healthcare, Agriculture, and Environmental Sustainability (pp. 318-324). CRC Press.

Gupta, S. K., Alemran, A., Ranjith, C. P., & Mohideen, M. S. K. (2024). Reliable Fingerprint Classification Based on Novel Deep Learning Approach. In Advancements in Science and Technology for Healthcare, Agriculture, and Environmental Sustainability (pp. 353-360). CRC Press.

Gupta, S. K., Natarajan, R., Pandey, A. K., & Singh, P. (2024). Integrated Model of Encryption and Steganography for Improving the Data Security in Communication Systems. In Advancements in Science and Technology for Healthcare, Agriculture, and Environmental Sustainability (pp. 333-338). CRC Press.

Gupta, S. K., Vohra, S. K., Hrybiuk, O., & Shukla, A. K. (2023). Public Service Strategy Empowered for Internet of Things Technologies and Its Challenges. In AI-Aided IoT Technologies and Applications for Smart Business and Production (pp. 308-321). CRC Press.

Gupta, A., Misra, S., Pathak, N., & Das, D. (2023). FedCare: Federated Learning for Resource-Constrained Healthcare Devices in IoMT System. *IEEE Transactions on Computational Social Systems*, 10(4), 1587–1596. DOI: 10.1109/TCSS.2022.3232192

Gupta, M. (2023). *A novel scheme to manage the e-healthcare system using cloud computing and the internet of things Computational Intelligence in Healthcare*. CRC Press.

Gupta, M., Sharma, P., & Kalra, R. (2024). *Federated learning and artificial intelligence in e-healthcare Federated Learning and AI for Healthcare 5.0*. IGI Global.

Gupta, R. (2023). Securing data transmission by cryptography using Rohit integral transform. *IACSIT International Journal of Engineering and Technology*, 12(2), 109–111.

Gupta, R., & Alam, T. (2022). Survey on Federated-Learning Approaches in Distributed Environment. *Wireless Personal Communications*, 125(2), 1631–1652. DOI: 10.1007/s11277-022-09624-y

Haan, M., Ongena, Y. P., Hommes, S., Kwee, T. C., & Yakar, D. (2021). Integration of artificial intelligence in radiology: Automated and standardized reporting. *Insights Into Imaging*, 12(1), 167. PMID: 34767092

Haddad, A., Habaebi, M. H., Islam, M. R., Hasbullah, N. F., & Zabidi, S. A. (2022). Systematic review on AI-blockchain based e-healthcare records management systems. *IEEE Access : Practical Innovations, Open Solutions*, 10, 94583–94615. DOI: 10.1109/ACCESS.2022.3201878

Haghayegh, F., Norouziazad, A., Haghani, E., Feygin, A. A., Rahimi, R. H., Ghavamabadi, H. A., & Felfeli, T. (2024). Revolutionary Point-of-Care Wearable Diagnostics for Early Disease Detection and Biomarker Discovery through Intelligent Technologies. *Advancement of Science*, 11(36), 2400595. DOI: 10.1002/advs.202400595 PMID: 38958517

Hardt, M., Price, E., & Srebro, N. (2016). Equality of opportunity in supervised learning. *Advances in Neural Information Processing Systems (NeurIPS).*

Heart, T., Ben-Assuli, O., & Shabtai, I. (2017). A review of PHR, EMR and EHR integration: A more personalized healthcare and public health policy. *Health Policy and Technology*, 6(1), 20–25. DOI: 10.1016/j.hlpt.2016.08.002

Heidari, A., & Jabraeil Jamali, M. A. (2023). Internet of Things intrusion detection systems: A comprehensive review and future directions. *Cluster Computing*, 26(6), 3753–3780. DOI: 10.1007/s10586-022-03776-z

He, R., Shen, L., Wang, Z., Wang, G., Qu, H., Hu, X., & Min, R. (2023). Optical fiber sensors for heart rate monitoring: A review of mechanisms and applications. *Results in Optics*, 11, 100386. DOI: 10.1016/j.rio.2023.100386

Hiwarekar, A. P. (2012). A new method of cryptography using Laplace transform. *International Journal of Mathematical Archive*, 3(3), 1193–1197.

Hoffman, K., Tom, S., Grierson, L., Greene, L., Rosenfeld, D., & Wong, A. (2023). Framework for evaluating bias in machine learning algorithms for health care. *Journal of the American Medical Informatics Association : JAMIA*, 30(5), 1094–1100.

Hon, K. (2024). *Artificial neural networks Technology and Security for Lawyers and Other Professionals*. Edward Elgar Publishing.

Hopfield, J. J. (1982). Neural networks and physical systems with emergent collective computational abilities. *Proceedings of the National Academy of Sciences of the United States of America*, 79(8), 2554–2558. DOI: 10.1073/pnas.79.8.2554 PMID: 6953413

Huifeng, W., Kadry, S. N., & Raj, E. D. (2020). Continuous health monitoring of sportsperson using IoT devices based wearable technology. *Computer Communications*, 160, 588–595. DOI: 10.1016/j.comcom.2020.04.025

Hu, K., Li, Y., Xia, M., Wu, J., Lu, M., Zhang, S., & Weng, L. (2021). Federated Learning: A Distributed Shared Machine Learning Method. *Complexity*, 8261663(1), 8261663. DOI: 10.1155/2021/8261663

Ibrahim, N. S., Rampal, S., Lee, W. L., Pek, E. W., & Suhaimi, A. (2024). Evaluation of wrist-worn photoplethysmography trackers with an electrocardiogram in patients with ischemic heart disease: A validation study. *Cardiovascular Engineering and Technology*, 15(1), 12–21. DOI: 10.1007/s13239-023-00693-z PMID: 37973701

Idoko, I. P., David-Olusa, A., Badu, S. G., Okereke, E. K., Agaba, J. A., & Bashiru, O. (2024). The dual impact of AI and renewable energy in enhancing medicine for better diagnostics, drug discovery, and public health. *Magna Scientia Advanced Biology and Pharmacy*, 12(2), 99–127.

Ijiga, A. C., Olola, T. M., Enyejo, L. A., Akpa, F. A., Olatunde, T. I., & Olajide, F. I. (2024). Advanced surveillance and detection systems using deep learning to combat human trafficking. *Magna Scientia Advanced Research and Reviews*, 11(01), 267–286.

Imoize, A. L., Balas, V. E., Solanki, V. K., Lee, C.-C., & Obaidat, M. S. (2023). *Handbook of Security and Privacy of AI-Enabled Healthcare Systems and Internet of Medical Things*. CRC Press.

Imteaj, A., Thakker, U., Wang, S., Li, J., & Hadi Amini, M. (2022). A Survey on Federated Learning for Resource-Constrained IoT Devices. *IEEE Internet of Things Journal*, 9(1), 1–24. DOI: 10.1109/JIOT.2021.3095077

Indra Priyadharshini, S., Padmavathy, T. V., & Ankith, S. R. (2023, October). Cybersecurity Threat Detection in SDN Clouds Using Attention Mechanism in RNN. In International Conference on Sustainable and Innovative Solutions for Current Challenges in Engineering & Technology (pp. 365-377). Singapore: Springer Nature Singapore.

Isad, S. N., & Hasan, R. (2024, March). Towards a Security Analysis of Radiological Medical Devices using the MITRE ATT&CK Framework. In SoutheastCon 2024 (pp. 1577-1582). IEEE.</conf>

Isibor, E. (2024). Regulation of Healthcare Data Security: Legal Obligations in A Digital Age. *Available atSSRN* 4957244. DOI: 10.2139/ssrn.4957244

Issa, A., & Kuffi, E. A. (2024). On the double integral transform (Complex EE Transform) and their properties and applications. *Ibn AL-Haitham Journal for Pure and Applied Sciences*, 37(1), 429–441. DOI: 10.30526/37.1.3329

Issac, B. M., & Kumar, S. N. (2024). Collaborative Federated Learning in Healthcare Systems. In Handbook on Federated Learning (pp. 226-244). CRC Press.

Jafleh, E. A., Alnaqbi, F. A., Almaeeni, H. A., Faqeeh, S., Alzaabi, M. A., & Al Zaman, K. (2024). The Role of Wearable Devices in Chronic Disease Monitoring and Patient Care: A Comprehensive Review. *Cureus*, 16(9). Advance online publication. DOI: 10.7759/cureus.68921 PMID: 39381470

Jain, P., Panesar, S. F., Talwar, B. F., & Sah, M. K. (2021). IoT-Based Solutions for Smart Healthcare. *Emerging Technologies for Healthcare: Internet of Things and Deep Learning Models*, 25-67.

Jamil, M. N., Schelén, O., Monrat, A. A., & Andersson, K. (2024). Enabling Industrial Internet of Things by Leveraging Distributed Edge-to-Cloud Computing: Challenges and Opportunities. *IEEE Access : Practical Innovations, Open Solutions*, 12, 127294–127308. DOI: 10.1109/ACCESS.2024.3454812

Jananee, M. G. (2023). SpO2 and temperature measurement device based on ATmega328p microcontroller chip with mobile connection for real-time monitoring (Master's thesis, İstanbul Gelişim Üniversitesi Lisansüstü Eğitim Enstitüsü).

Javaid, H. A. (2024). Improving Fraud Detection and Risk Assessment in Financial Service using Predictive Analytics and Data Mining. *Integrated Journal of Science and Technology, 1*(8).

Javaid, M., Haleem, A., Singh, R. P., & Suman, R. (2023). *5G technology for healthcare: Features, serviceable pillars, and applications.* Intelligent Pharmacy.

Jiang, F., & Jiang, Y.. (2017). Artificial intelligence in healthcare: Anticipating challenges to ethics, privacy, and bias. *Journal of Medical Internet Research*, 19(4), e139.

Jiang, Y., Ma, B., Wang, X., Yu, G., Yu, P., Wang, Z., Ni, W., & Liu, R. P. (2024). Blockchained federated learning for internet of things: A comprehensive survey. *ACM Computing Surveys*, 56(10), 1–37. DOI: 10.1145/3659099

Jimmy, F. (2024). Cyber security Vulnerabilities and Remediation Through Cloud Security Tools. *Journal of Artificial Intelligence General science (JAIGS) ISSN: 3006-4023, 2*(1), 129-171.

Jin, Q., Leaman, R., & Lu, Z. (2023). Retrieve, Summarize, and Verify: How Will ChatGPT Affect Information Seeking from the Medical Literature? *Journal of the American Society of Nephrology*, 34(8), 1302–1304. DOI: 10.1681/ASN.0000000000000166 PMID: 37254254

Johnson, D., Goodman, R., Patrinely, J., Stone, C., Zimmerman, E., Donald, R., Chang, S., Berkowitz, S., Finn, A., Jahangir, E., Scoville, E., Reese, T., Friedman, D., Bastarache, J., Heijden, Y. V. D., Wright, J., Carter, N., Alexander, M., Choe, J., & Wheless, L. (2023). *Assessing the Accuracy and Reliability of AI-Generated Medical Responses: An Evaluation of the Chat-GPT Model.* DOI: 10.21203/rs.3.rs-2566942/v1

Johnson, K. B., Wei, W. Q., Weeraratne, D., Frisse, M. E., Misulis, K., Rhee, K., & Snowdon, J. L. (2021). Precision medicine, AI, and the future of personalized health care. *Clinical and Translational Science*, 14(1), 86–93. DOI: 10.1111/cts.12884 PMID: 32961010

Kanna, G. P., Kumar, S. J. K. J., Kumar, Y., Changela, A., Woźniak, M., Shafi, J., & Ijaz, M. F. (2023). Author Correction: Advanced deep learning techniques for early disease prediction in cauliflower plants. *Scientific Reports*, 13(1), 13. DOI: 10.1038/s41598-023-47732-2 PMID: 38001261

Kashuri, A., & Fundo, A. (2013). A new integral transform. *Advances in Theoretical and Applied Mathematics*, 8(1), 27–43.

Kelaidonis, D., Vlacheas, P., Stavroulaki, V., Georgoulas, S., Moessner, K., Hashi, Y., . . . Demestichas, P. (2017). Cloud internet of things framework for enabling services in smart cities. *Designing, Developing, and Facilitating Smart Cities: Urban Design to IoT Solutions*, 163-191.

Kelly, C. J., Karthikesalingam, A., Suleyman, M., Corrado, G., & King, D. (2019). Key challenges for delivering clinical impact with artificial intelligence. *BMC Medicine*, 17(1), 195. DOI: 10.1186/s12916-019-1426-2 PMID: 31665002

Khairuddin, M. A., Isa, M. R. M., Shukran, M. A. M., Ismail, M. N., & Maskat, K. (2024). Detecting Distributed Denial-of-Service (DDoS) Attacks Through the Log Consolidation Processing (LCP) Framework. *JOIV: International Journal on Informatics Visualization*, 8(3), 1064. DOI: 10.62527/joiv.8.3.2184

Khalid, N., Qayyum, A., Bilal, M., Al-Fuqaha, A., & Qadir, J. (2023). Privacy-Preserving Artificial Intelligence in Healthcare: Techniques and Applications. *Computers in Biology and Medicine*, 158, 106848. DOI: 10.1016/j.compbiomed.2023.106848 PMID: 37044052

Khan, D., Jung, L. T., & Hashmani, M. A. (2021). Systematic literature review of challenges in blockchain scalability. *Applied Sciences (Basel, Switzerland)*, 11(20), 9372. DOI: 10.3390/app11209372

Khang, A., & Gupta, S. K. (2024, March). 36 Traffic Management and Decision Support System Based on the Internet of Things. In Advancements in Business for Integrating Diversity, and Sustainability: International Analytics Conference 2023| IAC 2023 February 2& 3, 2023| Virtual Conference (p. 210). Taylor & Francis.

Khang, A., Misra, A., Gupta, S. K., & Shah, V. (Eds.). (2023). *AI-Aided IoT Technologies and Applications for Smart Business and Production*. CRC Press.

Khanh, H. H., & Khang, A. (2021). The role of artificial intelligence in blockchain applications. In *Reinventing Manufacturing and Business Processes through Artificial Intelligence* (pp. 19–38). CRC Press. DOI: 10.1201/9781003145011-2

Khan, I. A., Razzak, I., Pi, D., Khan, N., Hussain, Y., Li, B., & Kousar, T. (2024). Fed-inforce-fusion: A federated reinforcement-based fusion model for security and privacy protection of IoMT networks against cyber-attacks. *Information Fusion*, 101, 102002. DOI: 10.1016/j.inffus.2023.102002

Khan, M. F., & Abaoud, M. (2023). Blockchain-Integrated Security for Real-Time Patient Monitoring in the Internet of Medical Things Using Federated Learning. *IEEE Access : Practical Innovations, Open Solutions*, 11, 117826–117850. DOI: 10.1109/ACCESS.2023.3326155

Khanna, A., & Gochhait, S. (Eds.). (2024). *Green AI-powered intelligent systems for disease prognosis*. IGI Global. DOI: 10.4018/979-8-3693-1243-8

Kharche, A., Badholia, S., & Upadhyay, R. K. (2024). Implementation of blockchain technology in integrated IoT networks for constructing scalable ITS systems in India. *Blockchain: Research and Applications*, 100188.

Kharde, U. D. (2017). An application of the Elzaki Transform in cryptography. *Journal for Advanced Research in Applied Sciences*, 4(5), 86–89.

Khujamatov, K., Khasanov, D., Reypnazarov, E., & Akhmedov, N. (2021). Existing technologies and solutions in 5G-enabled IoT for industrial automation. *Blockchain for 5G-Enabled IoT: The new wave for Industrial Automation*, 181-221.

Kim, H., Park, J., Bennis, M., & Kim, S.-L. (2019). Blockchained on-device federated learning. *IEEE Communications Letters*, 24(6), 1279–1283. DOI: 10.1109/LCOMM.2019.2921755

Kirkpatrick, K. (2023). *The carbon footprint of artificial intelligence*. ACM New York. DOI: 10.1145/3603746

Knosp, B. M., Craven, C. K., Dorr, D. A., Bernstam, E. V., & Campion, T. R.Jr. (2022). Understanding enterprise data warehouses to support clinical and translational research: Enterprise information technology relationships, data governance, workforce, and cloud computing. *Journal of the American Medical Informatics Association : JAMIA*, 29(4), 671–676. DOI: 10.1093/jamia/ocab256 PMID: 35289370

Kolosov, D., Kelefouras, V., Kourtessis, P., & Mporas, I. (2023). Contactless Camera-Based Heart Rate and Respiratory Rate Monitoring Using AI on Hardware. *Sensors (Basel)*, 23(9), 4550. DOI: 10.3390/s23094550 PMID: 37177754

Kuffi, E. A., Mehdi, S. A., & Mansour, E. A. (2022, August). Color image encryption based on new integral transform SEE. [IOP Publishing.]. *Journal of Physics: Conference Series*, 2322(1), 012016. DOI: 10.1088/1742-6596/2322/1/012016

Kumar, P. M., Vedantham, K., Selvaraj, J., & Kavin, B. P. (2024, February). Enhanced Network Intrusion Detection System Using PCGSO-Optimized BI-GRU Model in AI-Driven Cybersecurity. In 2024 IEEE 3rd International Conference on AI in Cybersecurity (ICAIC) (pp. 1-6). IEEE.

Kumar, A., Bansal, S. H., & Aggarwal, S. (2021). A new novel integral transform "Anuj Transform" with application. *Design Engineering (London)*, (9), 12741–12751.

Kumaresan, M., Gopal, R., Mathivanan, M., & Poongodi, T. (2022). *Amalgamation of blockchain, IoT, and 5G to improve security and privacy of smart healthcare systems Blockchain Applications for Healthcare Informatics*. Elsevier.

Kumari, P., & Jain, A. K. (2023). A comprehensive study of DDoS attacks over IoT network and their countermeasures. *Computers & Security*, 127, 103096. DOI: 10.1016/j.cose.2023.103096

Kung, T. H., Cheatham, M., Medenilla, A., Sillos, C., Leon, L. D., Elepaño, C., Madriaga, M., Aggabao, R., Diaz-Candido, G., Maningo, J., & Tseng, V. (2023). Performance of ChatGPT on USMLE: Potential for AI-assisted medical education using large language models. *PLOS Digital Health*, 2(2), e0000198. DOI: 10.1371/journal.pdig.0000198 PMID: 36812645

Lacity, M. C., Khan, S. A., & Yan, A. (2017). *Review of the empirical business services sourcing literature: an update and future directions Outsourcing and offshoring business services*. Springer.

Lack, A., Kwon, S., Duflo, E., McCarthy, M., Baker, S., Tsalatsanis, A., & Denker, M. (2023). Advancing health equity through artificial intelligence: Recommendations for policymakers. *Health Affairs*, 42(7), 112–120.

Lakshmi, G. N., Kumar, B. R., & Sekhar, A. C. (2011). A cryptographic scheme of Laplace transforms. *International Journal of Mathematical Archive*, 2, 2515–2519.

Lanza, C., Lahmadi, A., & François, J. (2024). *Ransomware Analysis: Knowledge Extraction and Classification for Advanced Cyber Threat Intelligence*. CRC Press. DOI: 10.1201/9781003528999

Lee, T., & Chen, Y. (2023). The role of AI in enhancing medical device cybersecurity. *International Journal of Medical Informatics*, 125, 23–30.

Lee, T., & Chen, Y. (2023). The Role of AI in Enhancing Medical Device Cybersecurity. *International Journal of Medical Informatics*, 125, 23–30.

Li, W., Tan, J., & Wang, Y. (2020). *A framework of blockchain-based collaborative intrusion detection in software defined networking*. Paper presented at the Network and System Security: 14th International Conference, NSS 2020, Melbourne, VIC, Australia, November 25–27, 2020, Proceedings 14. DOI: 10.1007/978-3-030-65745-1_15

Li, K., Cardoso, C., Moctezuma-Ramirez, A., Elgalad, A., & Perin, E. (2023). Heart Rate Variability Measurement through a Smart Wearable Device: Another Breakthrough for Personal Health Monitoring? *International Journal of Environmental Research and Public Health*, 20(24), 7146. DOI: 10.3390/ijerph20247146 PMID: 38131698

Lim, W. Y. B., Luong, N. C., Hoang, D. T., Jiao, Y., Liang, Y.-C., Yang, Q., Niyato, D., & Miao, C. (2020). Federated Learning in Mobile Edge Networks: A Comprehensive Survey. *IEEE Communications Surveys and Tutorials*, 22(3), 2031–2063. DOI: 10.1109/COMST.2020.2986024

Lipton, Z. C. (2018). The mythos of model interpretability. *Communications of the ACM*, 61(10), 36–43. DOI: 10.1145/3233231

Liu, H., Crespo, R. G., & Martínez, O. S. (2020). *Enhancing privacy and data security across healthcare applications using blockchain and distributed ledger concepts*. Paper presented at the Healthcare. DOI: 10.3390/healthcare8030243

Liu, Z., Zhang, J., Hou, Y., Zhang, X., Li, G., & Xiang, Y. (2022). *Machine learning for multimodal electronic health records-based research: Challenges and perspectives.* Paper presented at the China Health Information Processing Conference.

Liu, S., Wang, Z., Kumari, S., Lv, J., & Chen, C. M. (2024). Provably Secure Anti-Phishing Scheme for Medical Information in Smart Healthcare. *IEEE Internet of Things Journal*, 11(23), 38086–38097. DOI: 10.1109/JIOT.2024.3445375

Li, X., Hu, Y., Zeng, L., An, Y., Yang, J., & Xiao, X. (2024). Blockchain-based federated learning approaches in internet of things applications. *Security and Privacy*, 7(6), 435. DOI: 10.1002/spy2.435

Li, X., Lu, Y., Fu, X., & Qi, Y. (2021). Building the Internet of Things platform for smart maternal healthcare services with wearable devices and cloud computing. *Future Generation Computer Systems*, 118, 282–296. DOI: 10.1016/j.future.2021.01.016

Logeswaran, K., Savitha, S., Suresh, P., Prasanna Kumar, K. R., Gunasekar, M., Rajadevi, R., & Jayasurya, A. S. (2024). Unifying Technologies in Industry 4.0: Harnessing the Synergy of Internet of Things, Big Data, Augmented Reality/Virtual Reality, and Blockchain Technologies. *Topics in Artificial Intelligence Applied to Industry*, 4(0), 127–147. DOI: 10.1002/9781394216147.ch7

Logeswaran, K., Suresh, P., Savitha, S., Prasanna Kumar, K. R., Ponselvakumar, A. P., & Kannan, A. R. (2020). Data driven diagnosis of cervical cancer using association rule mining with trivial rule expulsion approach. *International Journal of Emerging Technologies*, 11(2), 110–115.

Lokmic-Tomkins, Z., Davies, S., Block, L. J., Cochrane, L., Dorin, A., von Gerich, H., Lozada-Perezmitre, E., Reid, L., & Peltonen, L.-M. (2022). Assessing the carbon footprint of digital health interventions: A scoping review. *Journal of the American Medical Informatics Association : JAMIA*, 29(12), 2128–2139. DOI: 10.1093/jamia/ocac196 PMID: 36314391

Lu, H. Y., Ding, X., Hirst, J. E., Yang, Y., Yang, J., MacKillop, L., & Clifton, D. A. (2024). Digital Health and Machine Learning Technologies for Blood Glucose Monitoring and Management of Gestational Diabetes. *IEEE Reviews in Biomedical Engineering*, 17, 98–117. DOI: 10.1109/RBME.2023.3242261 PMID: 37022834

Lu, Y., Huang, X., Dai, Y., Maharjan, S., & Zhang, Y. (2020). Federated learning for data privacy preservation in vehicular cyber-physical systems. *IEEE Network*, 34(3), 50–56. DOI: 10.1109/MNET.011.1900317

Lu, Y., Huang, X., Zhang, K., Maharjan, S., & Zhang, Y. (2020). Blockchain empowered asynchronous federated learning for secure data sharing in internet of vehicles. *IEEE Transactions on Vehicular Technology*, 69(4), 4298–4311. DOI: 10.1109/TVT.2020.2973651

Lu, Z., Pan, H., Dai, Y., Si, X., & Zhang, Y. (2024). Federated Learning with Non-IID Data: A Survey. *IEEE Internet of Things Journal*, 11(11), 19188–19209. DOI: 10.1109/JIOT.2024.3376548

Lyons, J. T., & Göçmen, T. (2021). Applied machine learning techniques for performance analysis in large wind farms. *Energies*, 14(13), 3756. DOI: 10.3390/en14133756

Lyu, L., Yu, H., Ma, X., Chen, C., Sun, L., Zhao, J., Yang, Q., & Yu, P. S. (2024). Privacy and Robustness in Federated Learning: Attacks and Defenses. *IEEE Transactions on Neural Networks and Learning Systems*, 35(7), 8726–8746. DOI: 10.1109/TNNLS.2022.3216981 PMID: 36355741

Madavarapu, J. B., Kasula, B. Y., Whig, P., & Kautish, S. (2024). AI-Powered Solutions Advancing UN Sustainable Development Goals: A Case Study in Tackling Humanity's Challenges. In *Digital Technologies to Implement the UN Sustainable Development Goals* (pp. 47–67). Springer Nature Switzerland. DOI: 10.1007/978-3-031-68427-2_3

Maddireddy, B. R., & Maddireddy, B. R. (2022). Real-Time Data Analytics with AI: Improving Security Event Monitoring and Management. *Unique Endeavor in Business & Social Sciences*, 1(2), 47–62.

Madhiarasan, M., & Louzazni, M. (2022). Analysis of artificial neural network: Architecture, types, and forecasting applications. *Journal of Electrical and Computer Engineering*, 2022, 2022. DOI: 10.1155/2022/5416722

Mahgoub, M. M. A. (2016). The new integral transform Mahgoub Transform. *Advances in Theoretical and Applied Mathematics*, 11(4), 391–398.

Majeed, U., & Hong, C. S. (2019). *FLchain: Federated learning via MEC-enabled blockchain network*. Paper presented at the 2019 20th Asia-Pacific Network Operations and Management Symposium (APNOMS).

Malallah, H. S., Qashi, R., Abdulrahman, L. M., Omer, M. A., & Yazdeen, A. A. (2023). Performance analysis of enterprise cloud computing: a review. *Journal of Applied Science and Technology Trends, 4*(01), 01-12.

Malik, H., & Anees, T. (2024). Federated Learning with Deep Convolutional Neural Networks for the Detection of Multiple Chest Diseases Using Chest X-Rays. *Multimedia Tools and Applications*, 83(23), 63017–63045. DOI: 10.1007/s11042-023-18065-z

Mallick, M. A. I., & Nath, R. (2024). Navigating the Cyber security Landscape: A Comprehensive Review of Cyber-Attacks, Emerging Trends, and Recent Developments. *World Scientific News*, 190(1), 1–69.

Mamdiwar, S. D., Shakruwala, Z., Chadha, U., Srinivasan, K., & Chang, C. Y. (2021). Recent advances on IoT-assisted wearable sensor systems for healthcare monitoring. *Biosensors (Basel)*, 11(10), 372. DOI: 10.3390/bios11100372 PMID: 34677328

Mandarino, V., Pappalardo, G., & Tramontana, E. (2024). A Blockchain-Based Electronic Health Record (EHR) System for Edge Computing Enhancing Security and Cost Efficiency. *Computers*, 13(6), 132. DOI: 10.3390/computers13060132

Manivannan, R. (2024). Improved restricted Boltzmann machine-based optimization model for the network security system in cloud environment. *Engineering Research Express*, 6(2), 025313. DOI: 10.1088/2631-8695/ad3f77

Manjula, V., Chillara, V. P. V., Rao, T. P. R. C., Varma, N. S. V. A., & Vulapalli, P. R. V. (2024). Cyber Threats and Vulnerabilities in Connected Medical Devices: A Review. Cybersecurity and Data Management Innovations for Revolutionizing Healthcare, 148-174.

Mansour, E. A., Kuffi, E. A., & Mehdi, S. A. (2022). Applying SEE integral transform in cryptography. [IOP Publishing.]. *Journal of Physics: Conference Series*, 2322(1), 012016.

Mansour, M., Darweesh, M. S., & Soltan, A. (2024). Wearable Devices for Glucose Monitoring: A Review of State-of-the-Art Technologies and Emerging Trends. *Alexandria Engineering Journal*, 89, 224–243. DOI: 10.1016/j.aej.2024.01.021

Martínez-Suárez, F., García-Limón, J. A., Baños-Bautista, J. E., Alvarado-Serrano, C., & Casas, O. (2023). Low-power long-term ambulatory electrocardiography monitor of three leads with beat-to-beat heart rate measurement in real time. *Sensors (Basel)*, 23(19), 8303. DOI: 10.3390/s23198303 PMID: 37837133

Mathew, U. O., Rodriguez, D. Z., Rosa, R. L., Ayub, M. S., & Adasme, P. (2024). *Advancing Healthcare 5.0 through Federated Learning: Opportunity for Security Enforcement using Blockchain.* Paper presented at the 2024 International Conference on Software, Telecommunications and Computer Networks (SoftCOM). DOI: 10.23919/SoftCOM62040.2024.10722012

Mathivanan, S. K., Shivahare, B. D., Chandan, R. R., & Shah, M. A. (2024). A comprehensive health assessment approach using ensemble deep learning model for remote patient monitoring with IoT. *Scientific Reports*, 14(1), 15661.

Mathur, P. (2024). Cloud computing infrastructure, platforms, and software for scientific research. *High Performance Computing in Biomimetics: Modeling, Architecture and Applications*, 89-127.

Matthew, U. O., Aderinola, M., Shuaibu, I., Kazaure, J. S., Ohabuiro, J., Daniel, O. O., & Nwamouh, U. C. (2023). Device to Device Communication Using Optimized Frequency Spectrum Reuse (OFSR) in Multi-Layered Cellular Network. *HAFED POLY Journal of Science. Management and Technology*, 5(2), 172–191.

Matthew, U. O., Asuni, O., & Fatai, L. O. (2024). *Green Software Engineering Development Paradigm: An Approach to a Sustainable Renewable Energy Future Advancing Software Engineering Through AI, Federated Learning, and Large Language Models*. IGI Global. DOI: 10.4018/979-8-3693-3502-4.ch018

Matthew, U. O., & Kazaure, J. S. (2021). Chemical polarization effects of electromagnetic field radiation from the novel 5G network deployment at ultra high frequency. *Health and Technology*, 11(2), 305–317. DOI: 10.1007/s12553-020-00501-x PMID: 33527067

Matthew, U. O., Kazaure, J. S., Amaonwu, O., Adamu, U. A., Hassan, I. M., Kazaure, A. A., & Ubochi, C. N. (2021). *Role of internet of health things (IoHTs) and innovative internet of 5G medical robotic things (IIo-5GMRTs) in COVID-19 global health risk management and logistics planning Intelligent Data Analysis for COVID-19 Pandemic*. Springer.

Matthew, U. O., Kazaure, J. S., John, O., & Haruna, K. (2021). Telecommunication Business Information System and Investment Ecosystem in a Growing Economy: A Review of Telecom Investment in Nigeria. [IJICTHD]. *International Journal of Information Communication Technologies and Human Development*, 13(2), 1–20. DOI: 10.4018/IJICTHD.2021040101

Matthew, U. O., Kazaure, J. S., & Okafor, N. U. (2021). Contemporary development in E-Learning education, cloud computing technology & internet of things. *EAI Endorsed Transactions on Cloud Systems*, 7(20), e3–e3.

Matthew, U. O., Kazaure, J. S., & Okochi, P. I. (2022). 5G Mid-Range Electromagnetic Spectrum Implementation for Critical Infrastructure Development: Electromagnetic Spectrum Sustainability. [IJITN]. *International Journal of Interdisciplinary Telecommunications and Networking*, 14(1), 1–26. DOI: 10.4018/IJITN.307103

Matthew, U. O., Onumaku, V. C., Fatai, L. O., Adekunle, T. S., Waliu, A. O., Nduk-wu, C. C., & Ebong, G. N. (2024). *E-Healthcare Data Warehouse Design and Data Mining Using ML Approach Reshaping Healthcare with Cutting-Edge Biomedical Advancements*. IGI Global.

Mavromatis, A., Colman-Meixner, C., Silva, A. P., Vasilakos, X., Nejabati, R., & Simeonidou, D. (2019). A software-defined IoT device management framework for edge and cloud computing. *IEEE Internet of Things Journal*, 7(3), 1718–1735. DOI: 10.1109/JIOT.2019.2949629

Mazhar, T., Irfan, H. M., Haq, I., Ullah, I., Ashraf, M., Shloul, T. A., Ghadi, Y. Y., Imran, , & Elkamchouchi, D. H. (2023). Analysis of Challenges and Solutions of IoT in Smart Grids Using AI and Machine Learning Techniques: A Review. *Electronics (Basel)*, 12(1), 242. DOI: 10.3390/electronics12010242

Mbatha, S. Z., Mulaudzi, T. V., Mbita, Z., Adeola, H. A., Batra, J., Blenman, K. R., & Dlamini, Z. (2023). *Artificial Intelligence–Enhanced Drug Discovery and the Achievement of Next-Generation Human-Centered Health System Society 5.0 and Next Generation Healthcare: Patient-Focused and Technology-Assisted Precision Therapies*. Springer.

McMahan, B.. (2017). Communication-efficient learning of deep networks from decentralized data. In *Artificial intelligence and statistics*. PMLR.

Mehrabi, N., Morstatter, F., Saxena, N., Lerman, K., & Galstyan, A. (2022). A Survey on Bias and Fairness in Machine Learning. *ACM Computing Surveys*, 54(6), 1–35. DOI: 10.1145/3457607

Meza, C., Juega, J., Francisco, J., Santos, A., Duran, L., Rodriguez, M., Alvarez-Sabin, J., Sero, L., Ustrell, X., Bashir, S., Serena, J., Silva, Y., Molina, C., & Pagola, J. (2023). Accuracy of a Smartwatch to Assess Heart Rate Monitoring and Atrial Fibrillation in Stroke Patients. *Sensors (Basel)*, 23(10), 4632. DOI: 10.3390/s23104632 PMID: 37430546

Miller, A. J., & Johnson, M. R. (2022). Blockchain applications in healthcare: Security and privacy implications. *Journal of Healthcare Information Management*, 36(4), 15–29.

Miller, A. J., & Johnson, M. R. (2022). Blockchain Applications in Healthcare: Security and Privacy Implications. *Journal of Healthcare Information Management*, 36(4), 15–29.

Mishra, V., Gupta, K., Saxena, D., & Singh, A. K. (2024). A Global Medical Data Security and Privacy Preserving Standards Identification Framework for Electronic Healthcare Consumers. *IEEE Transactions on Consumer Electronics*, 70(1), 4379–4387. DOI: 10.1109/TCE.2024.3373912

Mittal, S., Singh, P. K., Gochhait, S., Gaur, N., & Kumar, S. (2024). AI-Powered Clinical Trial Design With Translational Bioinformatics. In Khanna, A., & Gochhait, S. (Eds.), *Green AI-Powered Intelligent Systems for Disease Prognosis* (pp. 57–72). IGI Global Scientific Publishing., DOI: 10.4018/979-8-3693-1243-8.ch004

Möller, D. P. (2023). *Threats and threat intelligence Guide to Cybersecurity in Digital Transformation: Trends, Methods, Technologies, Applications and Best Practices*. Springer.

Molo, M. J., Badejo, J. A., Adetiba, E., Nzanzu, V. P., Noma-Osaghae, E., Oguntosin, V., Baraka, M. O., Takenga, C., Suraju, S., & Adebiyi, E. F. (2021). A Review of Evolutionary Trends in Cloud Computing and Applications to the Healthcare Ecosystem. *Applied Computational Intelligence and Soft Computing*, 2021(1), 1843671. DOI: 10.1155/2021/1843671

Motsi-Omoijiade, I., & Kharlamov, A. (2021). Blockchain for healthcare applications and use cases. In *Blockchain and Public Law* (pp. 157–190). Edward Elgar Publishing. DOI: 10.4337/9781839100796.00015

Mukhopadhyay, B., Bose, R., & Roy, S. (2020). A novel approach to load balancing and cloud computing security using SSL in IaaS environment. *International Journal (Toronto, Ont.)*, 9(2).

Mumuni, A., & Mumuni, F. (2021). CNN architectures for geometric transformation-invariant feature representation in computer vision: A review. *SN Computer Science*, 2(5), 340. DOI: 10.1007/s42979-021-00735-0

Nadella, G. S., Meduri, K., Gonaygunta, H., Addula, S. R., Satish, S., Harish, M., & Maturi, S. (2024). Advancing Edge Computing with Federated Deep Learning: Strategies and Challenges. *International Journal for Research in Applied Science and Engineering Technology*, 12(4), 3422–3434. DOI: 10.22214/ijraset.2024.60602

Nafea, A. A., Hamdi, M. M., saad Abdulhakeem, B., Shakir, A. T., Alsumaidaie, M. S. I., & Shaban, A. M. 2024, April. Detection Systems for Distributed Denial-of-Service DDoS Attack Based on Time Series: Review, A. In 2024 21st International Multi-Conference on Systems, Signals & Devices (SSD) (pp. 43-48). IEEE.

Nagendran, M., Chen, Y., Lovejoy, C. A., Gordon, A. C., Komorowski, M., Harvey, H., Topol, E. J., Ioannidis, J. P. A., Collins, G. S., & Maruthappu, M. (2020). Artificial intelligence versus clinicians: Systematic review of design, reporting standards, and claims of deep learning studies. *BMJ (Clinical Research Ed.)*, m689, m689. DOI: 10.1136/bmj.m689 PMID: 32213531

Nahavandi, D., Alizadehsani, R., Khosravi, A., & Rajendra Acharya, U. (2022). Application of Artificial Intelligence in Wearable Devices: Opportunities and Challenges. *Computer Methods and Programs in Biomedicine*, 213, 106541. DOI: 10.1016/j.cmpb.2021.106541 PMID: 34837860

Naik, K., Goyal, R. K., Foschini, L., Chak, C. W., Thielscher, C., Zhu, H., Lu, J., Lehár, J., Pacanoswki, M. A., Terranova, N., Mehta, N., Korsbo, N., Fakhouri, T., Liu, Q., & Gobburu, J. (2024). Current Status and Future Directions: The Application of Artificial Intelligence/Machine Learning for Precision Medicine. *Clinical Pharmacology and Therapeutics*, 115(4), 673–686. DOI: 10.1002/cpt.3152 PMID: 38103204

Nair, M. M., & Tyagi, A. K. (2023). *AI, IoT, blockchain, and cloud computing: The necessity of the future Distributed Computing to Blockchain*. Elsevier.

Naithani, K., Raiwani, Y. P., Tiwari, S., & Chauhan, A. S. (2024). Artificial Intelligence Techniques Based on Federated Learning in Smart Healthcare. In Federated Learning for Smart Communication Using IoT Application (pp. 81-108). Chapman and Hall/CRC.

Naithani, K., Raiwani, Y., Tiwari, S., & Chauhan, A. S. (2024). *Artificial Intelligence Techniques Based on Federated Learning in Smart Healthcare Federated Learning for Smart Communication using IoT Application*. Chapman and Hall/CRC.

Najjar, R. (2023). Redefining radiology: A review of artificial intelligence integration in medical imaging. *Diagnostics (Basel)*, 13(17), 2760.

Nasir, S., Khan, R. A., & Bai, S. (2024). Ethical framework for harnessing the power of AI in healthcare and beyond. *IEEE Access : Practical Innovations, Open Solutions*, 12, 31014–31035. DOI: 10.1109/ACCESS.2024.3369912

Nath, V. G., Bharath, S. P., Dsouza, A., & Subramanian, A. (2024). Machine Learning Algorithms for Smart Gas Sensor Arrays. *Nanostructured Materials for Electronic Nose*, 185-225.

National Institute of Standards and Technology. (2022). Framework for improving critical infrastructure cybersecurity. NIST Special Publication 800-53.

National Institute of Standards and Technology. (2022). Framework for Improving Critical Infrastructure Cybersecurity. NIST Special Publication 800-53.

Nazir, S., & Kaleem, M. (2023). Federated learning for medical image analysis with deep neural networks. *Diagnostics (Basel)*, 13(9), 1532.

Nekui, O. D., Wang, W., Liu, C., Wang, Z., & Ding, B. (2024). IoT-Based Heartbeat Rate-Monitoring Device Powered by Harvested Kinetic Energy. *Sensors (Basel)*, 24(13), 4249. DOI: 10.3390/s24134249 PMID: 39001027

Nifakos, S., Chandramouli, K., Nikolaou, C. K., Papachristou, P., Koch, S., Panaousis, E., & Bonacina, S. (2021). Influence of human factors on cyber security within healthcare organisations: A systematic review. *Sensors (Basel)*, 21(15), 5119. DOI: 10.3390/s21155119 PMID: 34372354

Ni, L., Huang, P., Wei, Y., Shu, M., & Zhang, J. (2021). Federated Learning Model with Adaptive Differential Privacy Protection in Medical IoT. *Wireless Communications and Mobile Computing*, 8967819(1), 8967819. DOI: 10.1155/2021/8967819

Nwanakwaugwu, A. C., Matthew, U. O., Kazaure, A. A., & Haruna, K. (2023). *Data Mining Business Intelligence Applications in Retail Services Using Artificial Neural Networks Handbook of Research on Cybersecurity Risk in Contemporary Business Systems*. IGI Global.

Obermeyer, Z., Powers, B., Vogeli, C., & Mullainathan, S. (2019). Dissecting racial bias in an algorithm used to manage the health of populations. *Science*, 366(6464), 447–453. DOI: 10.1126/science.aax2342 PMID: 31649194

Ogundokun, R. O., Misra, S., Maskeliunas, R., & Damasevicius, R. (2022). A review on federated learning and machine learning approaches: Categorization, application areas, and blockchain technology. *Information (Basel)*, 13(5), 263.

Ohalete, N. C., Aderibigbe, A. O., Ani, E. C., Ohenhen, P. E., Daraojimba, D. O., & Odulaja, B. A. (2023). AI-driven solutions in renewable energy: A review of data science applications in solar and wind energy optimization. *World Journal of Advanced Research and Reviews*, 20(3), 401–417.

Oh, S.-R., Seo, Y.-D., Lee, E., & Kim, Y.-G. (2021). A Comprehensive Survey on Security and Privacy for Electronic Health Data. *International Journal of Environmental Research and Public Health*, 18(18), 9668. DOI: 10.3390/ijerph18189668 PMID: 34574593

Okafor, C. M., Kolade, A., Onunka, T., Daraojimba, C., Eyo-Udo, N. L., Onunka, O., & Omotosho, A. (2023). Mitigating cybersecurity risks in the US healthcare sector. [IJRSI]. *International Journal of Research and Scientific Innovation*, 10(9), 177–193.

Okafor, N., Ingle, R., Matthew, U., Saunders, M., & Delaney, D. (2024). Assessing and Improving IoT Sensor Data Quality in Environmental Monitoring Networks: A Focus on Peatlands. *IEEE Internet of Things Journal*, 11(24), 40727–40742. DOI: 10.1109/JIOT.2024.3454241

Omidian, H. (2024). Synergizing blockchain and artificial intelligence to enhance healthcare. *Drug Discovery Today*, 29(9), 104111. DOI: 10.1016/j.drudis.2024.104111 PMID: 39034026

Onyebuchi, A., Matthew, U. O., Kazaure, J. S., Nwanagwaugwu, A. C., Nwamouh, U. C., & Adamu, U. A. (2022). Cloud based IoT Electronic Healthcare Data Warehouse Integration in emerging 5G Health Grid Ecosystem.

Onyebuchi, A., Matthew, U. O., Kazaure, J. S., Ebong, G. N., Ndukwu, C. C., Nwanakwaugwu, A. C., & Okey, O. D. (2024). *Cloud-Based IoT Data Warehousing Technology for E-Healthcare: A Comprehensive Guide to E-Health Grids Pioneering Smart Healthcare 5.0 with IoT, Federated Learning, and Cloud Security*. IGI Global.

Onyebuchi, A., Matthew, U. O., Kazaure, J. S., Okafor, N. U., Okey, O. D., Okochi, P. I., Taiwo, J. F., & Matthew, A. O. (2022). Business demand for a cloud enterprise data warehouse in electronic healthcare computing: Issues and developments in e-healthcare cloud computing. [IJCAC]. *International Journal of Cloud Applications and Computing*, 12(1), 1–22. DOI: 10.4018/IJCAC.297098

Ouadrhiri, A. E., & Abdelhadi, A. (2022). Differential Privacy for Deep and Federated Learning: A Survey. *IEEE Access : Practical Innovations, Open Solutions*, 10, 22359–22380. DOI: 10.1109/ACCESS.2022.3151670

Oyekunle, D. O. T., Okwudili Matthew, U., Preston, D., & Boohene, D. (2024). Trust beyond technology algorithms: A theoretical exploration of consumer trust and behavior in technological consumption and AI projects. *Journal of Computer and Communications, 12*(06), 10.4236.

Oyekunle, D. O., Esseme, A. C. B., Oladipupo, M. A., Oseni, V. E., Adebola, N. T., Nwaiku, M., & Matthew, U. O. (2025). *Artificial Neural Network Algorithm in Nutritional Assessment: Implication for Machine Learning Prediction in Nutritional Assessments Precision Health in the Digital Age: Harnessing AI for Personalized Care*. IGI Global Scientific Publishing.

Oyinloye, T. S., Arowolo, M. O., & Prasad, R. (2024). *Enhancing Cyber Threat Detection with an Improved Artificial Neural Network Model*. Data Science and Management.

Padmaja, K., & Seshadri, R. (2021). A real-time secure medical device authentication for personal E-Healthcare services on cloud computing. *International Journal of System Assurance Engineering and Management*, •••, 1–11. DOI: 10.1007/s13198-021-01148-1

Palakurti, N. R. (2024). Challenges and future directions in anomaly detection. In *Practical Applications of Data Processing, Algorithms, and Modeling* (pp. 269–284). IGI Global. DOI: 10.4018/979-8-3693-2909-2.ch020

Panch, T., Mattie, H., & Celi, L. A. (2023). The role of artificial intelligence in healthcare: A review of ethical and practical considerations. *The New England Journal of Medicine*, 389(2), 138–148.

Panimalar, S., & Gunasundari, S. (2023). *A survey based on privacy-preserving over health care data analysis.* Paper presented at the International Conference on Emerging Trends in Expert Applications & Security. DOI: 10.1007/978-981-99-1946-8_40

Pansara, R. R., Kasula, B. Y., Bhatia, A. B., & Whig, P. (2024, April). Enhancing Sustainable Development Through Machine Learning-Driven Master Data Management. In *International Conference on Sustainable Development through Machine Learning, AI and IoT* (pp. 332-341). Cham: Springer Nature Switzerland.

Pappas, H., & Frisch, P. (2022). *Leveraging technology as a response to the COVID pandemic: Adapting diverse technologies, workflow, and processes to optimize integrated clinical management*. CRC Press.

Park, J., & Lim, H. (2022). Privacy-preserving federated learning using homomorphic encryption. *Applied Sciences (Basel, Switzerland)*, 12(2), 734.

Patel, V., Kahn, C., Borovick, S., Denny, J., Kittner, S., & Kettler, J. (2023). Addressing inequities in AI applications in health care: Perspectives and strategies. *Journal of Health Policy*, 27(4), 504–512. https://doi.org/10.1016/j.jhe.2023.05.001

Pathan, A.-M. K., & Buyya, R. (2007). A taxonomy and survey of content delivery networks. *Grid computing and distributed systems laboratory, University of Melbourne. Technical Report*, 4, 70.

Patil, R. Y., Patil, Y. H., & Bannore, A. (2024). *Cybersecurity in medical Internet of Things: Issues, challenges, and future directions Security Implementation in Internet of Medical Things*. CRC Press.

Pengel, L. K., Robbers-Visser, D., Groenink, M., Winter, M. M., Schuuring, M. J., Bouma, B. J., & Bokma, J. P. (2023). A comparison of ECG-based home monitoring devices in adults with CHD. *Cardiology in the Young*, 33(7), 1129–1135. DOI: 10.1017/S1047951122002244 PMID: 35844104

Pfeifer, G. P., & Jin, S. G. (2024). Methods and Applications of Genome-Wide Profiling of DNA Damage and Rare Mutations. *Nature Reviews. Genetics*, 2024(12), 1–18. DOI: 10.1038/s41576-024-00748-4 PMID: 38918545

Pfohl, S. R., Dai, Y., & Ding, D. Y. (2021). Creating fair models of atrial fibrillation detection in diverse populations. *Nature Medicine*, 27(9), 1526–1534.

Phelan, J. C., & Link, B. G. (2015). Is racism a fundamental cause of inequalities in health? *Annual Review of Sociology*, 41(1), 311–330. DOI: 10.1146/annurev-soc-073014-112305

Platt, M., & McBurney, P. (2023). Sybil in the haystack: A comprehensive review of blockchain consensus mechanisms in search of strong Sybil attack resistance. *Algorithms*, 16(1), 34. DOI: 10.3390/a16010034

Prasad, V. K., Tanwar, S., & Bhavsar, M. D. (2021). Advance cloud data analytics for 5G enabled IoT. *Blockchain for 5G-Enabled IoT: The new wave for Industrial Automation*, 159-180.

Prasad, V. K., Bhattacharya, P., Maru, D., Tanwar, S., Verma, A., Singh, A., & Raboaca, M. S. (2022). Federated learning for the internet-of-medical-things: A survey. *Mathematics*, 11(1), 151.

Praseed, A., & Thilagam, P. S. (2022). HTTP request pattern based signatures for early application layer DDoS detection: A firewall agnostic approach. *Journal of Information Security and Applications*, 65, 103090. DOI: 10.1016/j.jisa.2021.103090

Price, W. N.II, & Cohen, I. G. (2019). Privacy in the age of medical big data. *Nature Medicine*, 25(1), 37–43. DOI: 10.1038/s41591-018-0272-7 PMID: 30617331

Pritee, Z. T., Anik, M. H., Alam, S. B., Jim, J. R., Kabir, M. M., & Mridha, M. F. (2024). Machine learning and deep learning for user authentication and authorization in cybersecurity: A state-of-the-art review. *Computers & Security*, 140, 103747. DOI: 10.1016/j.cose.2024.103747

Putra, K. T., Arrayyan, A. Z., Hayati, N., Damarjati, C., Bakar, A., & Chen, H. C. (2024). A Review on the Application of Internet of Medical Things in Wearable Personal Health Monitoring: A Cloud-Edge Artificial Intelligence Approach. *IEEE Access : Practical Innovations, Open Solutions*, 12, 21437–21452. DOI: 10.1109/ACCESS.2024.3358827

Qasem, A. A., Qutqut, M. H., Alhaj, F., & Kitana, A. (2024). SRFE: A stepwise recursive feature elimination approach for network intrusion detection systems. *Peer-to-Peer Networking and Applications*, 17(6), 3634–3649. DOI: 10.1007/s12083-024-01763-2

Qi, P., Chiaro, D., Guzzo, A., Ianni, M., Fortino, G., & Piccialli, F. (2024). Model Aggregation Techniques in Federated Learning: A Comprehensive Survey. *Future Generation Computer Systems*, 150, 272–293. DOI: 10.1016/j.future.2023.09.008

Radhakrishnan, L., Schenk, G., Muenzen, K., Oskotsky, B., Ashouri Choshali, H., Plunkett, T., Israni, S., & Butte, A. J. (2023). A certified de-identification system for all clinical text documents for information extraction at scale. *JAMIA Open*, 6(3), ooad045. DOI: 10.1093/jamiaopen/ooad045 PMID: 37416449

Raghavan, M., & Barocas, S.. (2020). Mitigating bias in algorithmic hiring: Evaluating claims and practices. *Proceedings of the 2020 Conference on Fairness, Accountability, and Transparency (FAT)*. DOI: 10.1145/3351095.3372828

Rahman, A., Hossain, M. S., Muhammad, G., Kundu, D., Debnath, T., Rahman, M., & Band, S. S. (2023). Federated learning-based AI approaches in smart healthcare: Concepts, taxonomies, challenges and open issues. *Cluster Computing*, 26(4), 2271–2311.

Rahman, M. H., Hossan, K. M. R., Uddin, M. K. S., & Hossain, M. D. (2024). Improving Collaborative Interactions Between Humans and Artificial Intelligence to Achieve Optimal Patient Outcomes in the Healthcare Industry. *Available atSSRN* 5029975. DOI: 10.2139/ssrn.5029975

Rahman, Z., Yi, X., & Khalil, I. (2022). Blockchain-based AI-enabled industry 4.0 CPS protection against advanced persistent threat. *IEEE Internet of Things Journal*, 10(8), 6769–6778. DOI: 10.1109/JIOT.2022.3147186

Rahnasto, J. (2023). Genetic data are not always personal—Disaggregating the identifiability and sensitivity of genetic data. *Journal of Law and the Biosciences*, 10(2), lsad029. DOI: 10.1093/jlb/lsad029 PMID: 38023689

Rai, N., Badrinath, A., Kamath, A., Kumar, V. A., & Gatti, R. R. (2024). *Security Challenges of IoT-Enabled Vehicular Communications and Their Countermeasures Communication Technologies and Security Challenges in IoT: Present and Future*. Springer.

Raji, I. D., & Buolamwini, J. (2019). Actionable auditing: Investigating the impact of publicly naming biased performance results of commercial AI products. In *Proceedings of the 2019 Conference on Fairness, Accountability, and Transparency* (pp. 1-12). DOI: 10.1145/3306618.3314244

Rajkomar, A., Hardt, M., Howell, M. D., Corrado, G., & Chin, M. H. (2018). Ensuring fairness in machine learning to advance health equity. *Annals of Internal Medicine*, 169(12), 866–872. DOI: 10.7326/M18-1990 PMID: 30508424

Rajput, A. R., Li, Q., & Ahvanooey, M. T. (2021). A Blockchain-Based Secret-Data Sharing Framework for Personal Health Records in Emergency Condition. *Healthcare (Basel)*, 9(2), 206. DOI: 10.3390/healthcare9020206 PMID: 33672991

Rani, S., Kataria, A., Kumar, S., & Tiwari, P. (2023). Federated Learning for Secure IoMT-Applications in Smart Healthcare Systems: A Comprehensive Review. *Knowledge-Based Systems*, 274, 110658. DOI: 10.1016/j.knosys.2023.110658

Rani, S., & Srivastava, G. (2024). Secure hierarchical fog computing-based architecture for industry 5.0 using an attribute-based encryption scheme. *Expert Systems with Applications*, 235, 121180. DOI: 10.1016/j.eswa.2023.121180

Ranjan, J., & Foropon, C. (2021). Big data analytics in building the competitive intelligence of organizations. *International Journal of Information Management*, 56, 102231. DOI: 10.1016/j.ijinfomgt.2020.102231

Ranjan, R., & Ch, B. (2024). A comprehensive roadmap for transforming healthcare from hospital-centric to patient-centric through healthcare internet of things (IoT). *Engineering and Science*, 30, 1175. DOI: 10.30919/es1175

Ratta, P., & Sharma, S. (2024). A blockchain-machine learning ecosystem for IoT-Based remote health monitoring of diabetic patients. *Healthcare Analytics*, 5, 100338. DOI: 10.1016/j.health.2024.100338

Raul, A. C. (2021). *The privacy, data protection and cybersecurity law review*. Law Business Research Limited.

Rauniyar, A., Hagos, D. H., Jha, D., Håkegård, J. E., Bagci, U., Rawat, D. B., & Vlassov, V. (2023). Federated learning for medical applications: A taxonomy, current trends, challenges, and future research directions. *IEEE Internet of Things Journal*.

Rauniyar, A., Hagos, D. H., Jha, D., Hakegard, J. E., Bagci, U., Rawat, D. B., & Vlassov, V. (2024). Federated Learning for Medical Applications: A Taxonomy, Current Trends, Challenges, and Future Research Directions. *IEEE Internet of Things Journal*, 11(5), 7374–7398. DOI: 10.1109/JIOT.2023.3329061

Reegu, F. A., Abas, H., Gulzar, Y., Xin, Q., Alwan, A. A., Jabbari, A., Sonkamble, R. G., & Dziyauddin, R. A. (2023). Blockchain-based framework for interoperable electronic health records for an improved healthcare system. *Sustainability (Basel)*, 15(8), 6337. DOI: 10.3390/su15086337

Ressi, D., Romanello, R., Piazza, C., & Rossi, S. (2024). AI-enhanced blockchain technology: A review of advancements and opportunities. *Journal of Network and Computer Applications*, 225, 103858. DOI: 10.1016/j.jnca.2024.103858

Rezayi, S., & Sharareh, R. (2022). Niakan Kalhori, and Soheila Saeedi. 2022. "Effectiveness of Artificial Intelligence for Personalized Medicine in Neoplasms: A Systematic Review.". *BioMed Research International*, 7842566(1), 7842566. DOI: 10.1155/2022/7842566 PMID: 35434134

Rieke, N., Hancox, J., Li, W., Milletari, F., Roth, H. R., Albarqouni, S., & Cardoso, M. J. (2020). The future of digital health with federated learning. *NPJ Digital Medicine*, 3(1), 1–7.

Rimal, B. P., & Choi, E. (2012). A service-oriented taxonomical spectrum, cloudy challenges and opportunities of cloud computing. *International Journal of Communication Systems*, 25(6), 796–819. DOI: 10.1002/dac.1279

Robert, L. (2023). AI-Driven Identity Access Management for Advanced Data Loss Prevention in Pharmaceutical Industries.

Roberts, K. E., & Martinez, S. (2023). Emerging trends in cybersecurity for healthcare systems. *Journal of Cybersecurity Research*, 18(1), 88–102.

Roberts, K. E., & Martinez, S. (2023). Emerging Trends in Cybersecurity for Healthcare Systems. *Journal of Cybersecurity Research*, 18(1), 88–102.

Romano, V., & Etim-Andy, M. (2023). An Examination of WHOOP Fitness Band Usage in College Athletics. *Journal of Coaching and Sports Science*, 2(2), 46–52. DOI: 10.58524/jcss.v2i2.220

Rosan, K. H. (2012). *Discrete mathematics and its applications*. McGraw Hill.

Saba Raoof, S., & Durai, M. (2022). A comprehensive review on smart health care: Applications, paradigms, and challenges with case studies. *Contrast Media & Molecular Imaging*, 2022(1), 2022. DOI: 10.1155/2022/4822235 PMID: 36247859

Sachin, D. N., Annappa, B., Ambasange, S., & Tony, A. E. (2023). A Multimodal Contrastive Federated Learning for Digital Healthcare. *SN Computer Science*, 4(5), 1–12. DOI: 10.1007/s42979-023-02124-1

Sachin, D. N., Annappa, B., & Ambesange, S. (2024). Federated Learning for Digital Healthcare: Concepts, Applications, Frameworks, and Challenges. *Computing*, 106(9), 3113–3150. DOI: 10.1007/s00607-024-01317-7

Sadhu, P. K., Yanambaka, V. P., & Abdelgawad, A. (2022). Internet of things: Security and solutions survey. *Sensors (Basel)*, 22(19), 7433. DOI: 10.3390/s22197433 PMID: 36236531

Saeed, H., Malik, H., Bashir, U., Ahmad, A., Riaz, S., Ilyas, M., & Khan, M. I. A. (2022). Blockchain technology in healthcare: A systematic review. *PLoS One*, 17(4), e0266462. DOI: 10.1371/journal.pone.0266462 PMID: 35404955

Saeed, S., Suayyid, S. A., Al-Ghamdi, M. S., Al-Muhaisen, H., & Almuhaideb, A. M. (2023). A systematic literature review on cyber threat intelligence for organizational cybersecurity resilience. *Sensors (Basel)*, 23(16), 7273. DOI: 10.3390/s23167273 PMID: 37631808

Saharan, S., & Gupta, V. (2024). Prevention of DDoS attacks: a comprehensive review and future directions. *Information Security Journal: A Global Perspective*, 1-33.

Sahu, M., Gupta, R., Ambasta, R. K., & Kumar, P. (2022). Artificial intelligence and machine learning in precision medicine: A paradigm shift in big data analysis. *Progress in Molecular Biology and Translational Science*, 190(1), 57–100. DOI: 10.1016/bs.pmbts.2022.03.002 PMID: 36008002

Sáinz-Pardo Díaz, J., & López García, Á. (2023). Study of the Performance and Scalability of Federated Learning for Medical Imaging with Intermittent Clients. *Neurocomputing*, 518, 142–154. DOI: 10.1016/j.neucom.2022.11.011

Salama, R., Al-Turjman, F., Chaudhary, P., & Yadav, S. P. (2023, April). (Benefits of Internet of Things (IoT) Applications in Health care-An Overview). In *2023 International Conference on Computational Intelligence, Communication Technology and Networking (CICTN)* (pp. 778-784). IEEE. DOI: 10.1109/CICTN57981.2023.10141452

Salim, S. J., & Ashruji, M. G. (2016). Application of Elzaki Transform in cryptography. *International Journal of Modern Sciences and Engineering Technology*, 3(3), 46–48.

Sallman, N. K. (2024). Integral transform of three parameters with its applications. *Kurdish Studies*, 12(1), 3743–3752.

Saminathan, K., Mulka, S. T. R., Damodharan, S., Maheswar, R., & Lorincz, J. (2023). An Artificial Neural Network Autoencoder for Insider Cyber Security Threat Detection. *Future Internet*, 15(12), 373. DOI: 10.3390/fi15120373

Samuel, A. L. (1959). Some Studies in Machine Learning Using the Game of Checkers. *IBM Journal of Research and Development*, 3(3), 210–229. DOI: 10.1147/rd.33.0210

Sandhu, S. S., Gorji, H. T., Tavakolian, P., Tavakolian, K., & Akhbardeh, A. (2023). Medical Imaging Applications of Federated Learning. *Diagnostics (Basel)*, 13(19), 3140.

Sardi, A., Rizzi, A., Sorano, E., & Guerrieri, A. (2020). Cyber risk in health facilities: A systematic literature review. *Sustainability (Basel)*, 12(17), 7002. DOI: 10.3390/su12177002

Sari, A., & Sopuru, J. (2021). E-Health Threat Intelligence Within Cyber-Defence Framework for E-Health Organizations. *Smart Systems for E-Health: WBAN Technologies, Security and Applications*, 161-179.

Savitha, S., Kannan, R., & Logeswaran, K. (2022). A Comprehensive Analysis of Machine Learning Algorithms in Diagnosis of Chronic Kidney Disease. In *2022 13th International Conference on Computing Communication and Networking Technologies (ICCCNT)* (pp. 1-5). IEEE.

Savitha, S., Sangana, C., Devendran, K., Pravin, L., Rajkumar, M., & Nirmal, C. (2023, February). Auto scaling infrastructure with monitoring tools using linux server on cloud. In 2023 7th International Conference on Computing Methodologies and Communication (ICCMC) (pp. 45-52). IEEE.

Savitha, S., & Rajiv Kannan, A. (2023). A novel technique based on mutual information weighted feature selection to predict chronic kidney disease. *Journal of Intelligent & Fuzzy Systems*, 45(1), 491–504. DOI: 10.3233/JIFS-222401

Schuurmans, A. A., De Looff, P., Nijhof, K. S., Rosada, C., Scholte, R. H., Popma, A., & Otten, R. (2020). Validity of the Empatica E4 wristband to measure heart rate variability (HRV) parameters: A comparison to electrocardiography (ECG). *Journal of Medical Systems*, 44(11), 1–11. DOI: 10.1007/s10916-020-01648-w PMID: 32965570

Sefati, S. S., & Halunga, S. (2023). Ultra-reliability and low-latency communications on the internet of things based on 5G network: Literature review, classification, and future research view. *Transactions on Emerging Telecommunications Technologies*, 34(6), e4770. DOI: 10.1002/ett.4770

Selvan, M. A. (2024). SVM-Enhanced Intrusion Detection System for Effective Cyber Attack Identification and Mitigation.

Sengan, S., Kamalam, G., Vellingiri, J., Gopal, J., Velayutham, P., & Subramaniyaswamy, V. (2020). Medical information retrieval systems for e-Health care records using fuzzy based machine learning model. *Microprocessors and Microsystems*, •••, 103344.

Sequeiros, J. B., Chimuco, F. T., Samaila, M. G., Freire, M. M., & Inácio, P. R. (2020). Attack and system modeling applied to IoT, cloud, and mobile ecosystems: Embedding security by design. *ACM Computing Surveys*, 53(2), 1–32. DOI: 10.1145/3376123

Setitra, M. A., Fan, M., & Bensalem, Z. E. A. (2023). An efficient approach to detect distributed denial of service attacks for software defined internet of things combining autoencoder and extreme gradient boosting with feature selection and hyperparameter tuning optimization. *Transactions on Emerging Telecommunications Technologies*, 34(9), e4827. DOI: 10.1002/ett.4827

Shaar, F., & Efe, A. (2018). DDoS attacks and impacts on various cloud computing components. *International Journal of Information Security Science*, 7(1), 26–48.

Shafiq, S., Rahman, M. S., Shaon, S. A., Mahmud, I., & Hosen, A. S. (2024). A Review on Software-Defined Networking for Internet of Things Inclusive of Distributed Computing, Blockchain, and Mobile Network Technology: Basics, Trends, Challenges, and Future Research Potentials. *International Journal of Distributed Sensor Networks*, 2024(1), 9006405. DOI: 10.1155/2024/9006405

Sharma, V., Singh, A., Saxena, A. K., & Saxena, V. (2023, December). A Logistic Regression Based Credit Risk Assessment Using WoE Bining and Enhanced Feature Engineering Approach ANOVA and Chi-Square. In 2023 12th International Conference on System Modeling & Advancement in Research Trends (SMART) (pp. 499-507). IEEE. DOI: 10.1109/SMART59791.2023.10428399

Sheikh, A., Anderson, M., Albala, S., Casadei, B., Franklin, B. D., Richards, M., Taylor, D., Tibble, H., & Mossialos, E. (2021). Health Information Technology and Digital Innovation for National Learning Health and Care Systems. *The Lancet. Digital Health*, 3(6), e383–e396. DOI: 10.1016/S2589-7500(21)00005-4 PMID: 33967002

Sheller, M. J., Edwards, B., Reina, G. A., Martin, J., Pati, S., Kotrotsou, A., & Colen, R. R. (2020). Federated learning in medicine: Facilitating multi-institutional collaborations without sharing patient data. *Scientific Reports*, 10(1), 12598. DOI: 10.1038/s41598-020-69250-1 PMID: 32724046

Shetty, R. S., & Shetty, R. S. (2021). 5G NSA Design and Deployment Strategy. *5G Mobile Core Network: Design, Deployment, Automation, and Testing Strategies*, 103-165.

Shrimali, R. (2020). How IoT is transforming the healthcare industry. Embedded Computing Design, Volansys LLC (accessed May 5, 2021) available at: https:// www. embeddedcomputing. com/application/healthcare/telehealth-healthcare-iot/ how-iot-is-transforming-the-healthcare-industry

Shrivastava, V., & Chaturvedi, A. K. (2024). A review on intrusion detection system for distributed network based on Machine Learning. *Journal of Integrated Science and Technology*, 12(2), 739–739.

Shukla, P., Krishna, C. R., & Patil, N. V. (2024). Iot traffic-based DDoS attacks detection mechanisms: A comprehensive review. *The Journal of Supercomputing*, 80(7), 9986–10043. DOI: 10.1007/s11227-023-05843-7

Silva, I., & Soto, M. (2022). Privacy-Preserving Data Sharing in Healthcare: An In-Depth Analysis of Big Data Solutions and Regulatory Compliance. *International Journal of Applied Health Care Analytics*, 7(1), 14–23.

Singh, B., & Kaunert, C. *(2024).Reinventing Artificial Intelligence and Blockchain for Preserving Medical Data.In Ethical Artificial Intelligence in Power Electronics (pp. 77-91).* CRC Press. DOI: 10.1201/9781032648323-6

Singh, L., & Singh, R. (2024). Comparative Analysis of Traditional Firewalls and Next-Generation Firewalls: A Review. Latest Trends in Engineering and Technology, 15-27.

Singh, O., Yadav, M., Yadav, P., & Rishiwal, V. (2021). AI-Based Renewable Energy with Emerging Applications: Issues and Challenges. In Introduction to AI Techniques for Renewable Energy System (pp. 29-42). CRC Press.

Singha, A., & Singhb, K. K. (2023). FedDDR: A Federated Improved DenseNet for Classification of Diabetic Retinopathy. Proceedings http://ceur-ws. org ISSN, 1613, 0073.

Singh, K., & Law, M. K. (2023). A Novel Enhanced Hybrid Clinical Decision Support System for Accurate Breast Cancer Prediction. *Measurement*, 221, 113525. DOI: 10.1016/j.measurement.2023.113525

Smith, R. L., & Thompson, J. (2023). Risk management in healthcare cybersecurity: Best practices and future directions. *Journal of Healthcare Risk Management*, 41(2), 72–85.

Smith, R. L., & Thompson, J. (2023). Risk Management in Healthcare Cybersecurity: Best Practices and Future Directions. *Journal of Healthcare Risk Management*, 41(2), 72–85.

Snehi, M., & Bhandari, A. (2021). Vulnerability retrospection of security solutions for software-defined Cyber–Physical System against DDoS and IoT-DDoS attacks. *Computer Science Review*, 40, 100371. DOI: 10.1016/j.cosrev.2021.100371

Song, H., Sui, S., Han, Q., Zhang, H., & Yang, Z. (2020). Autoregressive Integrated Moving Average Model–Based Secure Data Aggregation for Wireless Sensor Networks. *International Journal of Distributed Sensor Networks*, 16(3). Advance online publication. DOI: 10.1177/1550147720912958

Song, J., Wang, W., Gadekallu, T. R., Cao, J., & Liu, Y. (2023). EPPDA: An Efficient Privacy-Preserving Data Aggregation Federated Learning Scheme. *IEEE Transactions on Network Science and Engineering*, 10(5), 3047–3057. DOI: 10.1109/TNSE.2022.3153519

Soni, D., & Kumar, N. (2022). Machine learning techniques in emerging cloud computing integrated paradigms: A survey and taxonomy. *Journal of Network and Computer Applications*, 205, 103419. DOI: 10.1016/j.jnca.2022.103419

Sotthiwat, E., Zhen, L., Li, Z., & Zhang, C. (2021, May). Partially encrypted multi-party computation for federated learning. In 2021 IEEE/ACM 21st International Symposium on Cluster, Cloud and Internet Computing (CCGrid) (pp. 828-835). IEEE.

Sree, K. S., Karthik, J., Niharika, C., Srinivas, P. V. V. S., Ravinder, N., & Prasad, C. (2021, November). Optimized conversion of categorical and numerical features in machine learning models. In 2021 Fifth International Conference on I-SMAC (IoT in Social, Mobile, Analytics and Cloud)(I-SMAC) (pp. 294-299). IEEE.

Srinivas, V., & Jayanthi, C. H. (2020). Application of the new Integral "J-transform" in cryptography. *International Journal of Emering Technologies*, 11(2), 678–682.

Stallings, W. (2005). *Cryptography and network security* (4th ed.). Prentice Hall.

Stanoyevitch, A. (2002). *Introduction to cryptography with mathematical foundations and computer implementations*. CRC Press.

Strubell, E., Ganesh, A., & McCallum, A. (2020, April). Energy and policy considerations for modern deep learning research. *Proceedings of the AAAI Conference on Artificial Intelligence*, 34(09), 13693–13696.

Sufyan, A., Khan, K. B., Khashan, O. A., Mir, T., & Mir, U. (2023). From 5G to beyond 5G: A comprehensive survey of Wireless network evolution, challenges, and promising technologies. *Electronics (Basel)*, 12(10), 2200. DOI: 10.3390/electronics12102200

Suleski, T., Ahmed, M., Yang, W., & Wang, E. (2023). A review of multi-factor authentication in the Internet of Healthcare Things. *Digital Health*, 9, 20552076231177144. DOI: 10.1177/20552076231177144 PMID: 37252257

Sun, J., & Xia, Y. (2024). Pretreating and normalizing metabolomics data for statistical analysis. *Genes & Diseases*, 11(3), 100979. DOI: 10.1016/j.gendis.2023.04.018 PMID: 38299197

Sun, Y., Li, J., Xu, Y., Zhang, T., & Wang, X. (2023). Deep learning versus conventional methods for missing data imputation: A review and comparative study. *Expert Systems with Applications*, 227, 120201. DOI: 10.1016/j.eswa.2023.120201

Supriya, Y., & Gadekallu, T. R. (2023). A survey on soft computing techniques for federated learning-applications, challenges and future directions. *ACM Journal of Data and Information Quality*, 15(2), 1–28. DOI: 10.1145/3575810

Syed, K., Sleeman, W. C., Nalluri, J. J., Kapoor, R., Hagan, M., Palta, J., & Ghosh, P. (2020). Artificial intelligence methods in computer-aided diagnostic tools and decision support analytics for clinical informatics. In *Artificial Intelligence in Precision Health* (pp. 31–59). Elsevier., DOI: 10.1016/B978-0-12-817133-2.00002-1

Szalados, J. E. (2021). Medical Records and Confidentiality: Evolving Liability Issues Inherent in the Electronic Health Record, HIPAA, and Cybersecurity. *The Medical-Legal Aspects of Acute Care Medicine: A Resource for Clinicians, Administrators, and Risk Managers*, 315-342.

Tabaa, M., Monteiro, F., Bensag, H., & Dandache, A. (2020). Green Industrial Internet of Things from a smart industry perspectives. *Energy Reports*, 6, 430–446. DOI: 10.1016/j.egyr.2020.09.022

Tagde, P., Tagde, S., Bhattacharya, T., Tagde, P., Chopra, H., Akter, R., Kaushik, D., & Rahman, M. H. (2021). Blockchain and artificial intelligence technology in e-Health. *Environmental Science and Pollution Research International*, 28(38), 52810–52831. DOI: 10.1007/s11356-021-16223-0 PMID: 34476701

Taha, Z. K., Yaw, C. T., Koh, S. P., Tiong, S. K., Kadirgama, K., Benedict, F., Jian, D. T., & Balasubramaniam, Y. A. L. (2023). A Survey of Federated Learning From Data Perspective in the Healthcare Domain: Challenges, Methods, and Future Directions. *IEEE Access : Practical Innovations, Open Solutions*, 11, 45711–45735. DOI: 10.1109/ACCESS.2023.3267964

Tange, K., De Donno, M., Fafoutis, X., & Dragoni, N. (2020). A systematic survey of industrial Internet of Things security: Requirements and fog computing opportunities. *IEEE Communications Surveys and Tutorials*, 22(4), 2489–2520. DOI: 10.1109/COMST.2020.3011208

Thakur, S., Chao, P. C. P., & Tsai, C. H. (2023). Precision Heart Rate Estimation Using a PPG Sensor Patch Equipped with New Algorithms of Pre-Quality Checking and Hankel Decomposition. *Sensors (Basel)*, 23(13), 6180. DOI: 10.3390/s23136180 PMID: 37448029

Töberg, J. P. (2022). Modelling and Enforcing Access Control Requirements for Smart Contracts (Doctoral dissertation, Karlsruher Institut für Technologie (KIT)).

Tran, A. T., Luong, T.-D., Karnjana, J., & Huynh, V.-N. (2021). An Efficient Approach for Privacy Preserving Decentralized Deep Learning Models Based on Secure Multi-Party Computation. *Neurocomputing*, 422, 245–262. DOI: 10.1016/j.neucom.2020.10.014

Turner, R. J. (2007). Book review. *Journal of Minimally Invasive Gynecology*, 14(6), 776. DOI: 10.1016/j.jmig.2007.07.001

Tyagi, V., Saraswat, A., & Bansal, S. (2023). An Analysis of Securing Internet of Things (IoT) Devices from Man-in-the-Middle (MIMA) and Denial of Service (DoS). In Smart Cities (pp. 337-357). CRC Press.

U.S. Food and Drug Administration. (2021). *Cybersecurity for medical devices: FDA's role in improving device security*. FDA Guidance Document.

U.S. Food and Drug Administration. (2021). *Cybersecurity for Medical Devices: FDA's Role in Improving Device Security*. FDA Guidance Document.

Uddin, R., Kumar, S. A., & Chamola, V. (2024). Denial of service attacks in edge computing layers: Taxonomy, vulnerabilities, threats and solutions. *Ad Hoc Networks, 152*, 103322. ul Sami, I., Ahmad, M. B., Asif, M., & Ullah, R. (2018). DoS/DDoS detection for E-Healthcare in internet of things. *International Journal of Advanced Computer Science and Applications*, 9(1).

Upadhyaya, N. (2024a). AI-Augmented Dynamic Language Adaptation for Low-Resource Languages: A Transfer Learning Solution for Optimized NLP Performance. *International Research Journal of Advanced Engineering and Science*, 9(4), 89–94.

Upadhyaya, N. (2024b). Enhancing real-time customer service through adaptive machine learning. *Int. J. Adv. Res. Sci. Commun. Technol.*, 4(1), 630–636. DOI: 10.48175/IJARSCT-19381

Upadhyaya, N. (2024c). Artificial intelligence in web development: Enhancing automation, personalization, and decision-making. *Int. J. Adv. Res. Sci. Commun. Technol.*, 4(1), 534–540. DOI: 10.48175/IJARSCT-19367

Upadhyaya, N., Joshi, H., & Agrawal, C. (2025). Examining NLP for Smarter, Data-Driven Healthcare Solutions. In *Intelligent Systems and IoT Applications in Clinical Health* (pp. 393–420). IGI Global.

van Boven, L. S., Kusters, R. W., Tin, D., van Osch, F. H., De Cauwer, H., Ketelings, L., Rao, M., Dameff, C., & Barten, D. G. (2024). Hacking acute care: A qualitative study on the health care impacts of ransomware attacks against hospitals. *Annals of Emergency Medicine*, 83(1), 46–56. DOI: 10.1016/j.annemergmed.2023.04.025 PMID: 37318433

Van der Laak, J., Litjens, G., & Ciompi, F. (2021). Deep learning in histopathology: The path to the clinic. *Nature Medicine*, 27(5), 775–784.

Veale, M., & Borgesius, F. Z. (2021). Demystifying the Draft EU Artificial Intelligence Act. *Computer Law Review International*, 22(4), 97–112. DOI: 10.9785/cri-2021-220402

Vellela, S. S., Reddy, B. V., Chaitanya, K. K., & Rao, M. V. (2023). *An Integrated Approach to Improve E-Healthcare System using Dynamic Cloud Computing Platform.* Paper presented at the 2023 5th International Conference on Smart Systems and Inventive Technology (ICSSIT). DOI: 10.1109/ICSSIT55814.2023.10060945

Velmovitsky, P. E., Bublitz, F. M., Fadrique, L. X., & Morita, P. P. (2021). Blockchain applications in health care and public health: Increased transparency. *JMIR Medical Informatics*, 9(6), e20713. DOI: 10.2196/20713 PMID: 34100768

Vemulapalli, G., Yalamati, S., Palakurti, N. R., Alam, N., Samayamantri, S., & Whig, P. (2024, July). Predicting Obesity Trends Using Machine Learning from Big Data Analytics Approach. In *2024 Asia Pacific Conference on Innovation in Technology (APCIT)* (pp. 1-5). IEEE. DOI: 10.1109/APCIT62007.2024.10673429

Venkatachalam, K., Yang, Z., Trojovský, P., Bacanin, N., Deveci, M., & Ding, W. (2023). Bimodal HAR-An efficient approach to human activity analysis and recognition using bimodal hybrid classifiers. *Information Sciences*, 628, 542–557. DOI: 10.1016/j.ins.2023.01.121

Verma, S., & Rubin, J. (2018). Fairness definitions explained. *Proceedings of the 2018 IEEE/ACM International Workshop on Software Fairness (FairWare'18)*, 1-7.

Vilakazi, K., & Adebesin, F. (2023). A Systematic Literature Review on Cybersecurity Threats to Healthcare Data and Mitigation Strategies. *EPiC Series in Computing*, 93, 240–251. DOI: 10.29007/hf15

Voigt, P., & Von dem Bussche, A. (2017). The eu general data protection regulation (gdpr). A Practical Guide, 1st Ed., Cham: Springer International Publishing, 10(3152676), 10-5555.

Wang, B., Li, H., Guo, Y., & Wang, J. (2023). PPFLHE: A Privacy-Preserving Federated Learning Scheme with Homomorphic Encryption for Healthcare Data. *Applied Soft Computing*, 146, 110677. DOI: 10.1016/j.asoc.2023.110677

Wang, H., & Liu, Z. (2023). AI-driven threat detection in medical devices: Challenges and solutions. *Cybersecurity in Health Care*, 12(2), 32–47.

Wang, H., & Liu, Z. (2023). AI-Driven Threat Detection in Medical Devices: Challenges and Solutions. *Cybersecurity in Health Care*, 12(2), 32–47.

Wang, H., Zhang, X., Xia, Y., & Wu, X. (2023). An Intelligent Blockchain-Based Access Control Framework with Federated Learning for Genome-Wide Association Studies. *Computer Standards & Interfaces*, 84, 103694. DOI: 10.1016/j.csi.2022.103694

Wang, J., Zhu, H., Wang, S. H., & Zhang, Y. D. (2021). A review of deep learning on medical image analysis. *Mobile Networks and Applications*, 26(1), 351–380. DOI: 10.1007/s11036-020-01672-7

Wang, X., Hu, J., Lin, H., Liu, W., Moon, H., & Piran, M. J. (2023). Federated Learning-Empowered Disease Diagnosis Mechanism in the Internet of Medical Things: From the Privacy-Preservation Perspective. *IEEE Transactions on Industrial Informatics*, 19(7), 7905–7913. DOI: 10.1109/TII.2022.3210597

Wang, Z., Ma, J., Wang, X., Hu, J., Qin, Z., & Ren, K. (2022). Threats to Training: A Survey of Poisoning Attacks and Defenses on Machine Learning Systems. *ACM Computing Surveys*, 55(7), 1–36. Advance online publication. DOI: 10.1145/3538707

Watson, D. S., Krutzinna, J., Bruce, I. N., Griffiths, C. E., McInnes, I. B., Barnes, M. R., & Floridi, L. (2019). Clinical applications of machine learning algorithms: Beyond the black box. *BMJ (Clinical Research Ed.)*, 364, l886. DOI: 10.1136/bmj.l886 PMID: 30862612

Weber, K., & Kleine, N. (2020). Cybersecurity in health care. *The Ethics of Cybersecurity*, 21, 139–156. DOI: 10.1007/978-3-030-29053-5_7

Weibel, R. P., Kerr, J. I., Naegelin, M., Ferrario, A., Schinazi, V. R., La Marca, R., Hoelscher, C., Nater, U. M., & von Wangenheim, F. (2023). Virtual reality-supported biofeedback for stress management: Beneficial effects on heart rate variability and user experience. *Computers in Human Behavior*, 141, 107607. DOI: 10.1016/j.chb.2022.107607

Wei, G., Mu, W., Song, Y., & Dou, J. (2022). An improved and random synthetic minority oversampling technique for imbalanced data. *Knowledge-Based Systems*, 248, 108839. DOI: 10.1016/j.knosys.2022.108839

Weinberg, J., Goldhardt, J., Patterson, S., & Kepros, J. (2024). Assessment of accuracy of an early artificial intelligence large language model at summarizing medical literature: ChatGPT 3.5 vs. ChatGPT 4.0. *Journal of Medical Artificial Intelligence*, 7(0), 33. Advance online publication. DOI: 10.21037/jmai-24-48

Wen, J., Yiu, S. M., & Hui, L. C. (2021, July). Defending against model inversion attack by adversarial examples. In *2021 IEEE International Conference on Cyber Security and Resilience (CSR)* (pp. 551-556). IEEE.

Wen, J., Zhang, Z., Lan, Y., Cui, Z., Cai, J., & Zhang, W. (2023). A survey on federated learning: Challenges and applications. *International Journal of Machine Learning and Cybernetics*, 14(2), 513–535.

Whig, P., Kouser, S., Bhatia, A. B., Purohit, K., & Modhugu, V. R. (2024). 9 Intelligent Control for Energy Management. *Microgrid: Design, Optimization, and Applications*, 137.

Whig, P., Madavarapu, J. B., Yathiraju, N., & Thatikonda, R. (2024). 3 IoT Healthcare's. *Evolution of Machine Learning and Internet of Things Applications in Biomedical Engineering*, 41.

Whig, P., Yathiraju, N., Modhugu, V. R., & Bhatia, A. B. (2024). 13 Digital Twin for. *AI-Driven Digital Twin and Industry 4.0: A Conceptual Framework with Applications*, 202.

Whig, P., Madavarapu, J. B., Yathiraju, N., & Thatikonda, R. (2024). Managing Knowledge in the Era of Industry 4.0: Challenges and Strategies. *Knowledge Management and Industry Revolution*, 4(0), 239–273. DOI: 10.1002/9781394242641.ch9

Wiens, J., Saria, S., Sendak, M., Ghassemi, M., Liu, V. X., & Kale, D. (2019). Do no harm: A roadmap for responsible machine learning for health care. *Nature Medicine*, 25(9), 1337–1340. DOI: 10.1038/s41591-019-0548-6 PMID: 31427808

Wilhelm, C., Steckelberg, A., & Rebitschek, F. G. (2024). Is artificial intelligence for medical professionals serving the patients? Protocol for a mixed method systematic review on patient-relevant benefits and harms of algorithmic decision-making. DOI: 10.1101/2024.03.27.24304965

Williamson, S. M., & Prybutok, V. (2024). Balancing privacy and progress: A review of privacy challenges, systemic oversight, and patient perceptions in AI-driven healthcare. *Applied Sciences (Basel, Switzerland)*, 14(2), 675. DOI: 10.3390/app14020675

Wong, B. K. M., Vengusamy, S., & Bastrygina, T. (2024). *Healthcare digital transformation through the adoption of artificial intelligence Artificial Intelligence, big data, blockchain and 5G for the digital transformation of the healthcare industry*. Elsevier.

Worden, K., Tsialiamanis, G., Cross, E., & Rogers, T. (2023). *Artificial neural networks Machine Learning in Modeling and Simulation: Methods and Applications*. Springer.

Wu, W., Elgendi, M., Fletcher, R. R., Bomberg, H., Eichenberger, U., Guan, C., & Menon, C. (2023). Detection of heart rate using smartphone gyroscope data: A scoping review. *Frontiers in Cardiovascular Medicine*, 10, 1329290. DOI: 10.3389/fcvm.2023.1329290 PMID: 38164464

Xia, Q., Ye, W., Tao, Z., Wu, J., & Li, Q. (2021). A Survey of Federated Learning for Edge Computing: Research Problems and Solutions. *High-Confidence Computing*, 1(1), 100008. DOI: 10.1016/j.hcc.2021.100008

Xie, Q., Jiang, S., Jiang, L., Huang, Y., Zhao, Z., Khan, S., Dai, W., Liu, Z., & Wu, K. (2024). Efficiency Optimization Techniques in Privacy-Preserving Federated Learning With Homomorphic Encryption: A Brief Survey. *IEEE Internet of Things Journal*, 11(14), 24569–24580. DOI: 10.1109/JIOT.2024.3382875

Xu, H.-L., Gong, T.-T., Liu, F.-H., Chen, H.-Y., Xiao, Q., Hou, Y., Huang, Y., Sun, H.-Z., Shi, Y., Gao, S., Lou, Y., Chang, Q., Zhao, Y.-H., Gao, Q.-L., & Wu, Q.-J. (2022). Artificial intelligence performance in image-based ovarian cancer identification: A systematic review and meta-analysis. *EClinicalMedicine*, 53, 101662. DOI: 10.1016/j.eclinm.2022.101662 PMID: 36147628

Xu, J., Glicksberg, B. S., Su, C., Walker, P., Bian, J., & Wang, F. (2021). Federated Learning for Healthcare Informatics. *Journal of Healthcare Informatics Research*, 5(1), 1–19. DOI: 10.1007/s41666-020-00082-4 PMID: 33204939

Xu, Y., Peng, C., Tan, W., Tian, Y., Ma, M., & Niu, K. (2022). Non-Interactive Verifiable Privacy-Preserving Federated Learning. *Future Generation Computer Systems*, 128, 365–380. DOI: 10.1016/j.future.2021.10.017

Yang, J., Soltan, A. A. S., Eyre, D. W., Yang, Y., & Clifton, D. A. (2023). An adversarial training framework for mitigating algorithmic biases in clinical machine learning. *NPJ Digital Medicine*, 6(1), 55. DOI: 10.1038/s41746-023-00805-y PMID: 36991077

Yang, P., Xiong, N., & Ren, J. (2020). Data security and privacy protection for cloud storage: A survey. *IEEE Access : Practical Innovations, Open Solutions*, 8, 131723–131740. DOI: 10.1109/ACCESS.2020.3009876

Yaqoob, I., Salah, K., Jayaraman, R., & Al-Hammadi, Y. (2022). Blockchain for healthcare data management: Opportunities, challenges, and future recommendations. *Neural Computing & Applications*, 34(14), 1–16. DOI: 10.1007/s00521-020-05519-w

Ye, R., Wang, W., Chai, J., Li, D., Li, Z., Xu, Y., . . . Chen, S. (2024). *Openfedllm: Training large language models on decentralized private data via federated learning*. Paper presented at the Proceedings of the 30th ACM SIGKDD Conference on Knowledge Discovery and Data Mining. DOI: 10.1145/3637528.3671582

Zahid, H., Hina, S., Hayat, M. F., & Shah, G. A. (2023). Agentless approach for security information and event management in industrial iot. *Electronics (Basel)*, 12(8), 1831. DOI: 10.3390/electronics12081831

Zala, K., Thakkar, H. K., Dholakia, N., Shukla, M., & Thumar, D. (2024). Designing an Attribute-Based Encryption Scheme with an Enhanced Anonymity Model for Privacy Protection in E-Health. *SN Computer Science*, 5(2), 203. DOI: 10.1007/s42979-023-02541-2

Zhang, C., Xie, Y., Bai, H., Yu, B., Li, W., & Gao, Y. (2021). A Survey on Federated Learning. *Knowledge-Based Systems*, 216, 106775. DOI: 10.1016/j.knosys.2021.106775 PMID: 34909232

Zhang, M., Martin, P., Powley, W., & Chen, J. (2017). Workload management in database management systems: A taxonomy. *IEEE Transactions on Knowledge and Data Engineering*, 30(7), 1386–1402. DOI: 10.1109/TKDE.2017.2767044

Zhang, Z., Song, X., Liu, L., Yin, J., Wang, Y., & Lan, D. (2021). Recent advances in blockchain and artificial intelligence integration: Feasibility analysis, research issues, applications, challenges, and future work. *Security and Communication Networks*, 2021(1), 9991535. DOI: 10.1155/2021/9991535

Zhao, Q., & Lee, Y. (2022). The impact of regulatory compliance on medical device cybersecurity. *Journal of Medical Device Regulation*, 29(1), 54–66.

Zhao, Q., & Lee, Y. (2022). The Impact of Regulatory Compliance on Medical Device Cybersecurity. *Journal of Medical Device Regulation*, 29(1), 54–66.

Zhou, J., Wang, X., Li, Y., Yang, Y., & Shi, J. (2024). Federated-Learning-Based Prognosis Assessment Model for Acute Pulmonary Thromboembolism. *BMC Medical Informatics and Decision Making*, 24(1), 1–13. DOI: 10.1186/s12911-024-02543-x PMID: 38802861

Zhuang, Y., Shyu, C.-R., Hong, S., Li, P., & Zhang, L. (2023). Self-sovereign identity empowered non-fungible patient tokenization for health information exchange using blockchain technology. *Computers in Biology and Medicine*, 157, 106778. DOI: 10.1016/j.compbiomed.2023.106778 PMID: 36934533

About the Contributors

Shrikaant Kulkarni, Ph.D. is currently working as a Research Professor in the School of Engineering & Technology at Sanjivani University, Kopargaon, India, and an Adjunct Professor, at the Faculty of Business, Victorian Institute of Technology, Melbourne, Australia, and Adjunct Professor at Chitkara University, Punjab, India. Dr. Kulkarni has been a senior academician and researcher for over four decades. He has delivered invited lectures and conducted sessions at national and international conferences and faculty development programs. He has guided many major and minor projects in areas like engineering chemistry, green chemistry, nanotechnology, analytical chemistry, catalysis, chemical engineering materials, industrial organization, and management, Advanced AI, and Educational Technology. He has published over 100+ research papers in national and international journals and conferences of repute. He has edited 30+ books including four books in Advanced AI, and authored 100+ book chapters in books published by CRC, Springer Nature, Apple Academic Press, Elsevier, Wiley, and IET. He authored four textbooks in engineering chemistry too. Dr Kulkarni possesses MSc, MPhil, and PhD degrees in Chemistry and master's degrees in Economics, Business Management, and Political Science.. Two of his Patents have been published and two more are applied for grant. He was invited by UNESCO for an invited talk on "Green Chemistry Education for Sustainable Development" at the International Conference on Green Chemistry, Bangkok, and was well received by international Jury members and dignitaries from across the world.

Saikat Gochhait My academic background includes obtaining a Post Doctoral Fellowship in Entrepreneurship from the University of Extremadura in 2018 and a Post Doctoral Fellowship from the National Dong Hwa University in 2019. Finished my PhD in Marketing from Sambalpur University, India in 2014 after receiving the Doctoral Bursary Award from Coventry University in 2010. Additionally, I was awarded a DITA Fellowship from the University of Deusto in 2016, a MOFA

Taiwan Fellowship in 2019, and a Russian Fellowship in 2020 from the Samara State Medical University, Russia. Approximately 50 research publications and presentations in national and international journals, with citations to ABDC, Web of Science, Scopus, and Google. My credentials include the publication of five books indexed in Scopus and recommended by top universities around the world.In addition to speaking at several international conferences, I possess extensive experience in teaching, mentoring, and leading research projects. I have also received numerous awards and grants for my re-search and publications. My teaching experience includes 15 years in marketing, entrepreneurship, and information technology, as well as five years of manufacturing industry experience with Tata Groups and Bajoria Groups. I am happy to contribute to both research-led and methodological modules at undergradu-ate and postgraduate levels.Currently collaborated with over 40 universities for research and project collaborations in Artificial Intelligence (AI), Healthcare Technology, and Entrepreneurship. Developed a model patented and has re-ceived awards from the Department of Science and Industrial Research regarding the application of AI in 11/16/23, 3:25 PM Dr Saikat Gochhait (Honoris Causa) (0000-0003-4583-9208) - ORCID | Connecting Research and Researchers the energy sector. Headed Business Incubator (BI) funded by MSME from 2016-2017. Currently also working on my own startup idea AI-VIM, which is supported by the Department of Science and Industrial Research, Government of India, and has been awarded three patents.

***

Bamidele Olalekan Ademilua is a scholar at University of Salford, Manchester, United Kingdom Department: Cybersecurity threat intelligence and forensics/ Operations current Job title: information security Analyst

Adeyinka Kehinde Iyioluwa is a dedicated student pursuing a degree in Information and Communication Engineering. With a strong passion for artificial intelligence and technology, Adeyinka has authored several academic papers, focusing on topics such as AI applications and data security. Currently, Adeyinka is actively involved in research related to privacy and security management practices in computer science

Adeyinka Taye Iyinoluwa is a passionate researcher and academic with a strong background in Information and Communication Engineering. Known for a deep interest in technology and its transformative impact, Adeyinka is driven by a commitment to advancing innovative solutions in the field of education and beyond.

Edidiong Elijah Akpan is a versatile professional with a wide range of specialized and academic experiences. He obtained a bachelor's degree in Biochemistry, an MBA in Business Administration and a master's degree in Information Technology. These established a strong basis for scientific investigation and analysis. Edidiong had a prosperous career for himself in the banking industry, gaining ten years of experience there. His work in banking helped him hone his managerial, strategic planning, and operational efficiency skills, which highlights his ability to work with complicated data sets, draw conclusions, and use technology to address challenging issues. Edidiong is about to start a PhD program with an emphasis on artificial intelligence and machine learning. His goal of expanding his knowledge of cutting-edge technology and making a positive impact on the quickly developing field of artificial intelligence is consistent with this endeavor. Edidiong is in a unique position to bridge the gap between scientific research, commercial strategy, technology innovation, and medicine because of his multidisciplinary skills and experience. He is a member of Chattered Institute of Bankers of Nigeria (CIBN), National Society of Black Engineers (NSBE), Nigeria Society of Biochemistry and Molecular Biology (NSBMB).

Bah Esseme, Alain Claude, Bah Esseme is a seasoned Developer and Architect with a focus on optimizing business processes through Salesforce CRM and various other web frameworks such as Angular, React, and Node.js.. My expertise extends to mentoring aspiring tech professionals, equipping them with essential skills for a successful career. Originally trained as a medical doctor, my passion for technology led me to pursue a full-time career in the tech industry post-graduation. Since then, I have helped numerous businesses achieve significant improvements in efficiency by developing web applications and increasing their customer engagement through automation. As co-founder of PathwayToSalesforce.com, I am dedicated to delivering high-quality training programs that enhance technical capabilities. My proficiency in JavaScript, Java, HTML, and APEX, combined with my Salesforce CRM expertise, helps organizations build robust customer relationships. I am committed to professional excellence and social responsibility, blending technical expertise with mentorship and philanthropy. Additionally, I actively share knowledge through my personal blog and research articles, believing in the collective advancement of our global community.

Oluwaseun Adeyombo Cole holds a Bachelor of Science (B.Sc., Honours) degree in Physiology from the University of Ilorin, Nigeria, and a Master of Science (M.Sc.) degree in International Business with Data Analytics from University of Ulster, United Kingdom.Her interests include artificial intelligence, machine learning, and data-driven innovation.

Ogheneruona Maria Esegbona-Isikeh is a Data Journalist with years of experience in uncovering compelling stories through data analysis and visualization. She specializes in using Python, R, and SQL to mine large datasets and distill complex information into clear, engaging narratives. Ogheneruona's work often explores social justice, economic trends, and public policy, with a particular focus on making data accessible to a broad audience. Her investigative reporting has been featured in leading publications such as News agency of Nigeria (NAN), The Guardian, UrbanKapital Magazine agmonst others. She has written multiple health data stories. Ogheneruona holds a Master's degree in Data Journalism from Birmingham City University(BCU), United Kingdom and a Bachelor's degree in Mass Communication from Delta State University, Abraka In Nigeria.When she's not crunching numbers, Jane enjoys mentoring aspiring data journalists and speaking at industry conferences about the importance of transparency in data storytel

Oluwatosin Samuel Falebita earned a Bachelor of Science in Computer Science from the Nigeria Police Academy, Wudil, in 2018. He is currently pursuing a Master's degree in Computer Science at Colorado State University, Fort Collins. Since 2019, he has been involved in cybercrime investigations and digital forensics. Before joining RaysCyberLab as a cybersecurity researcher, he received specialized training in digital forensics and incident response from the FBI and Interpol. He is also a member of the International Information System Security Certification Consortium $(ISC)^2$. His research interests focus on AI security, the intersection of AI, machine learning, and cybersecurity, and developing innovative technologies to combat cybercrime and enhance cybersecurity.

Saikat Gochhait teaches at Symbiosis Institute of Digital & Telecom Management, Symbiosis International Deemed University Pune, India. He is Ph.D and Post-Doctoral Fellow from the UEx, Spain. He was Awarded DITA and MOFA Fellowship in 2017 and 2018. His research publication with foreign authors indexed in Scopus, ABDC, and Web of Science. He is an IEEE member.

Jabin Shiji Koshy is a student and researcher affiliated with Christ University, India. With a strong academic background and keen interest in the intersection of artificial intelligence and healthcare, he has contributed significantly to understanding the challenges and opportunities of securing AI algorithms in medical applications. His expertise lies in cybersecurity, ethical AI, and data privacy frameworks, particularly focusing on regulations such as GDPR and HIPAA. Residing in Ghaziabad, Uttar Pradesh, Jabin has actively pursued research and academic endeavors, addressing key issues such as algorithmic bias, adversarial attacks, and the ethical implications of AI in healthcare diagnostics. His work emphasizes collaboration among healthcare providers, developers, and policymakers to create secure and equitable AI-driven healthcare systems. Jabin can be reached at jabinesd@gmail.com for inquiries and collaborations in the fields of AI, healthcare, and cybersecurity.

Sangeetha M obtained her Bachelor of Engineering from Anna University, Chennai in 2008 and Master of Engineering from Anna University, Coimbatore in 2010. Her research interests lies on Machine Learning, Deep Learning and Graph Neural Networks. She is having 13 years of experience in engineering Colleges. Now she is working as an Assistant Professor (Selection Grade) in Dr.N.G.P. Institute of Technology, Coimbatore. She has filed 1 patent and also published 19 journals including SCI, Scopus journals and Scopus chapters. She also published 18 papers in various national and international conferences. She has published 11 books and completed 10 consultancy works. She is an active member of Computer Society of India.

Ugochukwu O. Matthew, presently is an Academic scholar with Hussaini Adamu Federal Polytechnic, Nigeria, in the Department of Computer Science with specialty in AI, Big Data Science, Cloud Computing, Internet of Things, Data Mining, Multimedia and E-Learning Education. A Member of Nigeria Computer Society (NCS), Nigeria Institute of Management (NIM), International Association of Computer Science & Information Technology (IACSIT), European Alliance for Innovation (EAI) and also a member of Teaching & Education Research Association (TERA). Ugochukwu O. Matthew hold Masters in Computer Applications from Bayero University Kano, Nigeria. Ugochukwu O. Matthew had reviewed several Journals and a member of Review Board Committee of Journals Indexed by Scopus and Web of Science including IEEE Access, SN Computer Science (Springer), International Journal of Information Communication Technologies & Human Development (IJICTHD), International Journal of Business Data Communications and Networking (IJBDCN), International Journal of Cloud Applications and Computing (IJCAC). Ugochukwu O. Matthew is a cofounder of U&J Digital Consult Limited, an IT and Educational Consulting Firm in Nigeria.

Morgan Nwaiku is a dedicated cybersecurity professional with a strong foundation in software development and a background in computer engineering. With a focus on building and monitoring systems that utilize anomaly detection and artificial intelligence, Morgan ensures that software products are both secure and user-friendly, balancing the critical aspects of security and usability. His passion for technology extends beyond his professional work, as he actively mentors aspiring tech enthusiasts and contributes to the tech community through volunteering and knowledge sharing. Morgan's expertise spans across various tools and technologies, including Azure cloud services, SQL and NoSQL databases, Python programming, application testing, and API. By integrating AI into their anomaly detection systems, Morgan stays at the cutting edge of cybersecurity innovation. This diverse skill set, coupled with a commitment to staying at the forefront of technological advancements, positions Morgan as a valuable asset in the technology space.

Chukwuka Oforgu is a data scientist and author specializing in the fields of machine learning, artificial intelligence, and data science. With a keen understanding of complex technological concepts, Chukwuka brings his expertise to the written page, making intricate topics accessible to both professionals and enthusiasts. His work focuses on exploring the cutting-edge developments in AI and data analysis, providing readers with insights into the rapidly evolving world of data-driven technologies. Through his writing, Chukwuka aims to bridge the gap between technical innovation and practical application, contributing to the growing body of knowledge in this dynamic field.

Hope Oladele Ayokunle earned a Bachelor of Science (B.Sc. Hons) degree in Architecture from Joseph Ayo Babalola University, Osun State, Nigeria, and a Master of Technology (M.Tech) degree in Architectural Technology from the Federal University of Technology, Akure, Nigeria. He recently completed a Master of Science (M.Sc.) degree in Sustainable Architecture and Healthy Buildings at the University of Derby. His primary research interests include human-centered design in sustainable education, as well as applications of data science, artificial intelligence, and machine learning. Email: oladelehopeayokunle@gmail.com

Amaonwu Onyebuchi is a lecturer in the Department of Computer Science, Hussaini Adamu Federal Polytechnic Kazaure, Jigawa State, Nigeria. Onyebuchi is a seasoned IT profession, registered with Nigeria Computer Society (NCS) with speciality in Artificial Intelligence, Cloud Technology Management, Information System Security, Internet of Things and E-Learning Education. Onyebuchi hold Masters of Science Degree in Computer Science from Kampala University Uganda.

Victor Onyenagubom is a Lecturer in Cybersecurity at Teesside University London, where he develops and delivers cybersecurity modules to students, fostering an engaging and inclusive learning environment. Victor has attended the Pre-Doctoral school organized by the Max Planck Institute of Software Systems in Germany, in partnership with the University of Maryland and Cornell University. He also volunteers as a Lead IT Trainer at CodeYourFuture, where he empowers refugees and asylum seekers with digital and cybersecurity skills.

Victor Nosakhare Oriakhi is a Design Engineer with specialized expertise in Electrical and Electronic Control, focusing on the integration of Artificial Intelligence (AI) into advanced engineering systems. He holds a Bachelor of Engineering (BEng) in Electrical and Electronic Engineering and a master's degree in Robotics and Automation. His research interests lie at the intersection of robotics, AI, and control systems engineering. Victor's research is centered on the development of innovative control systems and electronic circuits designed to optimize performance and enhance operational efficiency. His deep understanding of electrical and electronic control, coupled with proficiency in tools such as CAD, MATLAB, and various simulation software, allows him to address complex design challenges. By integrating AI into control systems, Victor is advancing automation, smart technology applications, and predictive maintenance strategies. Throughout his career, Victor has led a series of projects that h

R. Keerthana is an Assistant Professor in the Department of Computer Science and Engineering at K.S.R. College of Engineering. She completed her B.Tech in Information Technology and went on to earn her M.E. in Computer Science and Engineering, achieving a commendable 25th rank from Anna University. Currently, she is pursuing a Ph.D. as a part-time scholar at Anna University, focusing on advancing research in her field. With a robust academic background, R. Keerthana has actively contributed to the academic community as a conference reviewer for various conferences. Her dedication to research is further exemplified by her submission of four papers to peer-reviewed journals. She has also acted as a session chair, facilitating discussions on emerging trends and technologies. In addition to her research efforts, R. Keerthana has received several grants and patents, showcasing her innovative contributions to the field. She has published various book chapters with Elsevier, reinforcing her commitment to sharing knowledge and advancements in computer science.

Manjula Devi Ramasamy received her B.E degree in Computer Science and Engineering and M.E degree in Computer Science and Engineering during the year 2004 and 2006 from Bharathiyar University, Coimbatore and Anna University Chennai respectively. She then completed Ph.D. degree in Information and Communication Engineering from Anna University, Chennai during the year 2015 in the area of Soft Computing and Pattern Classification. She worked as Associate Professor in the Department of Computer Science and Engineering at Kongu Engineering College (Autonomous), Perundurai, Erode till February 2023. From March 2023 oonwards, she has been working as Professor in the Department of Computer Science and Engineering at KPR Institute of Engineering and Technology, Coimbatore. She published more than 50 research articles in well reputed and refereed international journals from Elsevier, Springer, IEEE, etc., She also published several research articles in National and International conference. She is also serving as Reviewer and Editorial Board member in reputed journals. She is authored more than 15 books edited by Charulatha Publications, Chennai. Her research interests are Machine Learning, Soft Computing, Image Processing, and Pattern Recognition.

Prabakaran Raghavendran, a dedicated mathematician specializing in Fractional Differential Equations, Integral Transforms, and Control Theory, holds a Ph.D. and a Master's degree in Mathematics from Vel Tech Rangarajan Dr. Sagunthala R&D Institute of Science and Technology, as well as a Bachelor's degree in Mathematics from Loyola College, Chennai. Mr. Raghavendran has made significant contributions to this field, evident through his publications in esteemed international journals and book chapters. He has authored numerous papers published in reputable Scopus, Web of Science, and SCI journals, further solidifying his impact in the academic community. Additionally, he has presented his work at various national and international conferences, where it has been well-received, earning him accolades such as the Best Paper Award at an International Conference. Mr. Raghavendran has also published patents, showcasing his innovative approach to mathematical research. His academic achievements, coupled with his passion for teaching and active participation in extracurricular activities, underscore his positive attitude, time management skills, and ability to foster relationships with students

S. Savitha is an Assistant Professor in the Department of Computer Science and Engineering, K.S.R. College of Engineering (Autonomous), India. She received her Master of Engineering degree in Computer Science and Engineering in 2012 from Anna University, Chennai, India. She is a Research scholar in Anna University, Chennai. She has published more than 15 papers in referred journals and conference proceedings. Her research interest includes Data Mining, Big Data, Cloud computing, Databases and Artificial Intelligence. She is a professional member of ISTE.

Dinesh Thakur is an Assistant Professor in the Department of Mathematics at the Bahra University, Waknaghat, District Solan, Himachal Pradesh, India.

Prakash Chand Thakur is an Associate Professor in the Department of Mathematics at the Bahra University, Waknagjat, District Solan, Himachal Pradesh, India.

Nitesh Upadhyaya is an Expert Solution Architect with over 15 years of experience in software development, architecture, and project management. He specializes in cutting-edge technologies such as AI, Machine Learning, Blockchain, and cloud computing. Nitesh has published numerous articles in leading technical journals, contributed to several research papers, and is a core program member at DZone, where he judges and reviews technical content. He is also a Certified Scrum Master (CSM) and AWS Cloud Practitioner, actively engaged in reviewing AI/ML books and speaking at industry conferences. Nitesh is committed to driving innovation through his research and thought leadership, with a focus on real-world applications in healthcare, cybersecurity, and distributed systems.

V. Vennila (Vennila Venkatachalam) Currently working as a Professor in the Department of Computer Science and Engineering, K.S.R. College of Engineering, Tiruchengode. She received her M.E. degree in Computer Science and Engineering from K.S.Rangaswamy College of Technology, Tiruchengode, India affiliated to Anna University, Chennai, India in 2008 and was awarded Ph.D. in Information and Communication Engineering from Anna University, Chennai, India in the year 2017. She has 15 years teaching experience. She has published numerous papers in reputed journals and conferences. Her research interests include Data Mining, Artificial Intelligence, Machine Learning, Big Data Analytics, Cloud Computing and Data Science.

Index

Symbols

A

B

C

D

E

F

H

I

J

M

N

P

R

S